Atlas of
FETAL ECHOCARDIOGRAPHY

System requirement:
- Windows XP or above
- Power DVD Player (Software)
- Windows Media Player 10.0 version or above (Software)

Accompanying **DVD-ROM** is playable only in Computer and not in **DVD** player.
CD/DVD has Autorun function—it may take few seconds to load on your computer. If it does not work for you, then follow the steps below to access the contents manually:
- Click on my computer
- Select the **CD/DVD** drive and after opening the drive, kindly double click the file **PPTVIEW.EXE**
- Select the file **echo.ppt** and click open.

DVD Contents

1. 4D Driving
2. 17 Weeks Fetal Heart with Zoom and without Zoom
3. 19 Weeks Hypoplastic Left Heart Syndrome
4. Aortic Arch
5. Aortic Arch with Power Doppler
6. Atrial Septal Defect (ASD)
7. Depth of the Heart and VSD
8. Dextro Hernia
9. Easy Sweep
10. Echocardiography
11. Heart Block
12. Focal Zone 1 to 4
13. Frame Rate 600 (High Frame Rate)
14. Harmonic Mid and High
15. High Frequency Probe
16. CINE Loop Ultrasound
17. Left Ventricular Outflow Tract (LVOT)
18. Normal ECHO 1 and 2
19. Persistence 1 and 2
20. Persistence Low
21. Rotation of the Probe
22. Right Ventricular Outflow Tract (RVOT)
23. Septal Defect
24. Single Sweep ECHO
25. Single Sweep Situs
26. Small-large View of the Heart
27. Speckle Reduction
28. Speckle Reduction + Compound Imaging
29. Tachycardia
30. Transposition of Great Arteries (TGA) 1 and 2
31. Tetralogy of Fallot (TOF) 1 and 2
32. Ventricular Septal Defect (VSD) Doppler 1 to 3
33. Ventricular Size Disproportionate
34. Ventricular Septal Defect 1 to 3
35. Zoom Image of the Four Chamber Heart
36. Zoom Image of the Four Chamber Heart in Grey Scale
37. View of Fetal Heart with Different Contrasts
38. Fetal Heart with 22 Weeks Pregnancy
39. Fetal Heart (22 Weeks with Chambers)
40. CINE Loop 2 and 3

Atlas of
FETAL ECHOCARDIOGRAPHY

Second Edition

Manish R Pandya
MD FICOG FICMCH (Gynecology) Endoscopy (CICE France)
ART (EART, Mumbai; CRM, Cleveland, Ohio, USA)
Professor and Head
Department of Obstetrics and Gynecology
CU Shah Medical College, Surendranagar, Gujarat, India
www.manishivf.com, www.drmanishpandya.com

Foreword
S Suresh FRCOG (Hon)

JAYPEE The Health Sciences Publisher
New Delhi | London | Philadelphia | Panama

Jaypee Brothers Medical Publishers (P) Ltd.

Headquarters

Jaypee Brothers Medical Publishers (P) Ltd.
4838/24, Ansari Road, Daryaganj
New Delhi 110 002, India
Phone: +91-11-43574357
Fax: +91-11-43574314
E-mail: jaypee@jaypeebrothers.com

Overseas Offices

J.P. Medical Ltd.
83, Victoria Street, London
SW1H 0HW (UK)
Phone: +44-20 3170 8910
Fax: +44 (0)-20 3008 6180
E-mail: info@jpmedpub.com

Jaypee-Highlights Medical Publishers Inc.
City of Knowledge, Bld. 237, Clayton
Panama City, Panama
Phone: +1 507-301-0496
Fax: +1 507-301-0499
E-mail: cservice@jphmedical.com

Jaypee Medical Inc.
The Bourse
111, South Independence Mall East
Suite 835, Philadelphia, PA 19106, USA
Phone: +1 267-519-9789
E-mail: jpmed.us@gmail.com

Jaypee Brothers Medical Publishers (P) Ltd.
17/1-B, Babar Road, Block-B, Shaymali
Mohammadpur, Dhaka-1207
Bangladesh
Mobile: +08801912003485
E-mail: jaypeedhaka@gmail.com

Jaypee Brothers Medical Publishers (P) Ltd.
Bhotahity, Kathmandu, Nepal
Phone: +977-9741283608
E-mail: kathmandu@jaypeebrothers.com

Website: www.jaypeebrothers.com
Website: www.jaypeedigital.com

Inquiries for bulk sales may be solicited at: jaypee@jaypeebrothers.com

Atlas of Fetal Echocardiography

First Edition: 2011
Second Edition: **2015**

ISBN 978-93-5152-476-2

Printed at: Ajanta Offset & Packagings Ltd., New Delhi

Dedicated to

My Patients
who kept full faith in me and
encouraged me indirectly
to write the book.

My family members
without whose constant inspiration
and
cooperation
this attempt would not have been completed.

Foreword

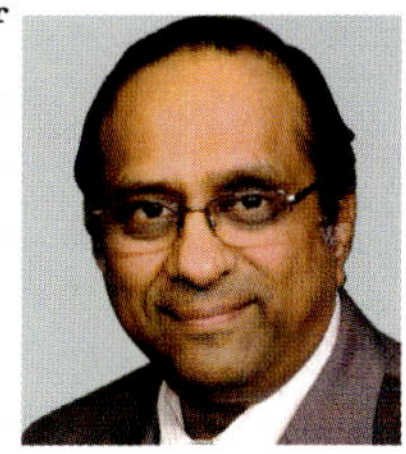

I am very happy to note that the second edition of *Atlas of Fetal Echocardiography* is being published. The author has taken efforts to compile a comprehensive book starting from the embryology of the heart to an illustrative frequently asked questions, chapter on cardiac anomalies which is easy to comprehend by the readers. For beginners, this illustrative book will serve as a guide to understand the various views in fetal echocardiography and also the normal and abnormal patterns. The author has made an effort to "Simplify" a complex subject and has placed emphasis on the importance of pattern recognition which is what an atlas is expected to do. The colorful line diagrams with explicit anatomical markings are easy-to-understand and help to retain concepts in memory. My best wishes to Dr Manish R Pandya for this effort and congratulate him on bringing out the second edition by which many students of this subject will benefit.

S Suresh FRCOG (Hon)
Director
MEDISCAN Systems
197, Dr Natesan Road, Mylapore
Chennai, Tamil Nadu, India

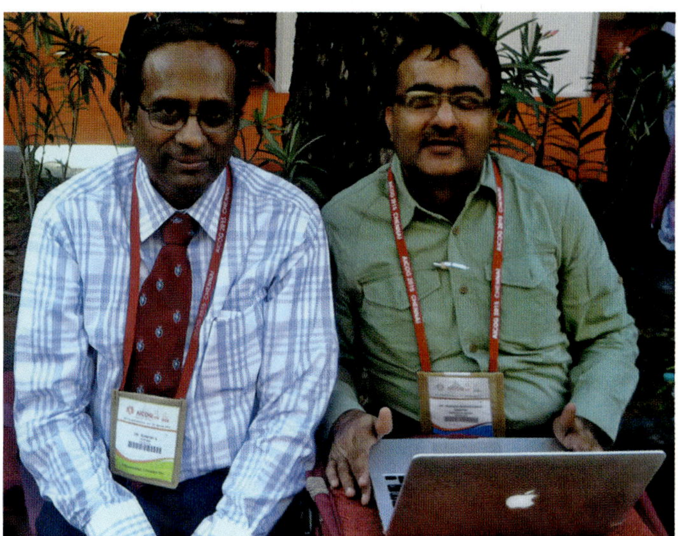

Preface

With the second edition, *Atlas of Fetal Echocardiography* completed four years of service to its readers.

Ultrasonography and echocardiography are two common tools for the obstetricians in their day-to-day practice. The use is limited to just biometry and routine use for detecting anomaly. The days have come now with lots of research and development in this particular field. With color Doppler high resolution machine spatiotemporal image correlation (STIC) and continuous wave Doppler, it is very easy to scan fetal heart and to detect anomalies.

With routine ultrasonography (USG) machine at least my goal to make sonographers to detect something is not normal in fetal heart... It makes us PASSS... in my efforts (Position, Axis, Size, Symmetry and Squeeze).

Advance technologies as well as increased capability of sonographers and sonologists have expanded use of USG as diagnostic tool for evaluation of fetal anatomy and fetal heart with the exception of the newly described "limited scan" a fetal survey has become an integral part of any basic or targeted (comprehensive) USG examination.

Today's need save for all care for all and with my machine, I am able to save one out of hundred babies born with congenital heart defect and many could be far better helped, if diagnosis is made earlier. It is not confident for anybody to give 100% accuracy in report but still we can diagnose major cardiac defect easily and guide patients accordingly.

The fetal heart undergoes complex developmental changes in the first few weeks of gestation and become fully developed by 8 weeks of embryonic life. Congenital heart disease (CHD) in fetus may be the result of abnormal cardiac development during embryonic life.

If we look at postnatal data, it shows frequency of chromosomal abnormalities has been estimated around 5–10%. Down syndrome associated with cardiac anomaly shows around 13%. The frequency of abnormal karyotype in fetus with cardiac defects is even higher. About 30–40%, chromosomal abnormalities are associated with cardiac defects.

Real-time imaging of the fetal heart first is considered feasible in the 1980s.

The addition of four-chamber view as a part of routine antenatal screening has helped clinicians a lot to diagnose complex cardiac anomalies.

The diagnosis of complex cardiac anomalies calls for considerable operator expertise and experience.

In the book, I have tried to explain the basic use of these new modalities and I am sure that it will be extremely useful to the newcomers entering in the new field of diagnostic procedures and also to those experienced obstetricians to give something new.

The second edition is updated and augmented with Nutshell at the end of each chapter for easy points to remember and one new chapter of abnormal heart presentations with tomographic ultrasound imaging (TUI) and 3D images for easy understanding.

There is always scope for improvements in any work and I will be highly obliged by suggestions and comments from learned teachers and students at *drmanish.pandya@gmail.com* or *www.manishivf.com* or *www.drmanishpandya.com*

I sincerely hope that this atlas will satisfy your academic success.

Manish R Pandya

Acknowledgments

I am thankful to:

- My idols and friends in this fraternity who encouraged me to pen the book. Particularly, Professor S Suresh and Mrs (Dr) Indrani Suresh who have given me guidance and support in journey of fetal echo.
- M/s Jaypee Brothers Medical Publishers (P) Ltd, New Delhi, India, for their constant encouragement and provoking me to write the book.
- My father, Rushi Kumar; my mother, Chandrikaben; my father-in-law, Dr Pravinbhai and my mother-in-law, Dr Shakuntala.
- My family members, for their constant inspiration, my lovely wife, Dr Nehal Pandya, my daughters Dhruti (Final year MBBS) and Rutvi (First year MBBS) (BJMC, Ahmedabad, Gujarat, India).
- Professor Rabih Chaoui for making my task easy while his visit to Chennai, Tamil Nadu, India.
- A number of other friends, postgraduate students, relatives and well-wishers who helped me to pen in many ways.

Contents

1

Fetal Embryology

Cardiovascular system in the fetus starts from the 3rd week of intrauterine life. Two vessel heart or paired endothelial cords called cardiogenic cords start forming and these cords canalize to form endocardial heart tubes. The embryology of fetal heart is illustrated in Figures 1.1A and B.

These later fuse to form a single tube that lies ventral to the foregut. Soon this heart tube gets elongated and develops alternate dilatations and constrictions which ultimately lead to formation of sinus venosus, atrium, ventricle, bulbus cordis and truncus arteriosus.

With the beginning of fetal circulation on day 22 and with contraction of the atrial muscles, blood is speeded through the ventricles just like peristalsis movement.

Later on, coordinated contractions become unidirectional and blood enters into the sinus venosus through three paired veins:

- Vitelline veins from the yolk sac
- Umbilical vein from the placenta
- Cardinal veins from the body of the embryo.

Blood flows through the atria, atrioventricular canal, ventricles, bulbus cordis and truncus arteriosus. The truncus arteriosus is continuous with the aortic sac. The aortic sac is connected to the dorsal aorta by the aortic arches.

FORMATION OF THE FETAL HEART

Formation of the fetal heart comprises of the following steps:

Heart Tube (Bending or Folding)

Bulbus cordis and the ventricular portion of the heart tube grows faster than the other organ so it leads to a bending of heart tube upon itself making the atrium and sinus venosus to lie dorsal to bulbus cordis, truncus arteriosus and the ventricles.

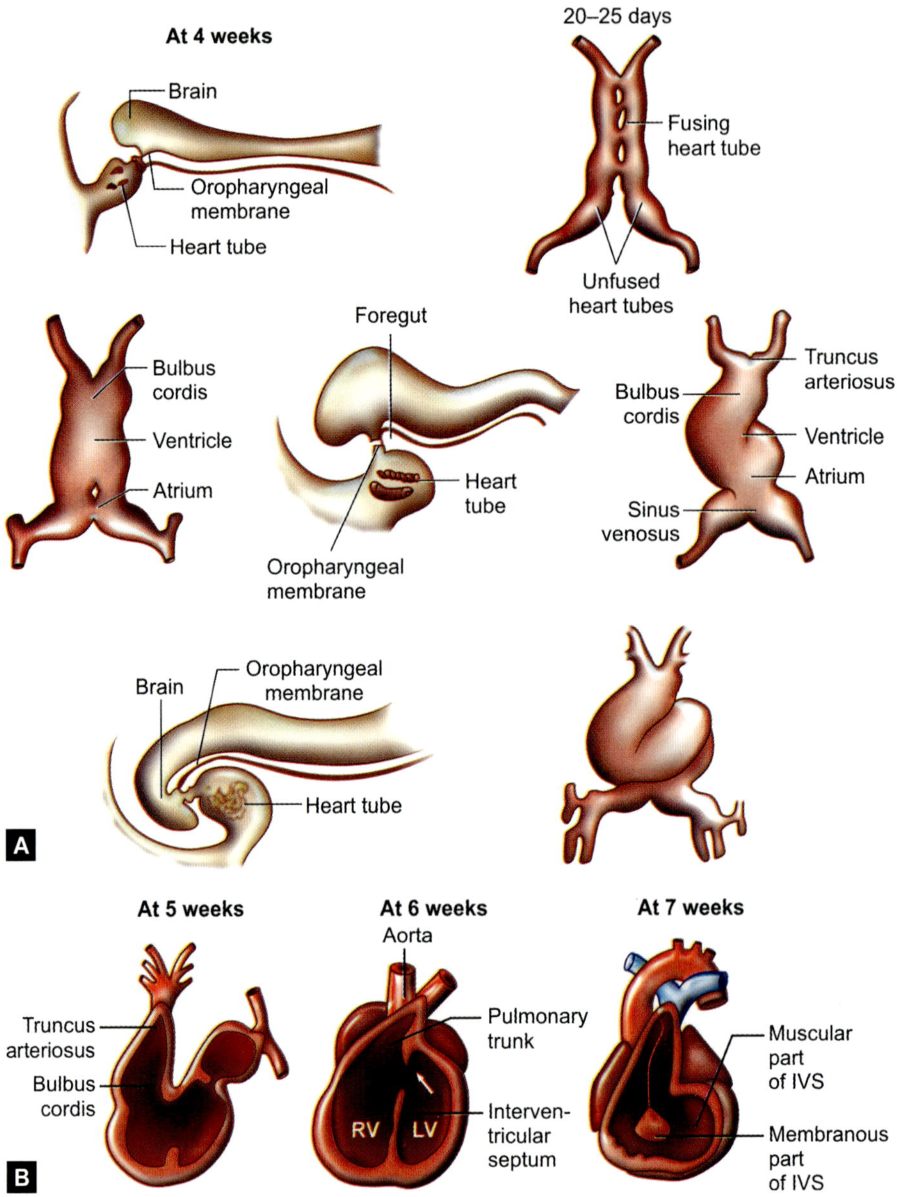

Figures 1.1A and B Embryology of the heart

Abbreviations: IVS, interventricular septum; LV, left ventricle; RV, right ventricle

Heart Partitioning

This involves the simultaneous partitioning of atrioventricular canal, atrium and ventricle and has been described here:

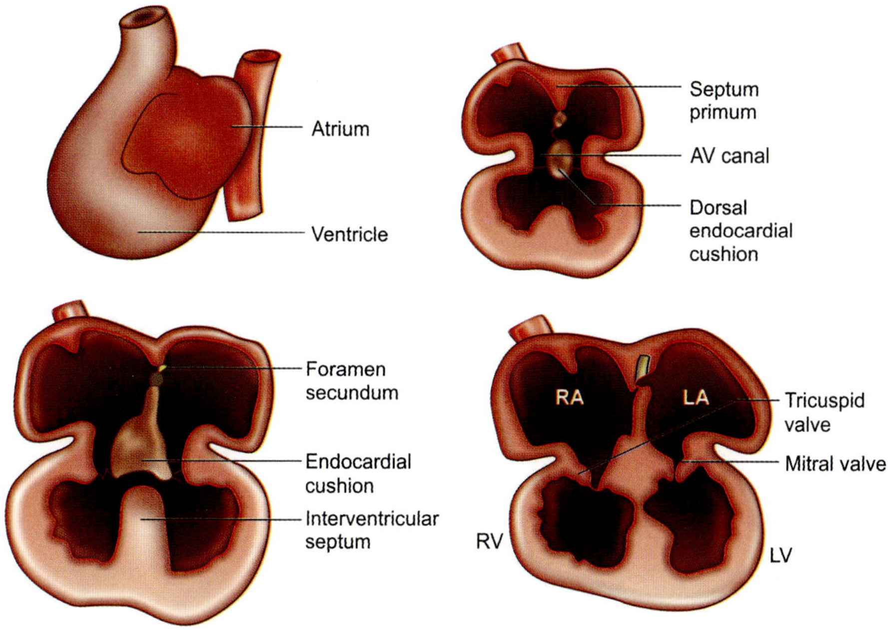

Figure 1.2 Partitioning of AV canal
Abbreviations: LA, left atrium; LV, left ventricle; RA, right atrium; RV, right ventricle

- **Partitioning of AV canal (Figure 1.2):** From the dorsal and ventral walls of the AV canal, two endocardial cushions appear. They approach to each other and fuse dividing the common canal into right and left AV canal.
- **Partitioning of the atrium (Figure 1.3):** The common atrium separates into a right and left atrium by two septae. From the roof of the atrium a thin septum, known as septum primum develops toward the endocardial cushion. Formation of septum primum results in the formation of foramen primum between septum primum and endocardial cushion. Foramen secundum is formed as a result of perforation in upper part of septum primum. The second septum or septum secundum is thick in nature and grows from the roof of atrium immediately to the right of the septum primum and overlaps the foramen secundum. This will eventually result in the formation of foramen ovale. The septum primum attached to the endocardial cushion forms—the flap of the foramen ovale (Figure 1.4). The foramen ovale allows flow of blood from the inferior vena cava (IVC) into the left atrium through the right atrium through the ductus venosus.
- **Partitioning of the ventricle (Figure 1.5):** There is formation of muscular ridge from the apex that grows toward the endocardial cushion and divides the ventricle. There is a crescent like opening between the edge of the ventricular septum and the endocardial cushion, the interventricular foramen. Closure of this foramen results due to growth of tissue from right and left bulbar ridges and the endocardial cushion. This is the membranous portion of ventricular septum.

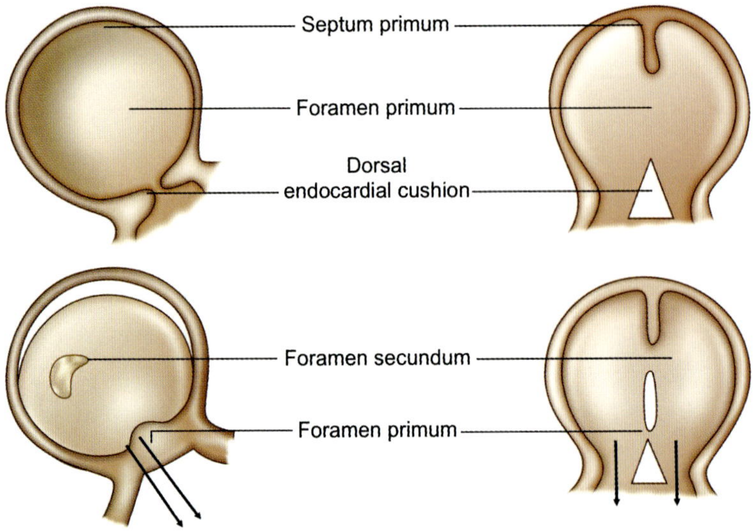

Figure 1.3 Partitioning of atrium

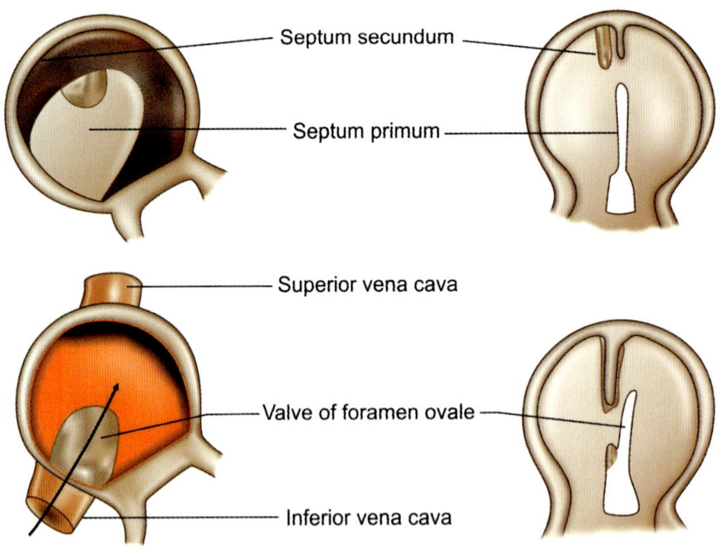

Figure 1.4 Formation of foramen ovale

- **Partitioning of the bulbus cordis and truncus arteriosus:** Bulbus cordis develops into bulbar ridge and truncus arteriosus develops from truncal ridge. These two fuse with each other and form aorticopulmonary septum. This is oriented in a spiral fashion. Bulbus cordis gives rise to a conical infundibulum on the right side and on the left side it gives rise to a narrow aortic vestibule. Truncus arteriosus gives rise to the posterior aorta and anterior pulmonary artery. The pulmonary artery wraps round the aorta due to spiraling of the aorticopulmonary septum.

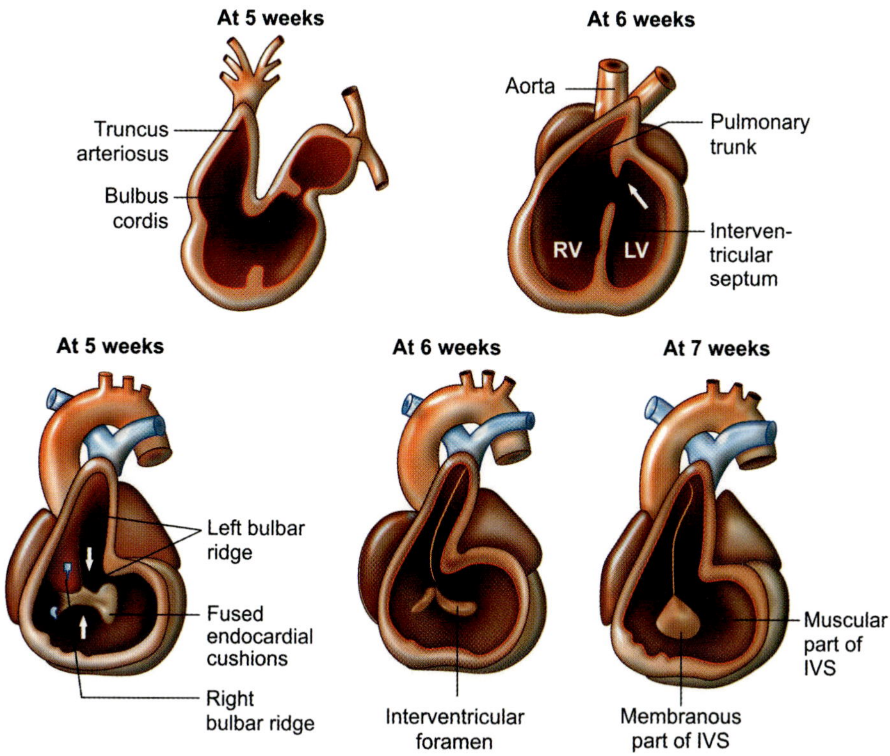

Figure 1.5 Partitioning of ventricle and formation of aorta and pulmonary artery

- **Development of the valves:** The mitral and tricuspid valves develop from the endocardial tissue at the atrioventricular orifice, while the semilunar valves develop from the endocardial tissue at the orifice of aorta and pulmonary arteries.
- **Development of conduction system:** In the beginning, temporary pacemaker of the heart is primitive atrium. Then there is formation of SA node from the walls of sinus venosus. The AV node and bundle of His develop from cells in the AV canal region. Soon they get innervated to form the specialized conduction system of the heart.

PHYSIOLOGY OF FETAL CIRCULATION

Almighty has designed beautiful system for fetal circulation. The physiology of fetal circulation is illustrated in Figures 1.6 and 1.7. There is equal pressure in the ventricles of both the sides. Blood coming from the umbilical vein through the placenta has high oxygen content and majority of it enters into right atrium via IVC and ductus venosus. As a result, the ductus venosus can be considered as the vessel of millennium for all practicing sonologists. It can be used for the prediction of fetal outcome.

Two major bypass routes in the fetal heart that prevent a major portion of the blood from entering the lungs are the foramen ovale and the ductus arteriosus.

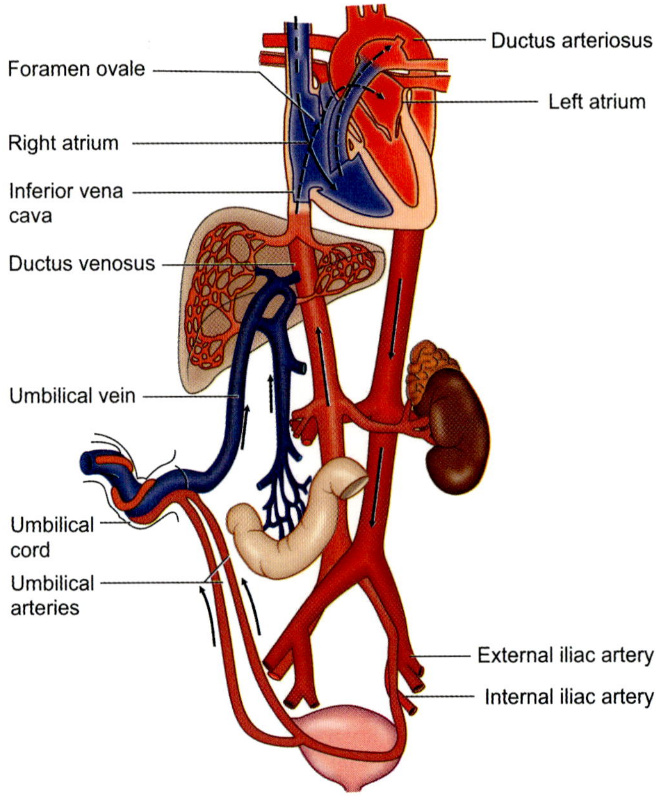

Figure 1.6 Fetal circulation with three shunts

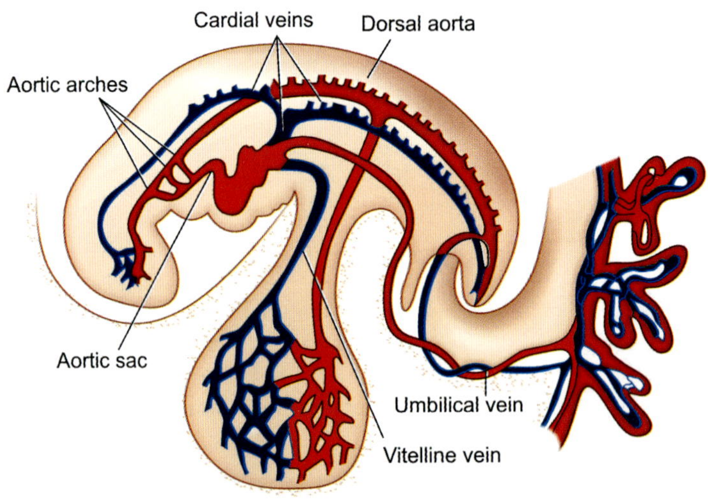

Figure 1.7 Fetal circulation

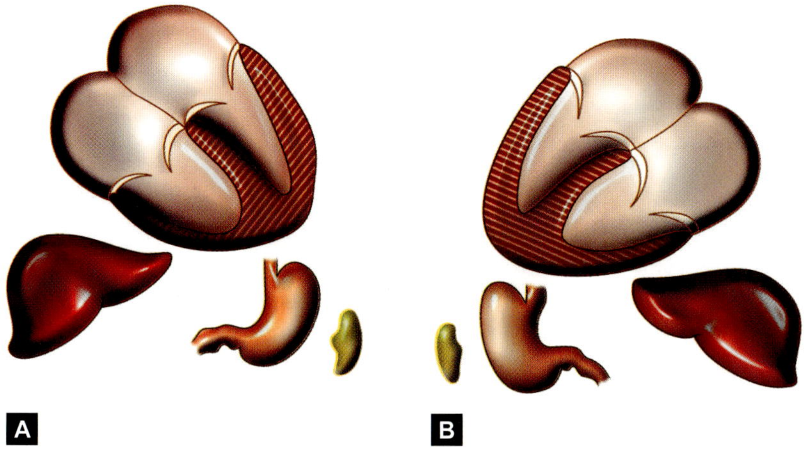

Figures 1.8A and B (A) Normal situs, (B) Situs inversus totalis

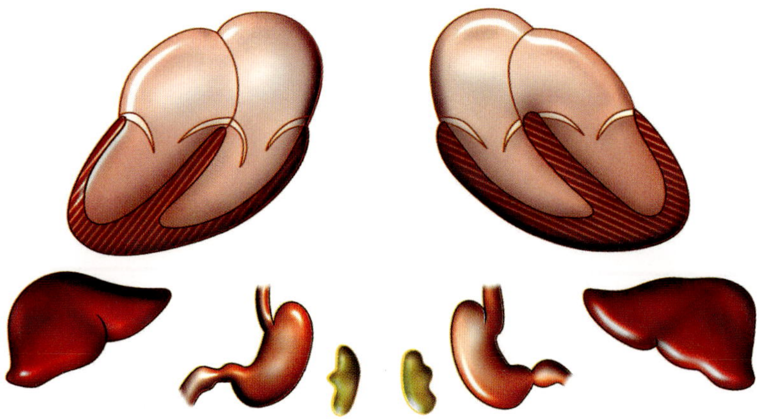

Figure 1.9 Situs ambiguous

Due to the presence of these two bypass mechanisms, only 30% of the fetal blood enters into fetal lungs. Blood gets entry into left atrium from right atrium via foramen ovale, which then gains entry into descending thoracic aorta via ductus arteriosus. First recipients of highly oxygenated blood are cardiac muscles and brain.

If we see fetal circulation in third trimester, there is prominence of pulmonary artery as right ventricular output is about 6% and left ventricular output is 34%.

If there is any change in hemodynamics, it may alter the shape and size of heart. Narrowing or obliteration of the inflow tracts (MV TV) or outflow tracts (AO and PA) will result in a redistribution of blood in cardiac chambers, altering the thickness of the ventricular walls and the function of the atria, ventricles and valves. Normal and abnormal positions of the heart have been illustrated in Figures 1.8 and 1.9, respectively.

NUTSHELL

1. This is the first system of the human race starts from 3rd week of intrauterine life and it last up to last breath and then shut down.
2. Circulation starts form 22nd days of intrauterine life through following three shunts
   A. Vitteline vein form yolk sac
   B. Umbilical vein from placenta
   C. Cardinal vein form embryo.
3. Heart tube is formed by fusion of two tubes and after bending there is formation of TBVAS (truncus arterious, bulbous cordis, primitive atria, primitive ventricle, and sinus venosus).
4. Endocardial cushion will separate atria form ventricle.
5. There are three things runs simultaneously:
   A. Formation of septum between two atria (interatrial septum)
   B. Formation of septum between two ventricle (interventricular septum)
   C. Formation of septum between truncus arterious (spiral septum, aortico-pulmonary septum).
6. Both mitral and tricuspid valves are formed from endocardial tissue between atria and ventricle.
7. Both semilunar valves are formed from endocardial tissue at origin from aorta and pulmonary artery.

2

Indications

INDICATIONS OF THE FETAL ECHO

Congenital heart disease (CHD) is a leading cause of infant mortality with an estimated incidence of about 4–13 per 1,000 livebirths. Between 1950 and 1994, 42% of infant deaths reported to the World Health Organization (WHO) were attributed to be due to cardiac defects. Structural cardiac anomalies were also among the abnormalities, most frequently missed by prenatal ultrasonologists. Prenatal detection of fetal cardiac anomalies helps in improving the outcome of pregnancies as nearly half of the cases of CHD are minor and may be easily corrected by surgery.

Nearly, 46% cases of CHDs are diagnosed by first week of life; 88% by first year and 98% by the age of 4 years. Incidence is typically increased after inclusion of bicuspid aortic valve disease as its incidence is estimated to be approximately 10 in 1,000 livebirths. In premature babies, cardiac defects such as patent ductus arteriosus (PDA) and ventricular septal defect (VSD) may be commonly encountered.

ETIOLOGY OF CARDIAC MALFORMATION

- Multifactorial mode of inheritance is a common cause of CVS anomalies. It could be associated with:
- Single gene disorders, such as autosomal recessive syndrome, e.g. hypoplastic left heart syndrome, Noonan syndrome and pulmonary stenosis.
- Chromosomal anomalies, e.g. Trisomy 21: (Atrial or ventricular septal defects); Trisomy 18 and 13: (ventricular septal defects)

During 1980 to 1990, it became a common practice to perform fetal echocardiography primarily in women who were considered to be at an increased risk of children having CHD. Some of these high-risk groups were as follows:

- Abnormal findings in the fetus on the routine obstetric study
- A family history or maternal disease associated with CHD

- Maternal indication:
  - Pre-existing metabolic diseases, such as diabetes, phenylketonuria, collagen vascular disease, etc.
  - Alcohol abuse
  - *Family history:* First degree relative of proband
  - *Maternal infections:* Parvovirus B19, rubella, coxsackie
  - *Cardiac teratogen exposure:* Retinoid, phenytoin, carbamazepine, lithium carbonate, valproic acid, etc.
  - *Maternal antibodies:* Anti-Ro (SSA), Anti-La (SSB)
- Fetal indication:
  - Nonimmune hydrops
  - Suspected fetal heart anomalies
  - Abnormal fetal karyotype
  - IUGR
  - Polyhydramnios
  - Increased nuchal translucency
  - Absent nasal bone
  - Fetal cardiac rate or rhythm disturbances, persistent bradycardia, persistent tachycardia, persistent irregular heart rhythm, etc.
- Familial risk factors:
  - Siblings history of cardiac defects
  - Cardiac defect in parents
  - Family history of cardiac defects.

There is always possibility of some type of cardiac anomalies in low-risk group of patients, especially where we see an abnormal four chamber view.

We prefer use of four chamber view as screening tool which helps in diagnosing at least one-third cases of CHDs. Prenatal detection of CHD depends on the following factors:

- Examiner's experience
- Maternal obesity
- Transducer frequency
- Abdominal scars
- Gestational age
- Amniotic fluid volume
- Fetal position.

The "basic" and "extended basic" cardiac ultrasound examinations are designed to maximize the detection of heart anomalies during second trimester scan and help in the visualization of the outflow tracts and great vessels.

We prefer to perform the initial transabdominal study of fetal heart between 16 and 20 weeks as at this gestational age, the valves are well developed, the size of heart is adequate for study and fetal size and position usually allow best access to fetal heart.

In some high-risk cases, early detection can be possible by 10–14 weeks with the help of TVS approach.

There are specific risk factors involved for CHD. Some of the fetal factors are enlisted here:

- Chromosomal abnormalities
- Extracardiac anatomical abnormalities
- Nonimmune hydrops fetalis
- Fetal cardiac arrhythmias
- Abnormal, cardiac scan on routine ultrasound examination

So many times, maternal history of congenital heart diseases and metabolic disorders, or exposure to some teratogenic agent may also lead to CHD.

On routine scan, if we see some anomaly per se such as nonimmune hydrops, we must always search for another anomaly and most of the times we may land up, detecting a CHD.

So, we must follow a rule that whenever we find some anomaly, we much definitely search for another one and usually it will be there.

In presence of fetal cardiac arrhythmias, we must think about some structural cardiac anomaly. If we look into statistics, we would find that more than 1% cases of CHD are associated with isolated extrasystole.

On fetal cardiac scan, if we see complete heart block, there are 50% chances of having cardiac anomalies.

Now, we have to observe every heart with suspicion and every pregnancy should be scanned because high level of suspicion will always pay in diagnosis of heart abnormalities. The incidence of maternal diabetes is now on a rise and more and more mothers having gestational diabetes are being encountered in clinical practice. Only, if we maintain a high level of suspicion at the time of routine ultrasound examinations, we would be able to pick-up fetal heart abnormalities. The incidence of CHD among diabetic mothers are five times higher in comparison to normal pregnant women; VSD and transposition of great vessels are very common and can be easily detected on targeted scanning.

In first trimester, high levels of glycosylated hemoglobin (HbA_{1C}) may sometimes result in the development of structural cardiac anomalies. So we must keep a strict watch for detecting the presence of cardiac anomalies in heart of the fetus of pregnant lady with high HBA_{1C} levels. This would enable us to give her best output in terms of normal fetal heart.

NUTSHELL

1. Congenital heart disease is a leading cause of infant mortality, structural anomaly were the most common and frequently missed by parental ultrasound.
2. Prenatal detection of fetal cardiac anomaly helps a lot because most of CHD are minor and may be corrected easily by surgery with very good outcome.
3. Multifactorial mode of inheritance is common cause of CVS anomaly. There will be indication for fetal cardiac evaluation on single gene or chromosomal anomaly, maternal and fetal indication as well as familial risk factors.
4. Examination of fetal heart will be dependent upon fetus as well as examiner's experience, maternal obesity, transducer frequency, abdominal scars, amniotic

fluid and most important is fetal position because if spine is anterior it will be very difficult to see fetal heart so cardiac conducive spine posterior fetus will be fine position.

5. Fetal cardiac examination is divided between two part basic and extended basic by International Society of Ultrasound in Obstetrics and Gynecology (ISUOG).
6. We can make sure after cardiac examination that this baby will require more comprehensive fetal echocardiography with detail examination of right ventricular outflow tract (RVOT), left ventricular outflow tract (LVOT), and tripple vessel and tracheal views.

3

Basics of Doppler

Nowadays, it has become a must for all of us to know about basics of Doppler as it is the study of blood flow in vessels and across valves in the heart. Obstetric Doppler ultrasound has gained a wide application in today's clinical practice.

FREQUENCY SHIFT

When there is relative motion between the source and observer, there occurs a change in the frequency of the sound waves and this change is known as the frequency shift.

DOPPLER SHIFT

When ultrasound waves are insolated on moving cells, such as the blood vessels, the backscattered echoes from the cells exhibit a different frequency in comparison to the transmitted frequency. The difference between the transmitted and the receiving frequency falls in the audible range and can be heard on a loudspeaker. The Doppler shift frequencies can also be recorded using frequency spectrum analyzers.

The waveform seen on the screen is known as a flow velocity waveform or a spectral waveform. With its use, it is possible to detect blood flow as well as its direction and velocity.

COLOR DOPPLER

This new modality of color Doppler helps to code the blood flow in color in a selected portion of vessels. The flow towards transducer is coded as red and flow away form the transducer is coded as blue (Figures 3.1A to C). Typical turbulent flow is shown as mosaic of colors.

This facility is very useful in segment selection of vessel and helps in judging the color flow pattern in particular segment. The fetal heart as visualized with color Doppler is shown in Figures 3.2 and 3.3.

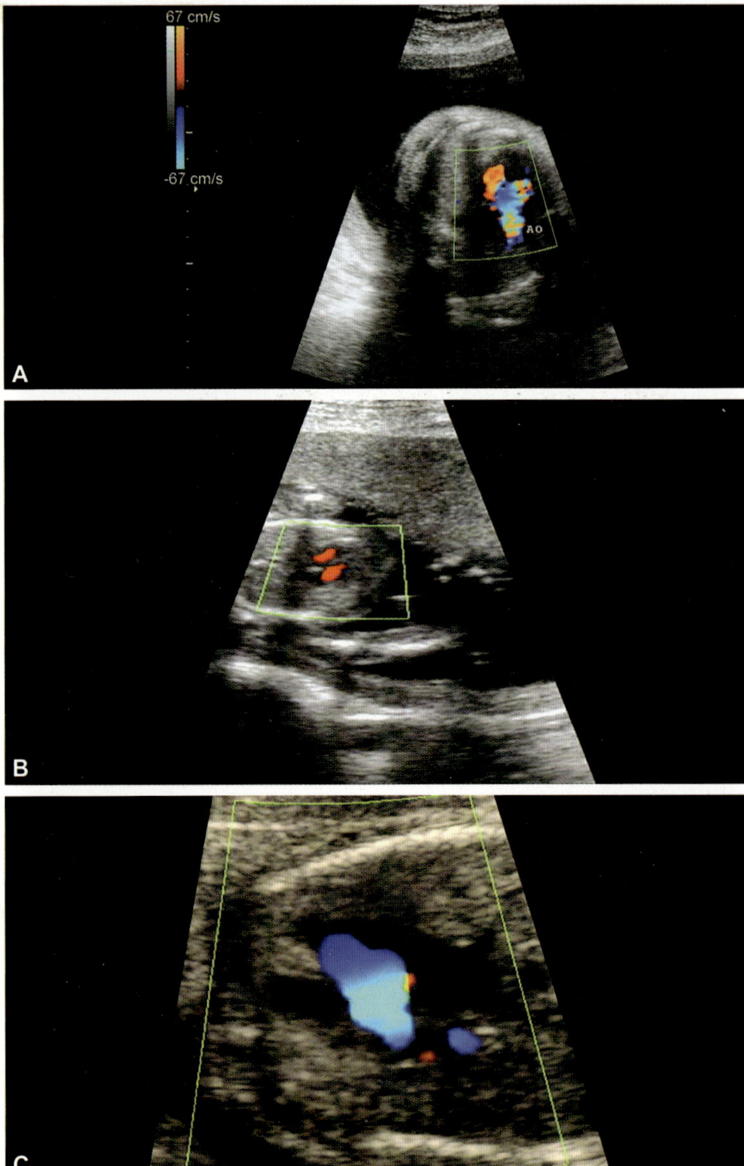

Figures 3.1A to C Difference in color on Doppler ultrasound in flow towards and away from transducer

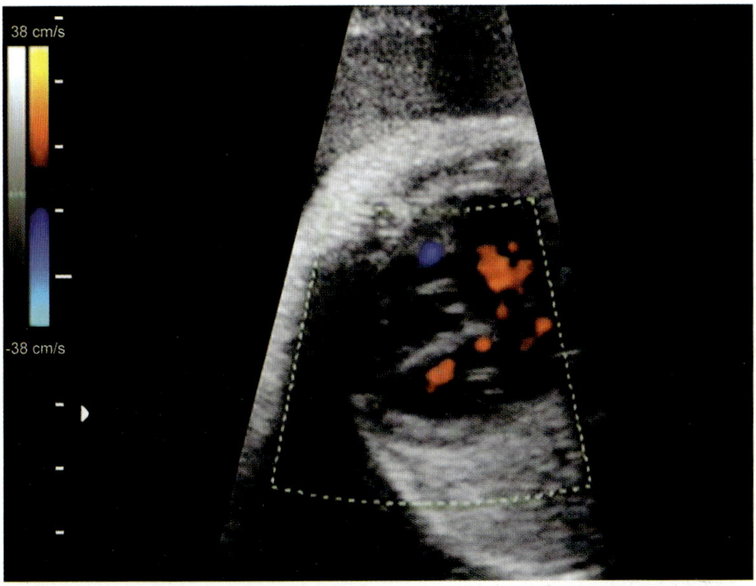

Figure 3.2 Fetal heart as seen with color Doppler

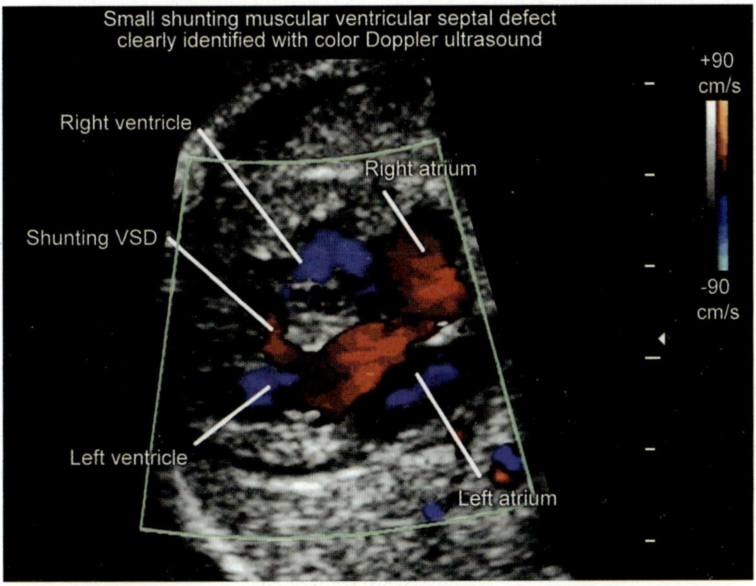

Figure 3.3 Labeled image of heart with color Doppler

Pulsed Wave (PW)

When the ultrasound beam passes through a vessel, the beam is reflected from the blood cells which are moving. By placing a marker within the lumen of the vessel, echosignals from moving cells can be processed and converted into a display as waveform on the screen which is also termed as a "spectral waveform" (Figure 3.4). The marker is called the "spectrum volume". The width and position of the sample volume is adjustable. By placement of the sample volume, the depth from which the Doppler information is obtained can be determined.

Duplex Ultrasound

The pulsed Doppler with the B mode is called the duplex ultrasound. This helps in visualizing the vessel with the B mode for precise placement of the sample volume for obtaining the Doppler shift. The Doppler shift thus determined is converted by the machine to three different kinds of output mainly:

1. Audio output on a loudspeaker
2. Recording on a zero crossing recorder
3. Spectral waveform by a specialized fast Fourier transform technique.

Continuous Wave (CW)

Ultrasound is continuously transmitted by one transducer and received by another. Doppler signals are received from all depths along the sound beam. Hence, when no depth resolution is possible, higher frequency of Doppler shifts can be detected.

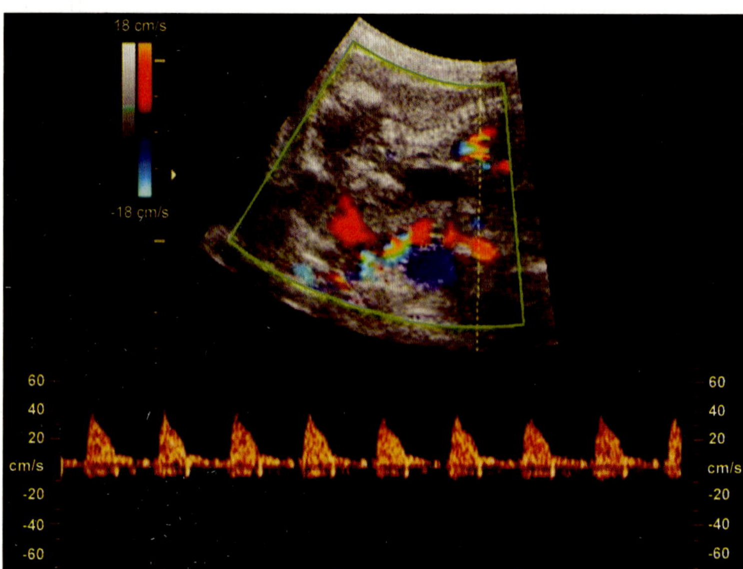

Figure 3.4 Spectral waveform

Two types of CW Doppler are as follows:

1. Directional Doppler with which flow direction can be detected
2. Nondirectional Doppler.

This mode is used for the study of blood vessel and flow across valves in the heart. It has wide application in echocardiography, peripheral vascular disease and in obstetrics.

Let us know a little bit about Doppler equations:

$$F_d = (2VF_o \cos \phi)/c$$

Where $F_d = F_o - F_r$ = Doppler shift frequency
F_o = Transmitted frequency
F_r = Received frequency
V = Average velocity of blood flow
c = Propagation speed of sound in blood
ϕ = Angle subtended by the Doppler beam to the direction of flow.

To obtain the maximum Doppler yield, it is imperative to maintain the Doppler angle between 45 and 60 degrees. As the angle approaches 90 degree, the cosine of 90 is 0 and hence no flow would be recorded.

The velocity of blood can be calculated when the Doppler shift frequency is known, i.e.

$$V = F_d \times c/F_o \cos \phi$$

Pulse Repetition Frequency (PRF)

This is the number of pulses occurring in a second and is expressed in Hertz (Hz) or kilohertz (kHz).

Nyquist Limits

An ultrasound pulse takes 6.5 msec to travel 1 cm of tissue. The deeper the pulse, more is the time taken to travel and hence the number of times a pulse is repeated in a second has to be less, i.e. the PRF reduces as the depth increases. The sampling theory states that if a wave has to be depicted accurately, it must be sampled by not less than twice its frequency. Thus, if a 2 kHz signal has to be detected, the PRF must be at least 4 kHz.

Aliasing

If the PRF is less than twice the Doppler shift, the detected Doppler shift will appear lower than the actual Doppler shift. This is known as aliasing (Figure 3.5). Aliasing can be avoided using CW Doppler.

Doppler Receiver Gain

It is ideal to have the maximum Doppler gain setting which is possible without producing "noise" on the screen. A high gain setting can produce "mirroring" of the Doppler signal and filling up of the spectral window.

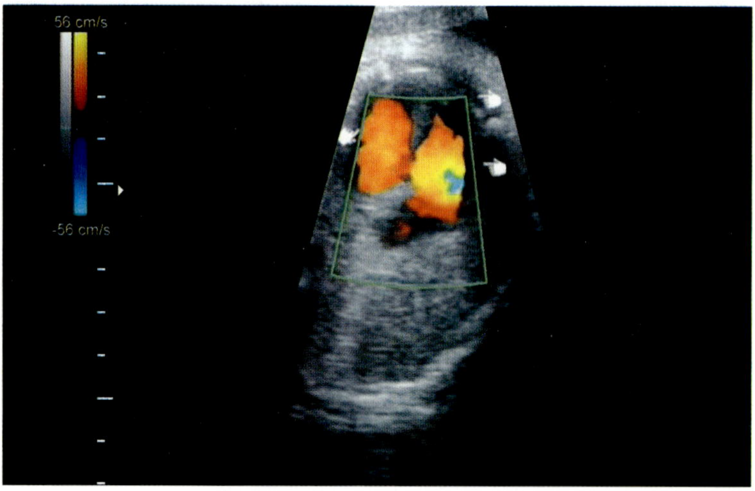

Figure 3.5 Aliasing in color Doppler

Sample Volume

The space from which Doppler information is obtained by a pulsed Doppler is called sample volume. The area of the sample volume is adjustable. It may also be positioned at the desired depth and location within the lumen of the vessel. Small sample volume is used to obtain Doppler information from precise points such as the center stream in the vessel, thereby eliminating noise from neighboring vessels.

Wall Filters

Wall filters or high pass filters are provided to eliminate low frequency Doppler signals in the spectral display. Wall filters are adjustable from 50–800 Hz. The lowest setting (50–100 Hz) is preferable unless the clutter from wall motion disturbs the spectral waveforms.

Spectral Broadening

When there is flow disturbance, the movement of blood cells is chaotic. This results in multiple velocities being present at any given time instant. These multiple velocities are depicted in the Doppler spectrum as a filling up of the spectral window and are termed as spectral broadening. Artifactual spectral broadening can also occur if the vessel is sampled very close to the wall and if the Doppler gain setting is very high.

Doppler audio signal are characteristic for each vessel and can be recognized easily. The spectral waveform also varies from vessel to vessel. The pattern of the waveform depends largely on the distal peripheral resistance and the compliance of the vessel. In a vessel such as the common femoral artery, where the distal resistance is quite high and the compliance of the vessel is good, a “triphasic waveform” is obtained with a sharp systolic peak, a brief period of flow in late systole and near zero flow during diastole. In a low resistance vessel such as the internal carotid artery, there is forward flow during systole and diastole.

KNOBOLOGY

It is mandatory for all of us to know our machine well. We must use all knobs of machine perfectly to get optimum result of image in order to scan well. We all are using only few buttons of machine in day-to-day ultrasound usage but in order to do echo, little bit more knowledge regarding different knobs is must.

We must know the frequency of our probe and for echo, higher frequency probe is must or we have to use the highest frequency probe we have.

Higher frequency probes will help in improving the likelihood of detecting subtle defects at an expense of reduced acoustic penetration.

We must know the trade off between penetration and resolution. We prefer 7.5 or 5 MHz transducer, but have also used a 3 MHz transducer, when deeper penetration is required.

Ideal machine for echo should be equipped with M mode, pulsed wave Doppler and continuous wave Doppler with color flow Doppler. Harmonics imaging may provide improved images especially for patients with increased maternal abdominal wall thickness during the third trimester of pregnancy. Gray scale is still better for imaging and reliable for fetal cardiac scanning. System setting should emphasize a high frame rate with increased contrast resolution. Low frame persistence, a single acoustic focal zone, and a relatively narrow image field should also be used for this purpose.

Figure 3.6 shows difference between native image without high contrast and we can see the difference with increased contrast. Figure 3.7 shows importance of focal zone where we have to see side arrow from where signals of ultrasound image are coming and best zone to visualize fetal heart is zone 4.

Now see the difference by using persistence, we can obtain fantastic clarity between heart walls (Figures 3.8A and B).

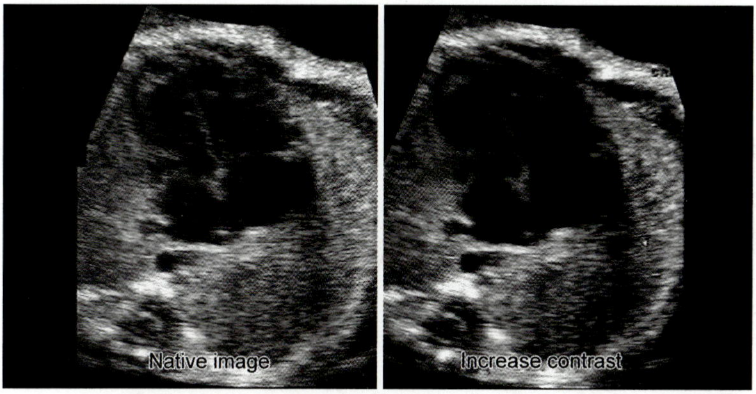

Figure 3.6 Difference between image qualities of the native image without high contrast and when seen with increase contrast

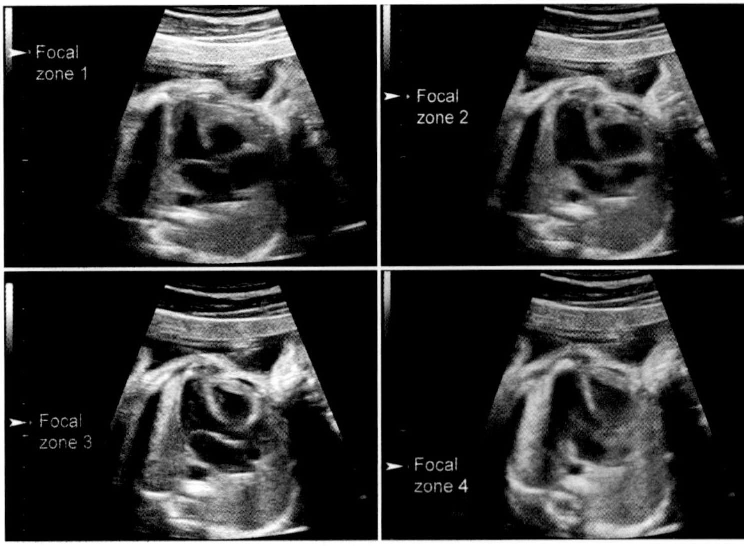

Figure 3.7 Importance of focal zone where we have to see side arrow from where signals of ultrasound image are coming and best zone to visualize fetal heart is zone 4

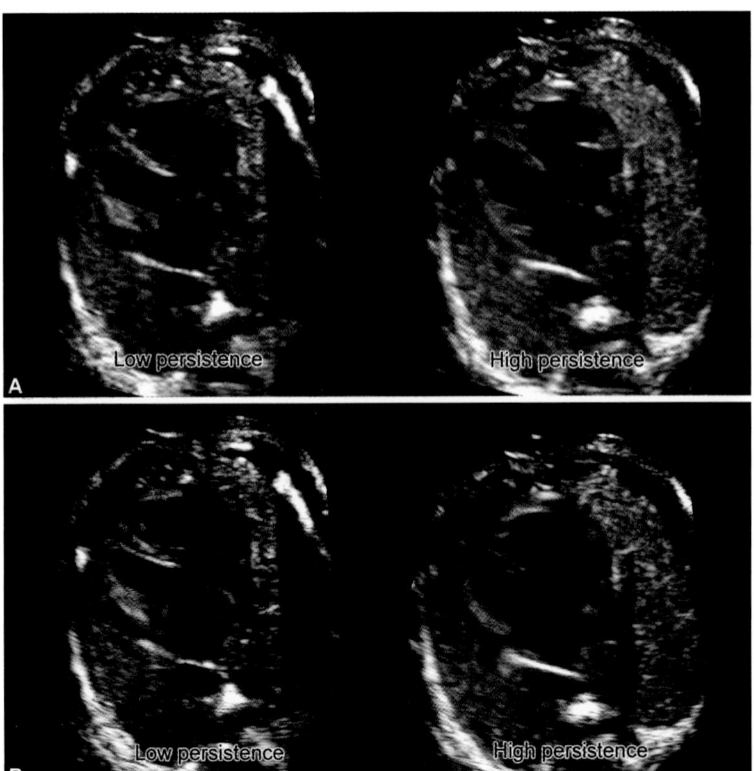

Figures 3.8A and B Difference in the image quality through the use of persistence

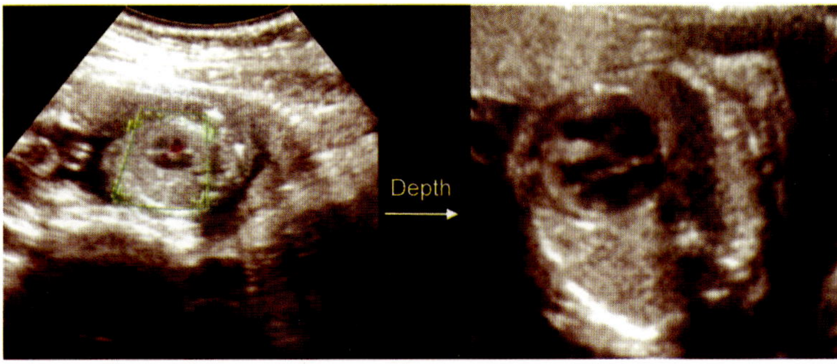

Figure 3.9 Use of depth view to visualize the fetal heart

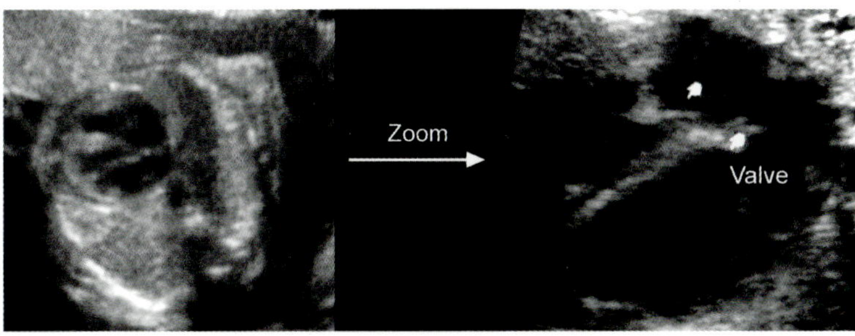

Figure 3.10 Zoom view for the heart

Zooming the image is best for cardiac scan and must be used enthusiastically by all the sonologists in order to get maximum output. Image should be magnified until the heart fills at least a third to one-half of the display screen. If available, a cine-loop feature can be used to assist in the evaluation of ventricular septal defect and heart valve leaflets throughout the cardiac cycle.

In routine ultrasound, we are visualizing image in low depth to get good resolution (Figure 3.9) but, in fetal echo we need to magnify the image. However, the most untouched button on the ultrasound screen is the zoom button. Zoom button on screen must be used more frequently in order to obtain best image of fetal heart. Yes, by zooming we can see the difference in image quality of heart (Figure 3.10).

NUTSHELL

1. Frequency shift is change in frequency of sound waves between source and observer.
2. Doppler shift is difference between frequency transmitted and frequency received and can be depicted as spectral waveforms.
3. Color Doppler will give us idea of flow towards to probe and flow away from the probe.

4. Pulsed wave is spectral waveform on screen by putting gate on moving cell in vessel.
5. Duplex wave form is pulsed Doppler with B mode and gives us audio output, recording on zero cross border and spectral waveforms.
6. Continuous wave is continues transmission by one transducer and received by another.
7. Pulsed repetitive frequency is number of pulse in a second and will be shown on screen as Hertz or Kilohertz and this have to be adjusted according to vessel for sample.
8. Knobology is must leaned by examiner as different machine will have different nobe, frequency of probe, focal length, brightness, contract, persistence, speckle reduction, depth and zoom.... is very much required for fetal heart examination.

4

Step-by-Step Approach to Fetal Heart

Anatomy of fetal heart makes fetal echo very easy to perform for scanning. It is very amazing to scan three dimensional heart using two dimensional ultrasound. Fetal heart occupies one-third of the thoracic cavity. In fetal life, the heart is seen in the mid-position with the apex to the left and is more horizontally placed. In postnatal life, heart is seen on the left side of thorax. The base of the heart is close to the spine and apex is close to the thoracic cage. Best position for fetal echo is spine posterior or posterolateral.

Fetal cardiac evaluation is done in following steps:

- Determination of cardiac situs
- Estimation of cardiac size and axis
- The four chamber view
- The outflow tracts
- Real time evaluation of valves, septae and contractility of ventricles
- M-mode studies
- Color flow and Doppler studies.

The 'basic' and 'extended basic' cardiac ultrasound examinations are designed to maximize the detection of heart anomalies during second trimester scan and to visualize the outflow tracts and great vessels.

We prefer to perform the initial transabdominal study of fetal heart between 16 and 20 weeks as at this gestational age the valves are well developed, the size of heart is adequate for study and fetal size and position usually allows best access to fetal heart.

In some high-risk cases, early detection can be possible with help of TVS approach by 10–14 weeks.

The sonologist must first acquire a four chamber view of the heart. While acquiring this view, the following points must be kept in mind:

- Transverse section must be obtained through the fetal thorax
- This corresponds to the four chamber apical view in the adult
- The atrium nearest to the spine is the left atrium

- The atrium nearest to the fetal anterior thoracic wall is the right, which is 45 + 20° towards the left
- Abnormal axis increases the risk of a cardiac malformation
- The heart may also be displaced from its normal position in diaphragmatic hernia or cystic adenomatoid malformations
- Fetus cephalic
- Probe marker to mother's left
- Fetal spine posterior.

BASIC FETAL CARDIAC EXAMINATION (FIGURE 4.1)

General

- Done on a four chamber view
- Heart mostly on the left side of the chest
- Occupies one-third of thoracic area
- Normal cardiac situs, axis and position
- No pericardial effusion.

Atria

- Both are same size
- *Lower end of atrial septum:* Septum primum is present
- *Lower end of septum:* Foramen ovale (Figure 4.2)
- Flap of foramen ovale opens in LA.

Ventricles

- Both are equal size
- Intact septum
- Moderator band identifies right ventricle.

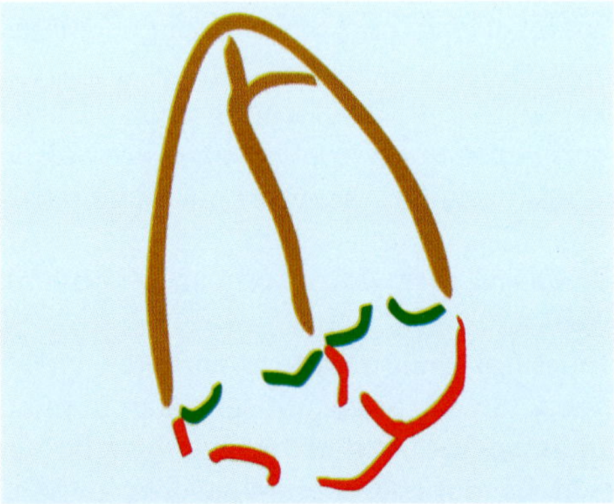

Figure 4.1 Structures to visualize the heart

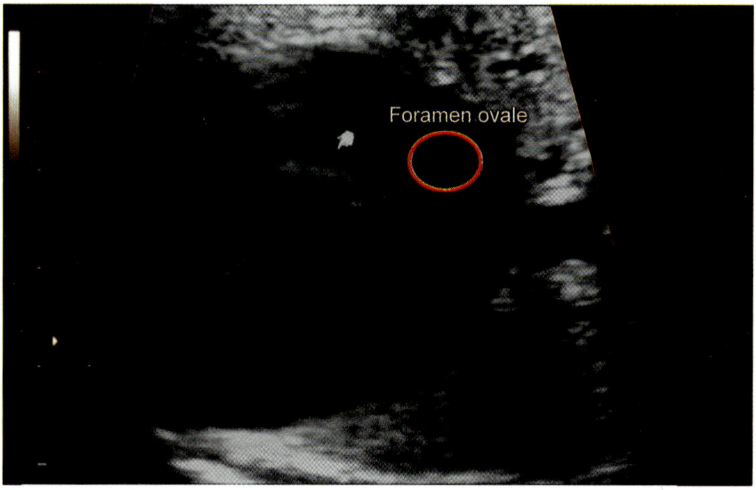

Figure 4.2 Foramen ovale

AV Valves

- Both valves move freely
- Tricuspid valve inserted more apically than mitral.

EXTENDED BASIC CARDIAC EXAMINATION

- The outflow tracts are imaged by tilting the probe towards the fetal head
- The great vessels should be of equal size and should cross at approximately 90° as they emerge from their respective ventricles.

Look for these:

- The outflow tracts cross each other at about 90° (Figures 4.3A and B)
- The anterior aortic root wall is continuous with the interventricular septum
- Bifurcation of pulmonary artery (Figure 4.4)
- The aortic and pulmonary valves move freely
- Both great vessels are of similar size, but the pulmonary artery tends to be slightly bigger.

The aortic arch (Figures 4.5A and B)

- The aortic arch can be identified
- The aortic cusps can be seen
- As the aortic arch is followed, the entire aorta (Figures 4.6A to F) can also be visualized.

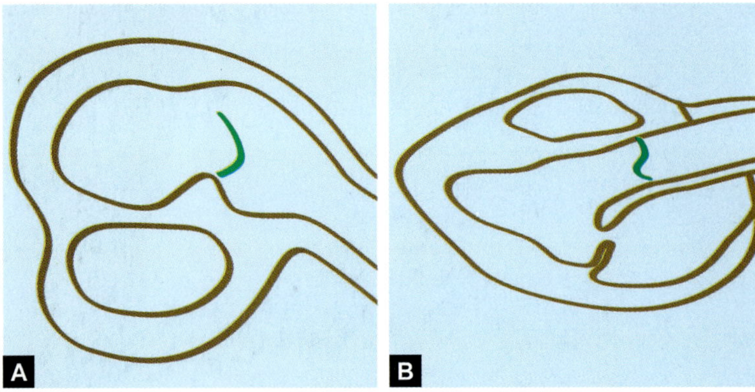

Figures 4.3A and B The outflow tracts crossing at around 90° (A) Pulmonary trunk; (B) Aortic arch

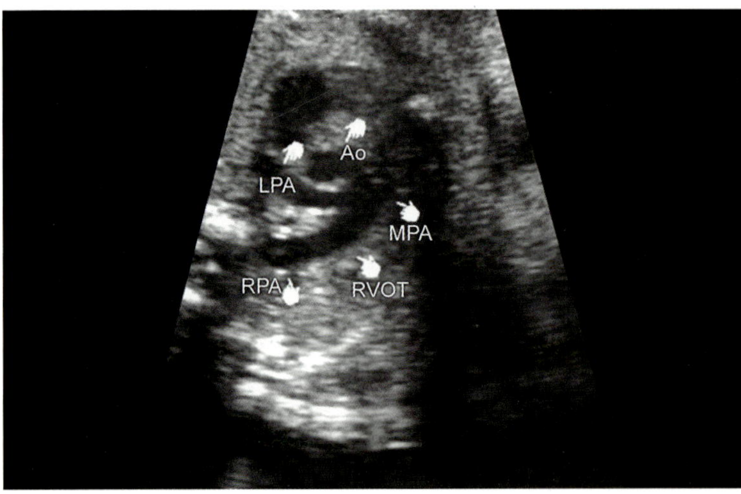

Figure 4.4 The pulmonary artery bifurcation
Abbreviations: Ao, aorta, LPA, left pulmonary artery; MPA, main pulmonary artery; RPA, right pulmonary artery; RVOT, right venticular outflow tract

ECHOGENIC INTRACARDIAC FOCUS (FIGURES 4.7A AND B)

- Can be seen in up to 6% of normal pregnancies
- Highly operator and machine dependent

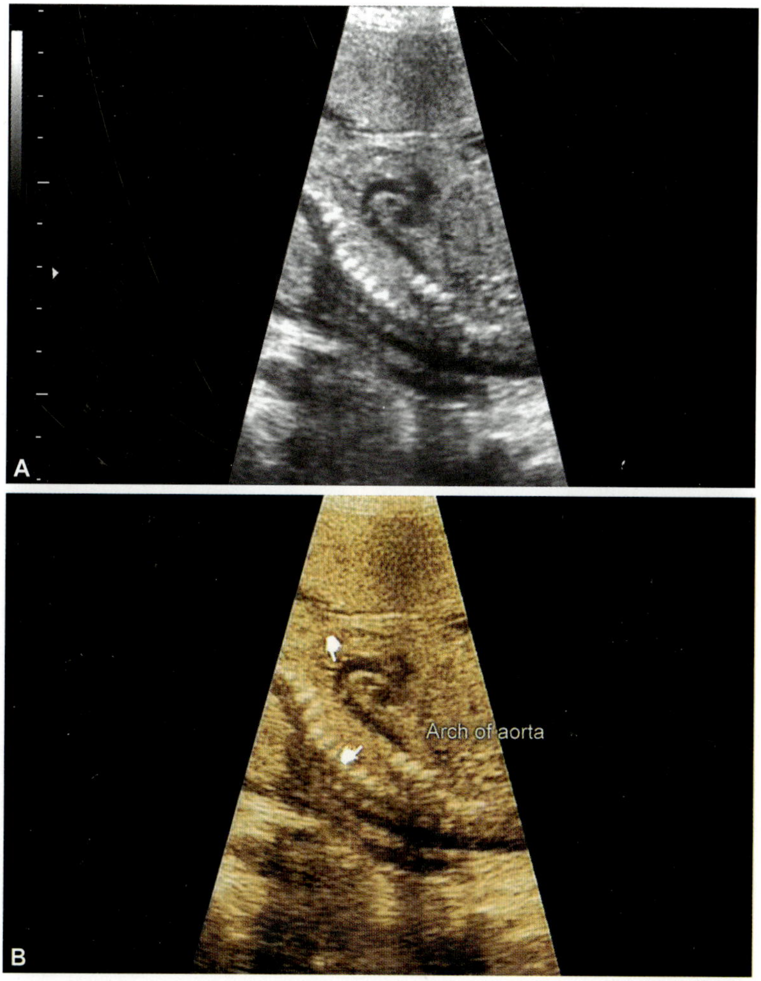

Figures 4.5A and B Arch of aorta

- Associated with cardiac and extracardiac anomalies
- Bilateral echogenic intracardiac focus (EIF) is more significant.

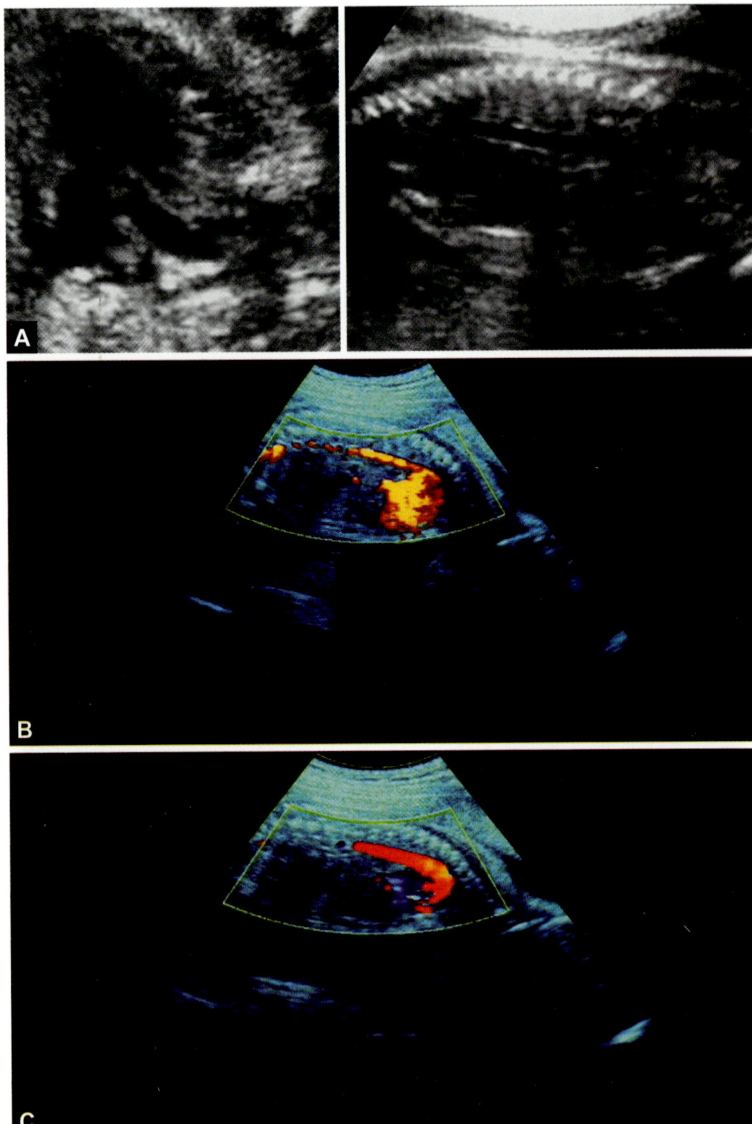

Figures 4.6A to C

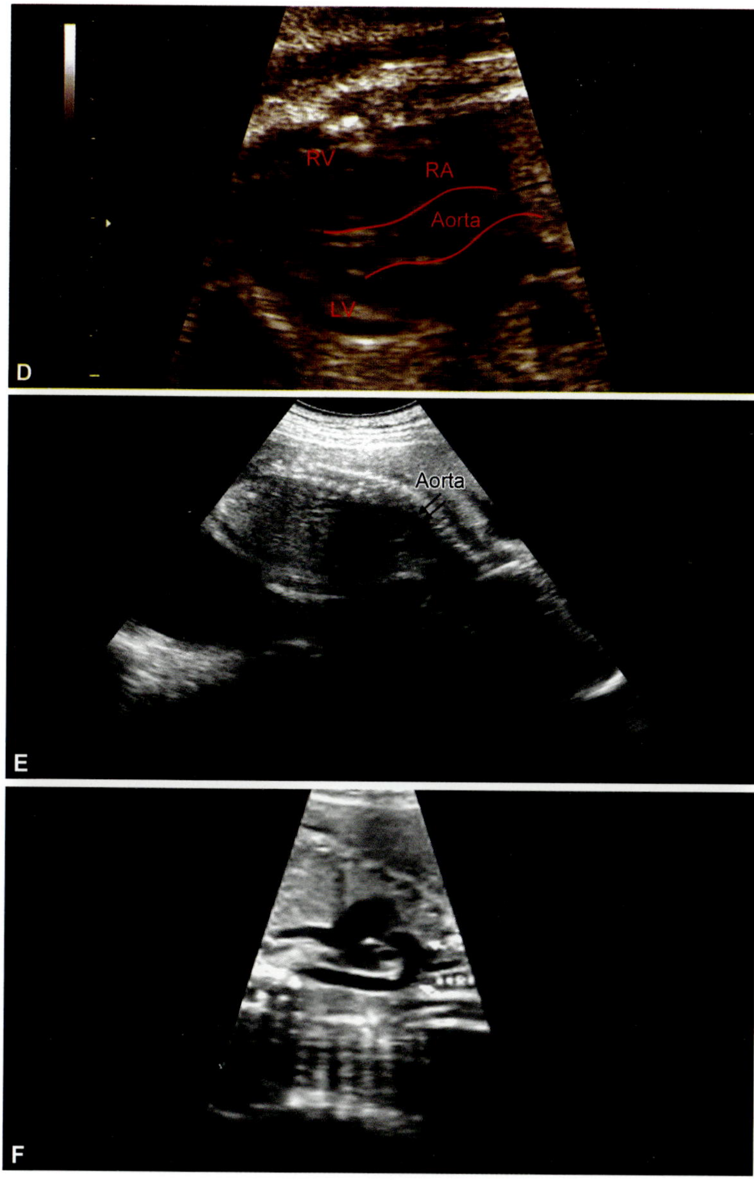

Figures 4.6D to F

Figures 4.6A to F Aorta

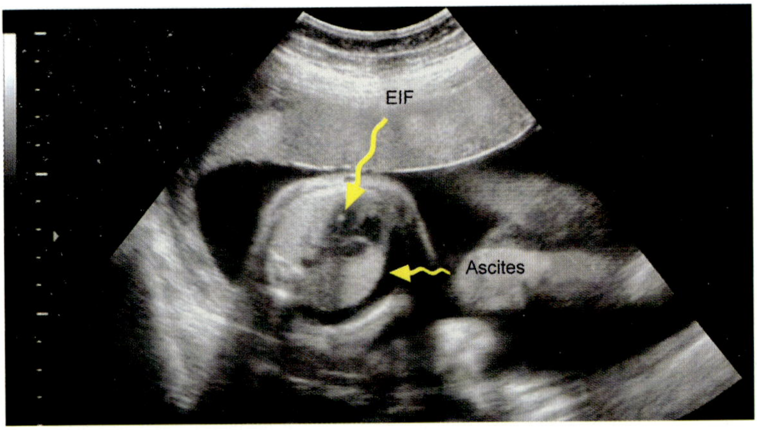

Figure 4.7A Echogenic intracardiac focus
Abbreviation: EIF, echogenic intracardiac focus

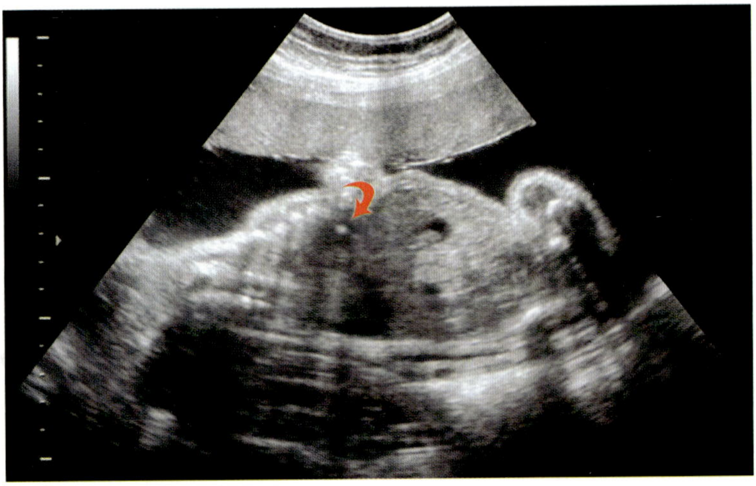

Figure 4.7B Echogenic intracardiac focus (Lateral view)

NUTSHELL

1. Heart is three-dimensional structure and we are examining it is two dimension with USG.
2. Heart occupied one third of thoracic cavity.
3. Best position of fetal heart examination is fetal spine posterior or posterolateral.
4. Heart should be examined stepwise like, determination of cardiac situs, estimation of cardiac size and axis, four chamber view, both outflow tract, i.e. LVOT and RVOT, movement of both valves, M mode study and color flow with Doppler study.
5. Fetal heart should be examined in both basic and extended basic examination.

5

Cardiac Examination

The basic cardiac screening examination relies on a four-chamber view of the fetal heart. We should not mistaken this as merely simple counting of the heart chambers, but it involves careful examination, taking into account the specific criteria and anatomical landmarks.

The best access to the heart is through the fetal abdomen but imaging is also possible through the rib cage and from the back because the fetal lungs are filled with fluid and are not a barrier to the passage of ultrasound, as they become so in the postnatal period.

In later period of gestation, fetal back is very much near to transducer and much of the ultrasonic energy is absorbed by the vertebral bodies, scapula and ribs which have become ossified, resulting in poorer imaging quality from the spine on the anterior side.

It may be sometimes necessary to turn mother to one side or elevate her chest or pelvis by pillow in order to improve the quality of scanning. Sometimes, we have to make mother walk around for some time and again examine her. At times, we may even have to postpone the scan for a day or a week.

In cases of polyhydramnios, the fetus sometimes lies away from the transducer when mother is recumbent. In these cases, the fetus can be made to lie close to transducer by asking the mother to put her knees in the genu position (mother has to rest on her knees and elbows, i.e. the knee-elbow position).

Once the fetal heart is located, only slight movements of the transducer are required to display the cardiac structures. A normal heart is usually no longer than one-third the area of the chest. Some views may reveal a small hypoechoic rim around the fetal heart that can be mistaken for a pericardial effusion. Figure 5.1 illustrates the pericardium in the normal four-chamber view.

Pericardial effusion may sometimes occur even in normal fetuses. An isolated finding of this type usually represents a normal variation. The four-chamber view of the heart is seen in a transverse section of the fetal thorax. Cardiac rate and rhythm should be confirmed as we all know that the normal range varies between 120 and 160 BPM. Mild bradycardia may be transiently observed in normal second

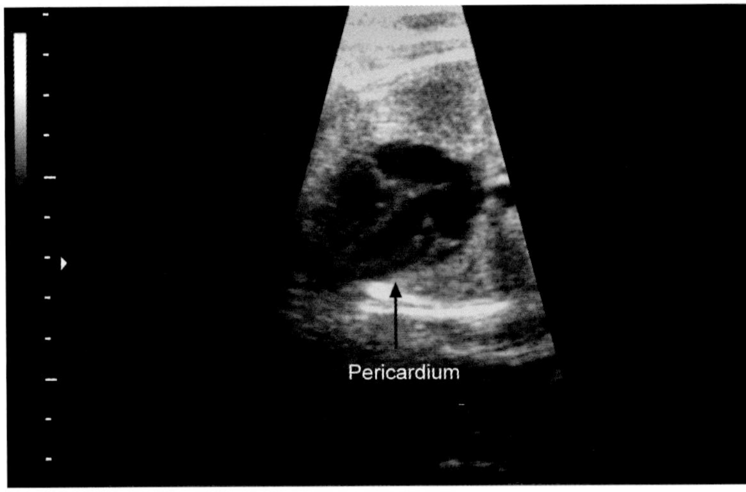

Figure 5.1 Pericardium in normal four-chamber view

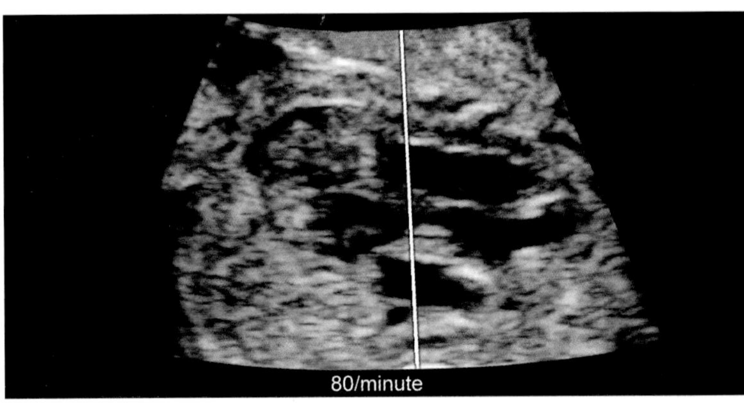

Figure 5.2 Bradycardia (heart rate < 100/min)

trimester fetuses. Fixed bradycardia, especially when it remains below 110 BPM, warns us to think of the possible underlying heart block (Figure 5.2).

If there is fetal distress, the heart may experience repetitive heart rate decelerations.

Occasional skipped beats are typically not associated with an increased risk of structural fetal heart disease. Mild tachycardia > 160 BPM (Figure 5.3) sometimes may occur because of fetal movements. However, persistent tachycardia must be further evaluated for possible fetal distress or more serious tachydysrhythmias.

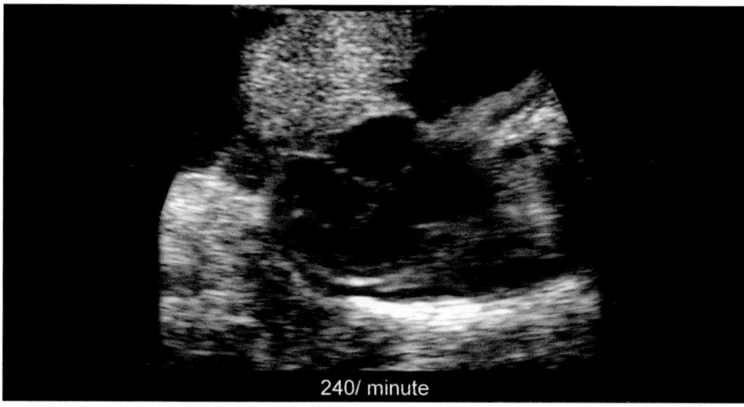

Figure 5.3 Tachycardia in a fetus (heart rate > 160/min)

The heart is normally deviated about 45 ± 20% (2 SD) towards left side. We must be very careful in measuring cardiac axis because this can be easily evaluated even if four-chamber view is not satisfactorily visualized. Situs abnormalities should be suspected when the fetal heart and/or stomach is not found on left side of baby. Abnormal axis increases the risk of a cardiac anomalies especially those of the outflow tract. Sometimes, the heart is abnormally displaced from its usual position in the anterior left central chest. Abnormal cardiac position can be caused by:

- Diaphragmatic hernia (Figures 5.4A and B).
- Space occupying lesion such as cystic adenomatoid malformation.

Position abnormalities can also be secondary to fetal lung hypoplasia or agenesis.

Both atrial chambers normally appear similar in size and foramen ovale flap should open into the left atrium (Figures 5.5A and B).

Pulmonary veins can often be seen entering the left atrium. However, their identification should not be considered as a mandatory part of basic cardiac screening examination.

The lower rim of atrial septal tissue called the septum primum should be present. A moderator band helps to identify the morphological right ventricle. Both ventricles should appear similar in size without evidence of thickened walls. However, mild ventricular disproportion may occur as normal variant. We must examine ventricular septum from apex to crux. It is very difficult to detect ventricular septal defect when angle of insonation is directly parallel to ventricular wall and may sometimes give false information regarding ventricular septal defect (VSD). Therefore, the sonologist must change the position of transducer and watch the septum carefully and put color on, in order to have a sense of security regarding the diagnosis. Figure 5.6 presents with a labeled image of all the structures to be visualized in an ultrasound examination of the normal heart.

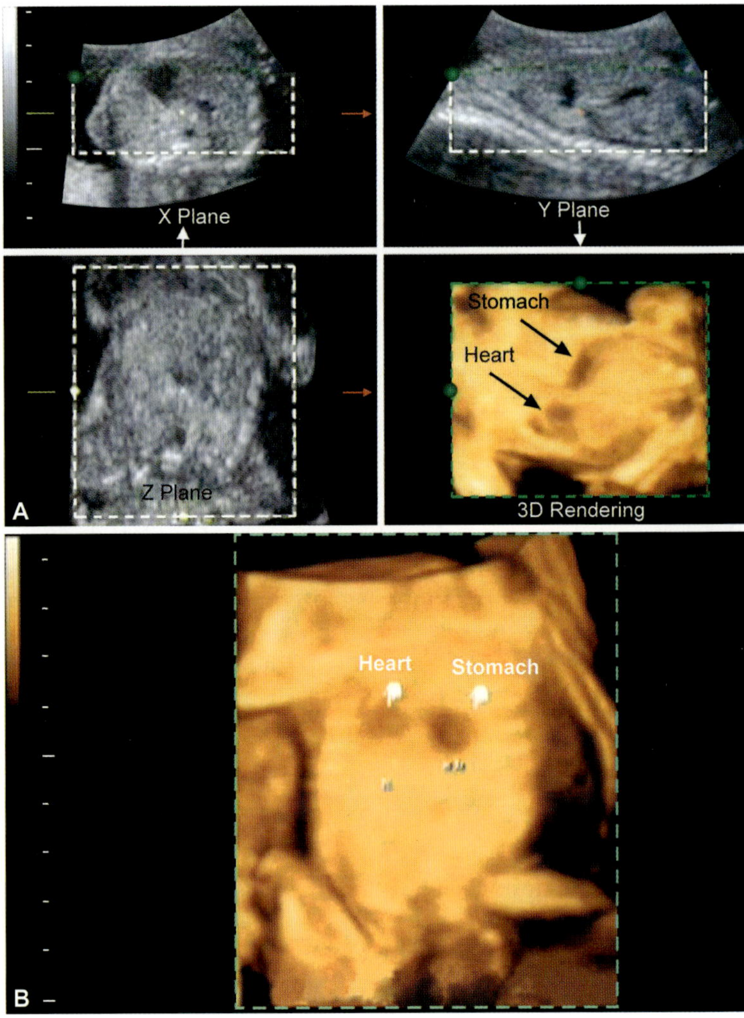

Figures 5.4A and B Diaphragmatic hernia

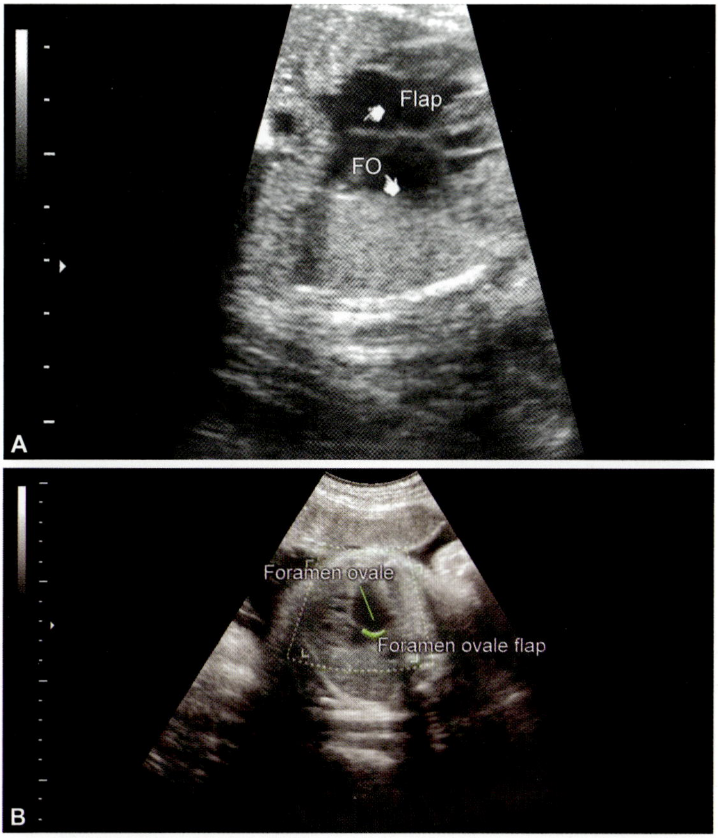

Figures 5.5A and B Labeled image of the foramen ovale flap
Abbreviation: FO, foramen ovale

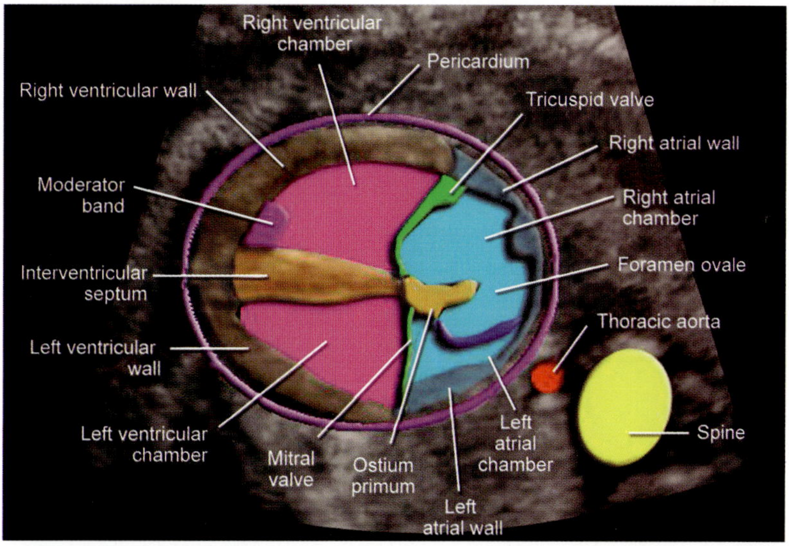

Figure 5.6 Labeled image of all the structures to be visualized in USG of the normal heart

NUTSHELL

1. Basic heart examination relies on four-chamber view, to get it, we must get proper view of fetal heart by moving mother to side, put pillow on one side, knee elbow position or postpond examination.
2. Cardiac axis is about 45 ± 20° (2 SD).
3. Heart occupy one-third of chest.
4. Both atrial should of equal size and foramen ovale open in LA (left atrium).
5. Both ventricles should be of equal size and moderator band should be seen in RV (right ventricle).
6. Both valves mitral and tricuspid should move freely.
7. Interventricular septum should be seen clearly form apex to crux.

6

Normal Situs

The very first step in ultrasonic evaluation of fetal heart is assessment of fetal situs.

Fetal situs establishes the accurate determination of the ventricular and atrial situs.

Three types of situs, which may exist are:

1. Situs solitus
2. Situs inversus (Figures 6.1A and B)
3. Situs ambiguous (Figure 6.2)

Clinical findings related to different types of situs are described in Table 6.1.

FETAL THORACIC ANATOMY

During embryogenesis, development of ribs occur from the mesenchymal costal process of the thoracic vertebrae. At the gestational age of 6.5 weeks, chondrification starts and well developed cartilaginous thoracic cage forms at

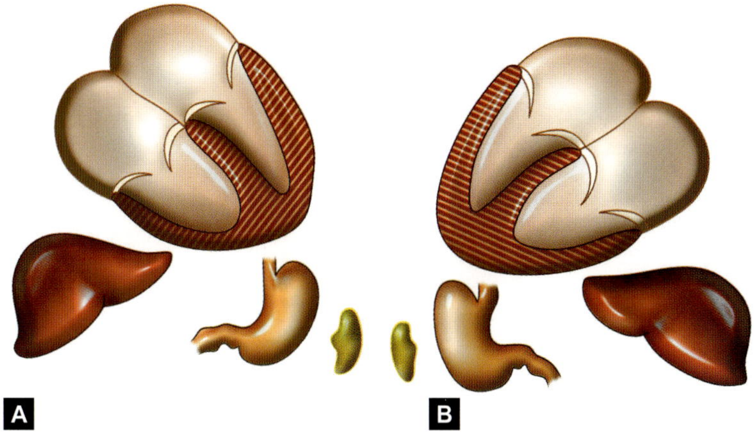

Figures 6.1A and B (A) Normal situs; (B) Situs inversus totalis

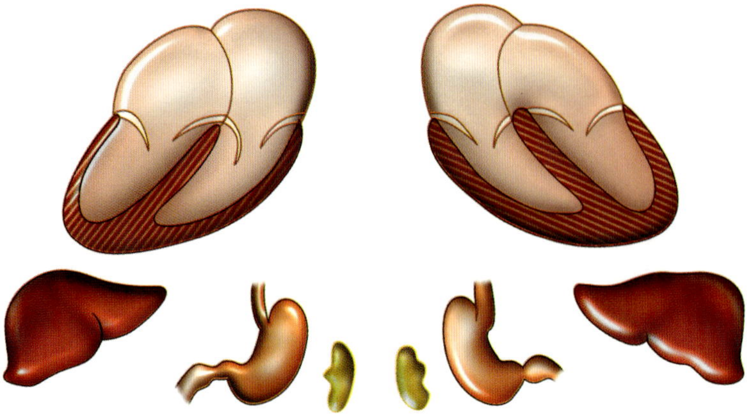

Figure 6.2 Situs ambiguous

Table 6.1 Clinical findings related to different types of situs

Situs	*Findings*	
	Right side	*Left side*
Solitus	Right atrium Major hepatic lobe Inferior vena cava Trilobed lung	Left atrium Stomach Descending aorta Bilobed lung
Inversus	Left atrium Stomach Descending aorta Bilobed lung	Right atrium Major hepatic lobe Inferior vena cava Trilobed lung
Ambiguous	Variable	Variable

the end of embryonic life. During the first trimester, endochondral ossification occurs. At the time of complete development, there is formation of thoracic cage, which consists of 12 thoracic vertebrae, 12 ribs and costal cartilage and sternum. During fetal life, ribs are more horizontally placed within the thoracic cavity.

STEP-BY-STEP APPROACH TO SITUS

Step 1

Step 1 involves locating the fetal head within the uterus and determining the presenting part, i.e. whether cephalic or breech (Figure 6.3).

Step 2

Step 2 involves determining the fetal lie within the uterus by obtaining a sagittal view of the fetal spine (Figures 6.4A and B). The lie is longitudinal when the fetal spine

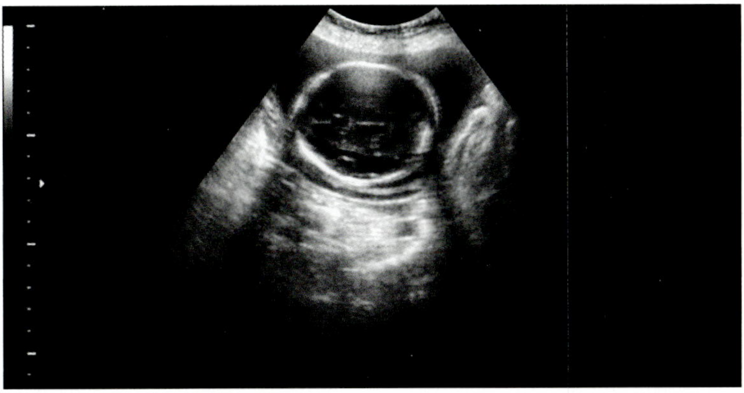

Figure 6.3 *Step 1:* Locating the fetal head within the uterus and determining the presenting part, i.e. cephalic or breech

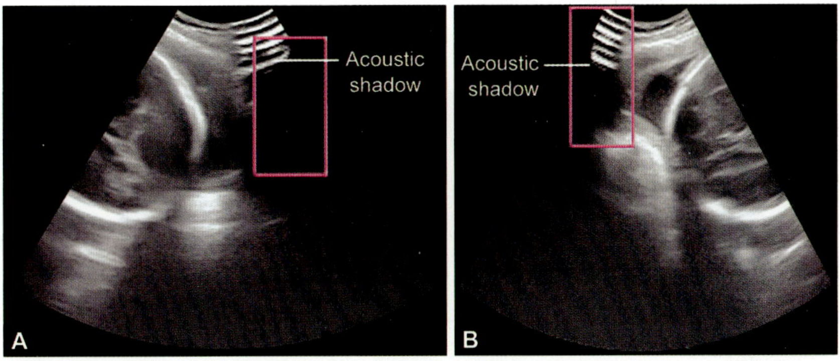

Figures 6.4A and B (A) As the examiner faces the transducer, the right edge of the transducer is lifted from the maternal abdomen and the corresponding acoustic shadow identified. If the shadow is on the same side, as the edge of the lifted transducer, then there is synchrony between the two; (B) If the examiner faces the transducer, the right edge of the transducer is lifted from the maternal abdomen and the acoustic shadow identified is on the other side of the screen, then the examiner need to rotate the transducer 180° so that there is synchrony between the transducer position and the ultrasound image

is parallel to the maternal spine; transverse when the fetal spine is perpendicular to the maternal spine; and oblique when the fetal spine is oblique to the maternal spine.

Step 3

After establishment of the exact position of the fetus with the help of step 1 and 2, the sonologist must then determine the location of the fetal left side with regards to the maternal abdomen (Figure 6.5) [fetal left side is anterior (closer to the transducer) or posterior (closer to the posterior uterine wall)].

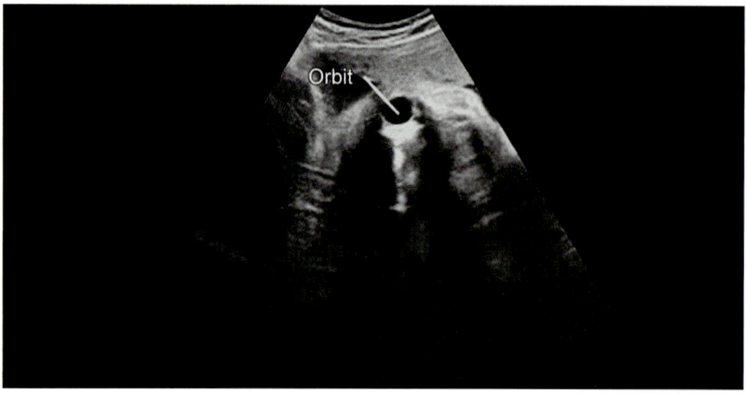

Figure 6.5 Once synchrony of the transducer and image are obtained, the examiner then rotates the transducer until either the cerebellum or the orbits of the eyes are identified. In this example, the orbits are identified on the examiner's left. This would imply that the fetal spine is on the right of the screen, with the left side of the fetus in the down position

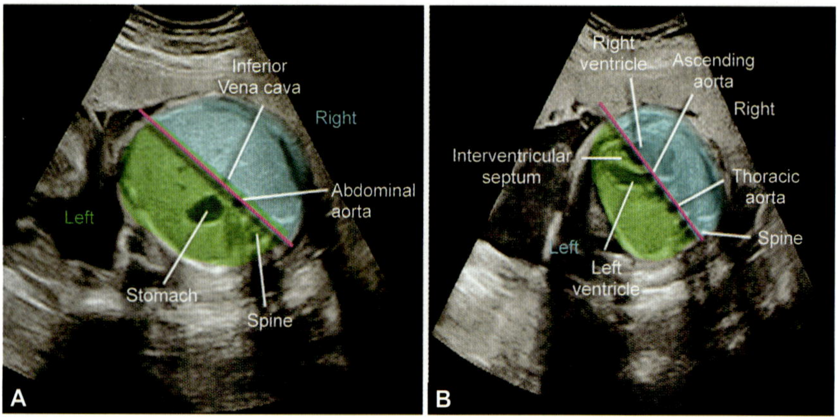

Figures 6.6A and B Step 4: Obtain a transverse view of the fetal abdomen by rotating the transducer 90° from the sagittal view of the lower thoracic spine; we must locate fetal stomach on left side of fetal abdomen

Step 4

Sonologist must then obtain a transverse view of the fetal abdomen by rotating the transducer 90° from the sagittal view of the lower thoracic spine (Figures 6.6A and B). We must locate fetal stomach on left side of the fetal abdomen.

By sliding the transducer towards the fetal chest, a four-chamber view of the heart is imaged. It is important for the sonologist to point out the apex of heart towards the left side of the chest. So, it becomes clear that in normal situs, we see fetal stomach and cardiac apex both towards the left side (Figure 6.7).

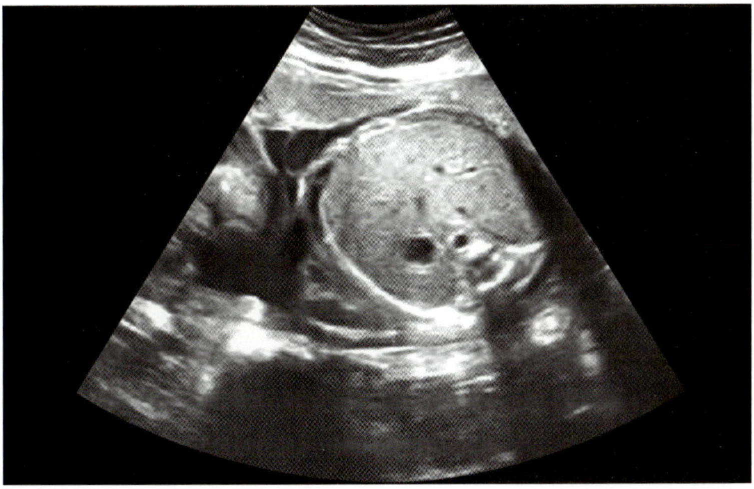

Figure 6.7 In normal situs, we must locate fetal stomach on left side of fetal abdomen; by sliding the transducer towards the fetal chest, a four-chamber view of the heart is imaged

FETAL CARDIAC AXIS

The fetal cardiac axis can be readily determined by obtaining a transverse view of the fetal chest at the level of four-chamber plane of the heart. A line drawn from the spine to the anterior chest wall divides the chest into two equal halves. The cardiac axis is the angle that the interventricular septum makes with this line.

- The heart is normally deviated about 45 ± 20° (2 SD) towards the left side of the fetus
- Careful attention should be given to cardiac axis and position because they can be easily evaluated even if the four-chamber view is not satisfactorily visualized.

Step 1

Step 1 involves the identification of fetal spine (Figure 6.8).

Step 2

In the step 2, a line is drawn parallel to the interventricular septum (Figure 6.9).

Step 3

In step 3, the line drawn from the spine to the anterior chest wall intersects the line parallel to the septum at 45° (Figures 6.10 and 6.11).

Studies show that wider cardiac axis was noted in fetuses with congenital heart disease compared to normal fetuses. The frequency of cardiac rotation was greater in fetuses with the following abnormalities:

- Truncus arteriosus
- Ebstein anomaly
- Pulmonary stenosis

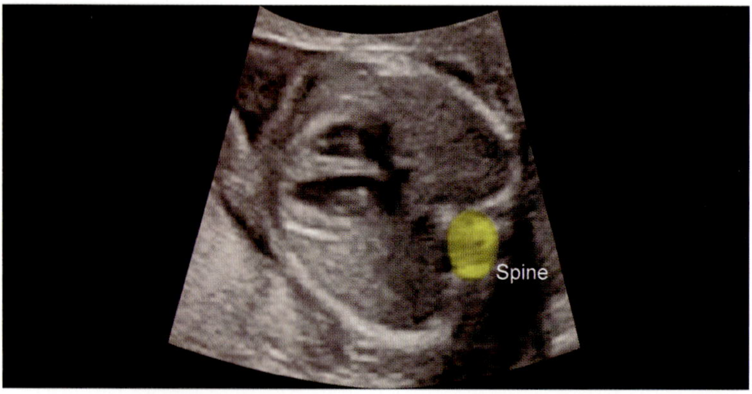

Figure 6.8 *Step 1:* Identification of the fetal spine

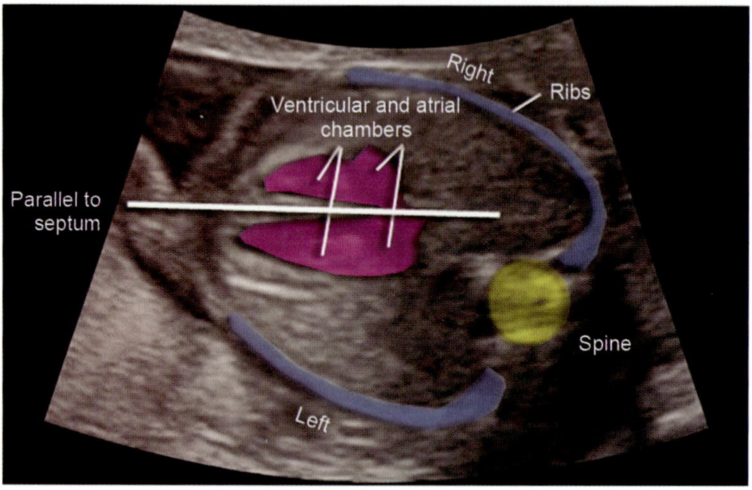

Figure 6.9 *Step 2:* A line parallel to the interventricular septum

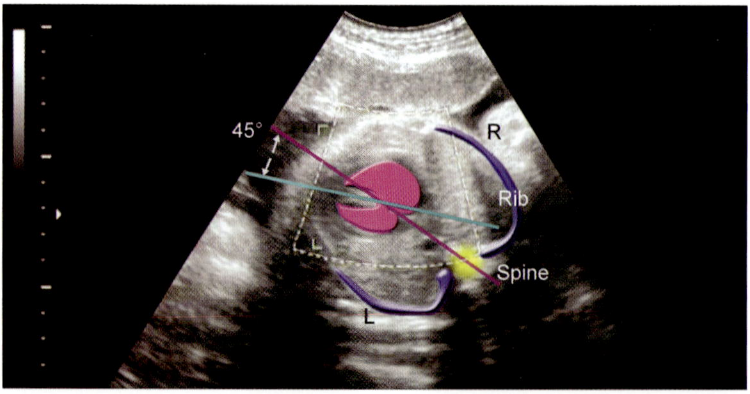

Figure 6.10 *Step 3:* The line drawn from the spine to the anterior chest wall intersects the line parallel to the septum at 45°

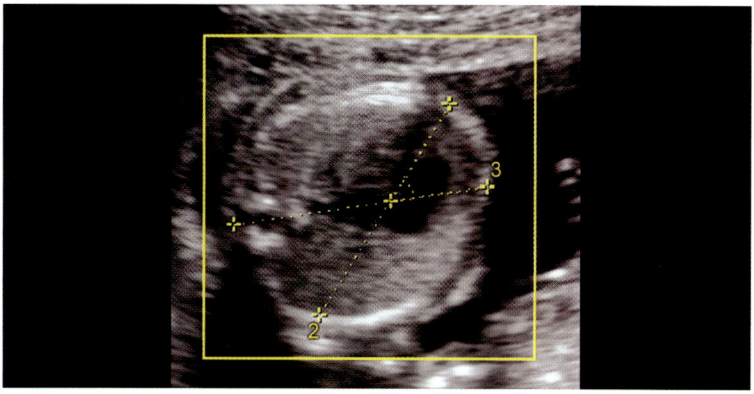

Figure 6.11 Demonstration of the cardiac axis

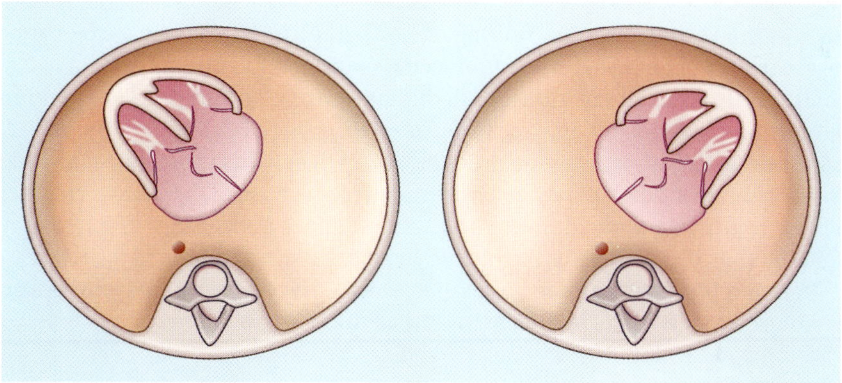

Figure 6.12 Diagrammatic presentation of dextrocardia

- Coarctation of the aorta
- Tetralogy of Fallot.

The embryonic event that results in an abnormal cardiac axis in some fetuses with cardiac abnormalities is not properly known, but it may be presumed that an over-rotation of the bulboventricular loop from right to left in early embryogenesis is the underlying mechanism.

Dextrocardia (Figure 6.12) is used to describe a condition when an anomaly of embryological development is present.

NUTSHELL

1. There are three types of situs—situs solitus means normal situs, situs inverses means everything will be reverse, situs ambiguous means variable changes.
2. Step by step approach for situs is easy and fast to get normal or abnormal situs.
3. Cardiac axis examination will be done in three steps.

7

Four-Chamber Heart

The most interesting and easy finding on sonography of fetal heart is the view of four-chambers of heart, seen in a transverse section of the thorax.

With widespread use of ultrasound, this view can be considered as a screening tool for ruling out most cases of chronic heart disease (CHD).

As such, to get this view we do not require much expertise and almost anybody can easily obtain this beautiful view in the transverse section of the thorax and watch the heart occupying approximately one-third of chest, and apex pointing towards left. Both lungs can be seen as echogenic structures on either side of the heart.

There is a big list of cardiac anomalies, which may be associated with normal four-chamber view of the fetal heart. Some of these are as follows:

- Tetralogy of Fallot
- Transposition of great vessels
- Double outlet right ventricle
- Small ventricular septal defect
- Small atrial septal defect
- Mild semilunar valve stenosis
- Mild coarctation of aorta.

The following list of abnormalities usually associated with abnormal four-chamber view of heart:

- Cardiac situs abnormalities
- Moderate to severe coarctation of aorta
- Ebstein anomaly
- Double outlet right ventricle (DORV)
- Valve stenosis
- Valve atresia
- Atrial septal defect (ASD) large
- Rhabdomyoma (cardiac tumors)
- Ventricular septal defect (VSD) large
- Single ventricle

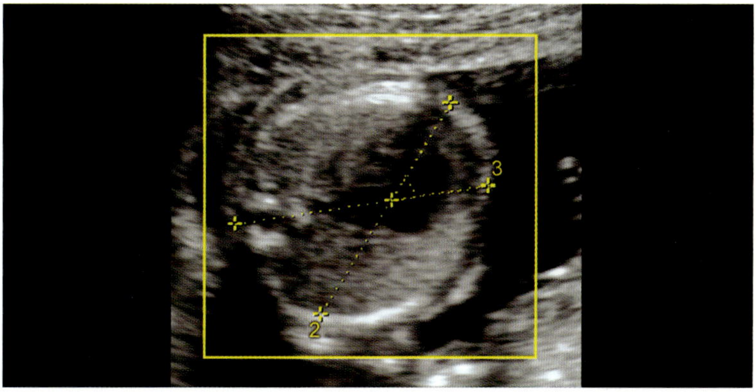

Figure 7.1 Cardiac axis

Table 7.1 Criteria for describing the normal four-chamber view of fetal heart	
General	• Normal cardiac situs, axis and position • Heart occupies a third of thoracic area • Majority of the heart lies on the left side of the chest • Four-chambers are present • No pericardial effusion or hypertrophy
Atria	• Atria are approximately equal in size • Foramen ovale flap open in left atrium • Atrial septum primum is present
Ventricle	• Ventricles are almost equal in size • No cardiac wall hypertrophy • Moderator band is present at the right ventricular apex • Ventricular septum is intact (apex to crux)
Atrioventricular valves	• Both atrioventricular valves open and move freely • Tricuspid valve leaflet inserts on ventricular septum closer to the cardiac apex than the mitral valve

- Hypoplastic right heart syndrome
- Hypoplastic left heart syndrome.

The apex of the heart lies at an angle of 30–45° to the line drawn from the spine to the anterior thoracic wall (Figure 7.1). This axis becomes abnormal due to the rotation of the heart in the presence of cardiac abnormalities. Normally, heart occupies one-third of chest, but if it occupies more than 50% of thoracic circumference, we have to diagnose it as cardiomegaly. A four-chamber view can be considered as normal, if it fulfills the criteria described in Table 7.1.

STEP BY STEP FOUR-CHAMBER VIEW OF THE HEART

The four-chamber view of fetal heart has been illustrated in Figures 7.2 and 7.3.

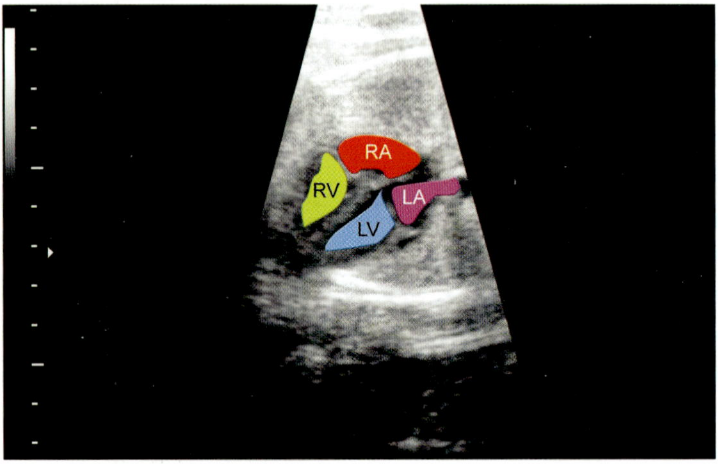

Figure 7.2 Labeled four-chamber view of fetal heart

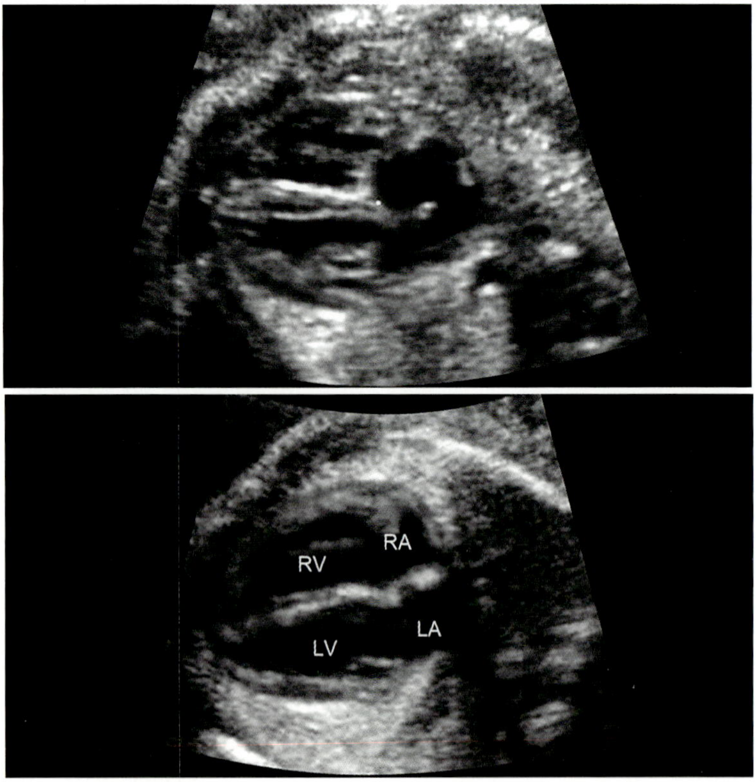

Figure 7.3A

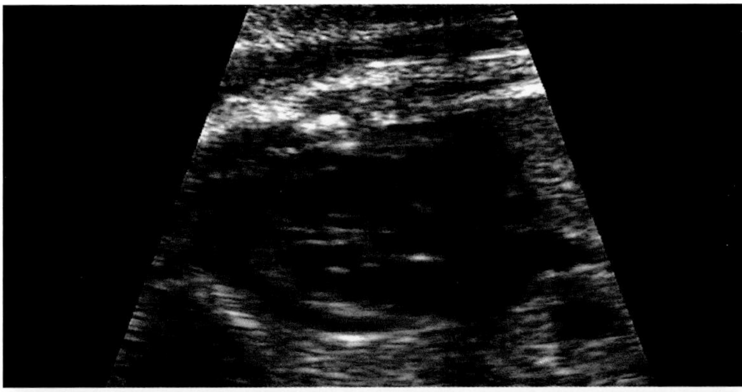

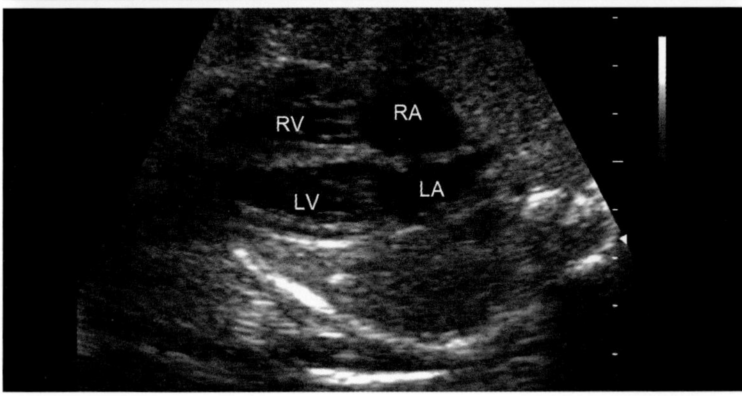

Figure 7.3B

Figures 7.3A and B Four-chamber view of the normal heart as visualized on ultrasound examination

Step 1

The right and left sides of the fetus are determined.

Step 2

A transverse view of the upper abdomen is taken at a point where the cross-section of the spine, stomach, portal vein and liver can be imaged.

Step 3

Cephalad angulations of the transducer will bring into focus the four-chamber view.

There are three different angles for imaging the four-chamber view, which are:

1. Apical
2. Basal
3. Lateral.

Apical View

Apical four-chamber view is obtained when the spine is posterior and the ultrasound beam is transverse from the apex to the base of the heart and is parallel to the interventricular septum. This is the best view for visualizing the cardiac axis, ventricular and atrial sizes, flap of the foramen ovale, and the atrioventricular valves (the position of the tricuspid valve is more apical than the mitral valve). Pulmonary veins (at least two) can also be seen entering the left atrium.

Basal View

When the spine in an anterolateral position, the sound beam enters through the right posterior chest wall and traverses from the base to the apex of the heart.

Lateral View

Lateral view is used when the fetal spine is to the right or left of the mother's spine. In this view, the sound beam is perpendicular to the interventricular septum.

NORMAL ORIENTATION OF THE FETAL HEART

Normal orientation of the fetal heart is as follows:

- Opposite to the spine → Sternum
- Just posterior to the sternum → Right ventricle
- Just anterior and left to the spine → Descending aorta
- Just anterior to the descending aorta → Left atrium.

Normal findings in a fetal four-chamber view are as follows:

- Heart covers one-third of the thoracic cross-section area
- Cardiac apex points towards the anterior left chest wall
- Atrial chambers are equal in size
- Ventricular chambers are also equal in size
- Thickness of the ventricular wall and septum is near equal
- At the apex, the right ventricle is coarse, the left ventricle is smooth
- The tricuspid valve is slightly more towards the apex in comparison to the mitral valve
- The junction of the AV valves with atrial and ventricular septum is intact
- Both AV valves function properly (open and close)
- Both ventricles contract equally well.

FIVE-CHAMBER VIEW OF THE FETAL HEART

This is a specific view of heart to improve screening for CHD (Figures 7.4 and 7.5).

This view demonstrates the four-chamber view, along with the aorta as it arises from the left ventricle and gets continuous with the interventricular septum. This is commonly known as the five-chamber view. As the five-chamber view also demonstrates LVOT, the sensitivity of predicting CHD will be more in comparison to the traditional four-chamber view. Though this view may be sometimes a little

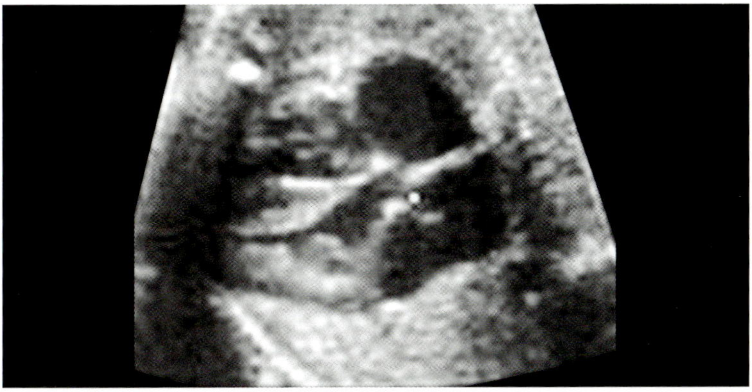

Figure 7.4 Five-chamber view of fetal heart

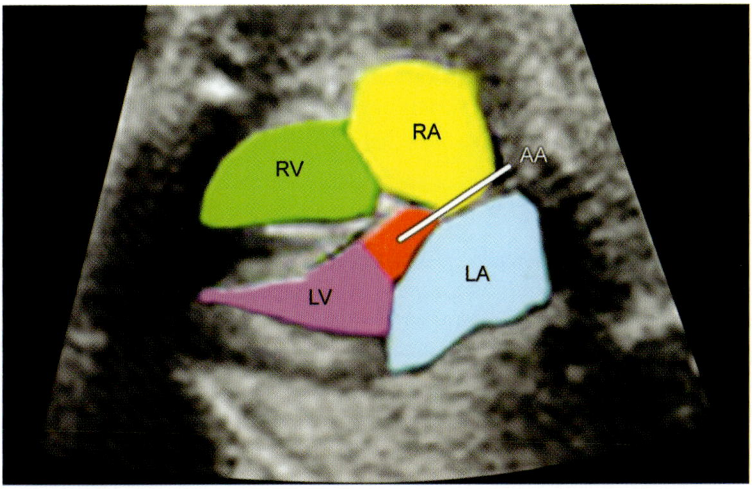

Figure 7.5 Labeled image of five-chamber view of fetal heart
Abbreviations: AA, ascending aorta; LA, left atrium; LV, left ventricular; RA, right atrium; RV, right ventricular

Table 7.2 Various studies describing the validity for five-chamber view

Author	*No. of study*	*Incidence of CHD*	*Risk status*	*Sensitivity*
Beinder	1600	25/1000	Low risk	81%
Kirk	5111	10/1000	Low risk	78%
Ott	1136	12/1000	Low risk	14.3%

difficult to obtain, but with some expertise we can obtain it easily. Studies also show data, which gives more validity for the five-chamber view (Table 7.2).

ANATOMICAL LANDMARKS AND FEATURES OF FOUR-CHAMBER VIEW

Ventricles

- Both ventricle should be of equal size
- Ventricular cavity of right side becomes slightly little larger than the left, with advancing gestational age
- Right ventricle is the cardiac chamber closest to anterior chest wall of fetus. The inlet and apical chamber of the right ventricle is heavily trabeculated
- The apical septoparietal muscle bundle known as moderator band is the characteristic point of right ventricle (Figure 7.6)
- Moderator band is well visualized with basal and apical four-chamber view
- In comparison to apical portion outflow portion, infundibulum of right ventricle is smooth
- Left ventricle lies posterior to the right ventricle
- Left ventricle is conical in shape and smooth in comparison to the right ventricle
- The left ventricle forms left border and apex of the heart
- An echogenic spot seen within left ventricular cavity is representative of the chordae tendinae or papillary muscles.

VENTRICULAR SEPTUM

Ventricular septum separates both the ventricles from each other (Figure 7.7). Lower two-thirds of ventricular septum is of muscular origin and upper one-third is of membranous origin. Atrioventricular (AV) canal defect is usually associated with membranous part of septum. So, it has two portions: one is thin and close to the crux of heart and known as membranous part and the second is thick and near the apex, known as muscular part. Best view of ventricular septum is in lateral four-chamber heart view.

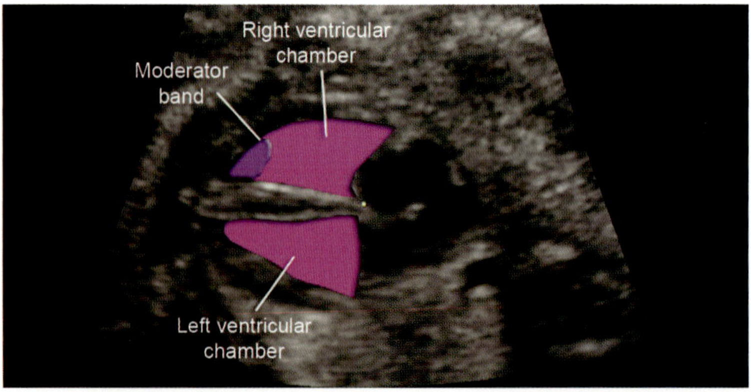

Figure 7.6 Both ventricular chambers with moderator band

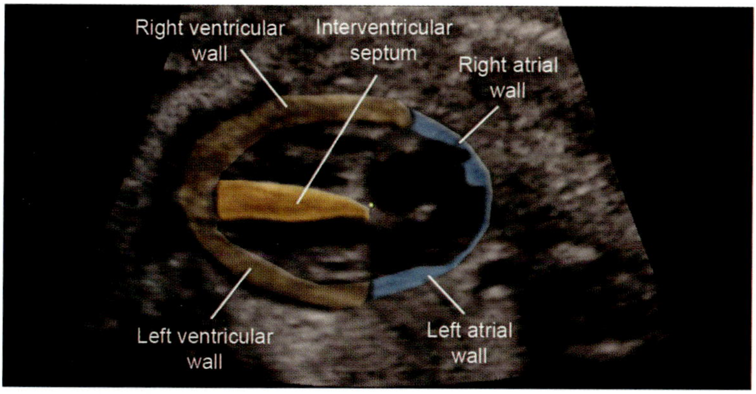

Figure 7.7 Four-chamber walls with interventricular septum

ATRIA

Both atria are of equal size and symmetry (Figure 7.8). Left atrium is the chamber near to the thoracic spine, posteriorly located and receives blood from right and left pulmonary veins; a total of four pulmonary veins enter into left atrium posteriorly, two from each side. In left atrium, foramen ovale flap is seen. Left atrium forms the base of the heart, is round and has smooth walls. Left atrial appendages are just like fingers and have got a very narrow base. Thoracic aorta is seen between the left atrium and the vertebral body.

Right atrium is anterior to the left atrium and forms the right border of the heart. Right atrial appendage is pyramidal in shape and has a broad base in comparison to finger-like base of the left; both appendages are not visualized routinely.

Cardiac anomalies usually change the hemodynamics of heart and open appendages and they are seen as prominent out pouches close to the atria. Right atrium receives the superior and inferior vena cava and the coronary sinus.

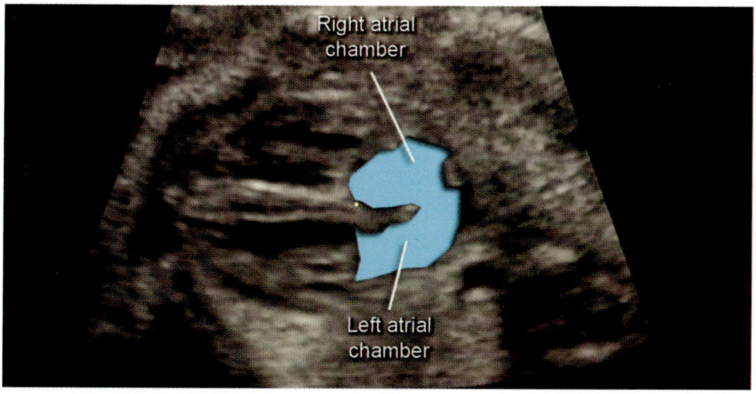

Figure 7.8 View showing both the atrial chambers

ATRIAL SEPTUM

- Two atria are separated by atrial septum (interatrial septum)
- Atrial septum has two compartments: Septum primum (Figure 7.9) and septum secundum
- The septum primum is the first to develop embryologically and it forms the valve of foramen ovale and is attached to the crux of the heart
- The septum has the shape of a distended pocket
- As a causative effect of ultrasound beams, the septum primum has the appearance of a flap or semicircular structure within the left atrium
- The septum secundum is seen to the right of primum and get attached at the roof of the atrium
- Foramen ovale (Figure 7.10) is present between the two septa and is formed as a result of perforation in septum secundum
- The flap of the foramen ovale is formed by the septum primum and is seen within the left atrium (Figure 7.10). It facilitates flow of blood from the right atrium to the left atrium

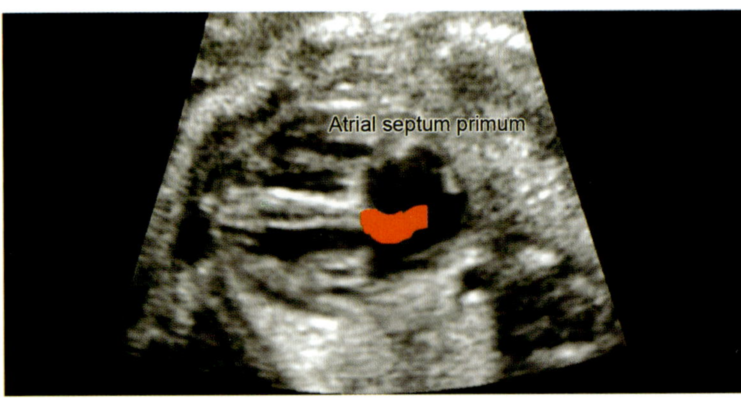

Figure 7.9 Atrial septum primum

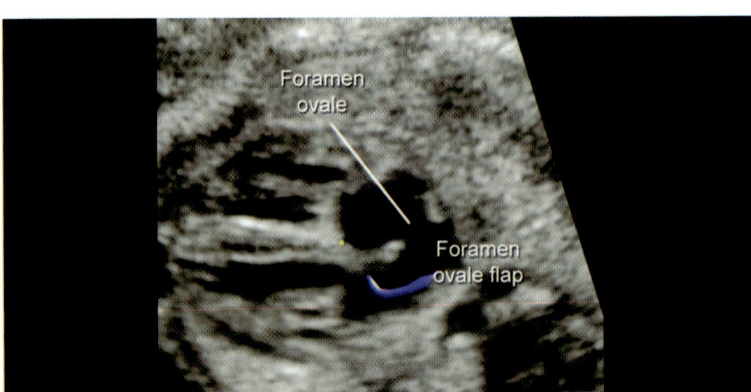

Figure 7.10 Foramen ovale flap

- Best visualization of foramen ovale is in the apical and lateral four-chamber view
- Apical four-chamber view also demonstrates at least 2–3 pulmonary veins entering into the left atrium.

ATRIOVENTRICULAR VALVES

Figure 7.11 shows both the atrioventricular valves present in the fetal heart. Other characteristic features of the heart valves are as follows:

- Mitral valve is in left ventricle and has got two cusps, namely anterior and posterior leaflets
- Mitral valve opens from the left atrium into the left ventricle
- Anterior leaflet is larger than the posterior leaflet
- Chordae tendineae from each leaflet inserts into the two papillary muscles (anterolateral and posteromedial) located within the left ventricle
- The anterior leaflet is in connection with aortic valve with fibrous continuity
- The left ventricular wall receives no direct chordae tendineae insertion from the mitral valve
- Tricuspid valve is in right ventricle and opens from right atrium into the right ventricle
- As name suggest, the tricuspid valve has got three cusps: Anterior, posterior and septal
- The tricuspid valve is more towards the apex on ventricular septum and offsets the insertion of the mitral valve
- In four-chamber view, only septal and anterior leaflets are visualized
- The tricuspid valve has one small anterior papillary muscle to which chordae tendineae from the anterior and septal leaflets attach
- The right ventricular wall receives chordae tendineous insertion from the tricuspid valve
- Tricuspid valve is separated from pulmonary valve by subpulmonic conus
- Both valves are best visualized in apical and basal four-chamber view

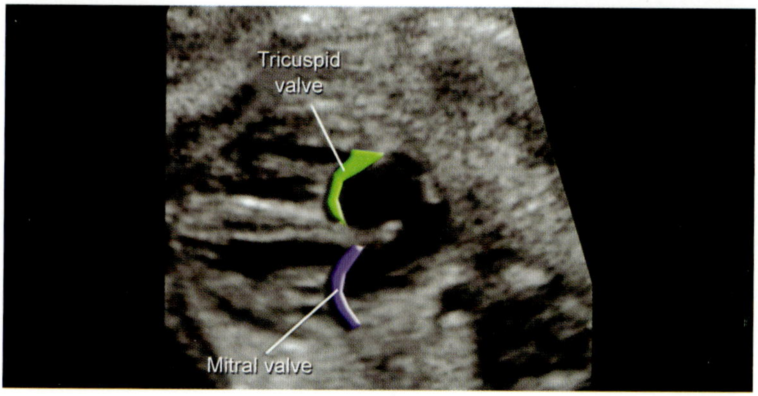

Figure 7.11 View of the heart showing both the atrioventricular valves

- We must evaluate valvular motion in the real time
- Crux of the heart (Figure 7.12) is made by two atrioventricular valves, and membranous portion of interventricular septum, which is best visualized in lateral view
- Any congenital anomaly related to crux must raise suspicion about presence of other defects.

SUMMARY

Labeled image of the normal heart with all the important structures is shown in Figure 7.13.

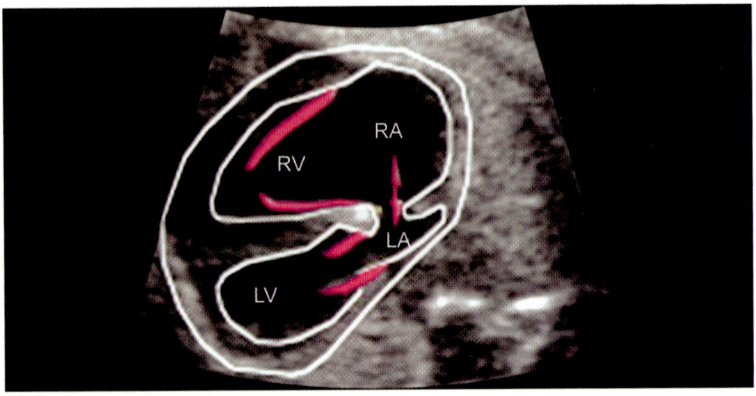

Figure 7.12 Crux of heart

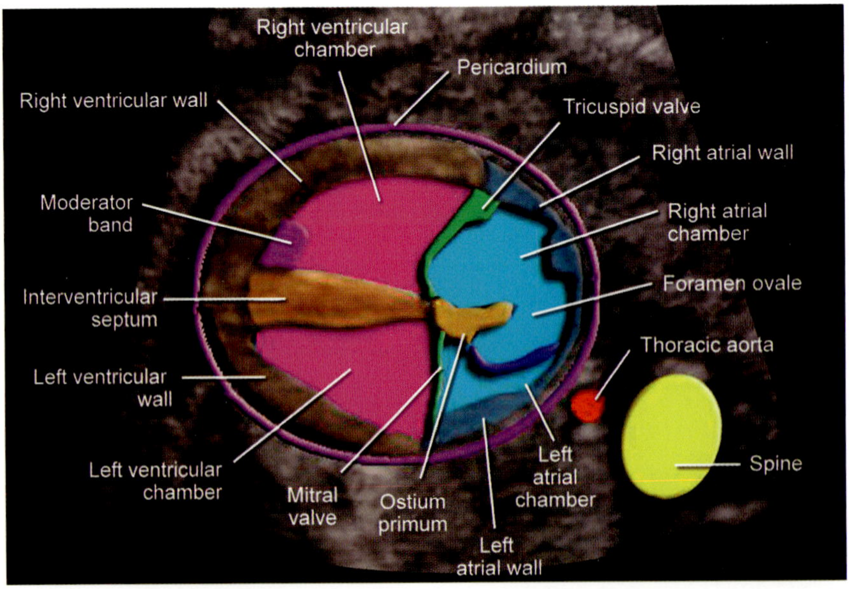

Figure 7.13 Labeled image of the normal heart with all the important structures

NUTSHELL

1. Four-chamber view is first step in fetal echocardiography examination and this can be obtained in transverse section of thorax, heart occupies one-third of chest apex pointing towards left. Both lungs can be seen as ecogenic structure on either side of the heart.
2. Step-by-step approach to four-chamber view, first determine side, take transverse view of upper abdomen, cross-section of spine, stomach, portal vein and liver, cephalad angulations brings four-chamber in view.
3. Apical four-chamber is best view obtained when spine is posterior and ultrasound beam is traveling from apex to base of heart and parallel to IVS (interventricular septum).
4. Basal view obtained when spine is an anterolateral position and ultrasound waves passes through right posterior chest wall from base to apex of the heart.
5. Lateral views is seen when fetal spine is to the right or left of the mother's spine and ultrasound waves are perpendicular to the IVS.
6. Both atria should be of equal size.
7. Both ventricles should be of equal size.
8. Both valve move freely and tricuspid valve is more apical then mitral valve.
9. IVS should be present from apex to crux.

8

Doppler Echocardiography

Basic concept of color and pulsed Doppler ultrasound is derived from the Doppler effects. This is based on the change in frequency of sound with motion. When an ultrasound wave with a certain frequency insonates a blood vessel, the frequency shift of the reflected ultrasound wave is directly proportional to the velocity of blood flow within this vessel. This frequency shift is also proportional to the cosine of the angle that the ultrasound beam makes with this vessel (the angle of incidence) and to the frequency of the insonating ultrasound wave. The Doppler frequency shift therefore reflects, but does not actually measure the velocity of blood flow.

Ideal time for initiation of fetal echocardiography is about 16–20 weeks. In recent times, there has been a lot of advancement in the field of imaging sciences due to good resolution images, use of color Doppler and introduction of TVS (Transvaginal ultrasound), which have made it possible to image cardiac hemodynamics in the embryonic heart during first trimester. These developments have opened up the area of early diagnosis in certain high-risk cases of congenital heart disease. Doppler shift is the difference in frequency of the transmitted sound and the reflected sound echoes. This frequency is in the range of audibility so that the sound of blood flow is heard. This Doppler shift frequency can be recorded in a frequency spectrum analyzer. Though the Doppler shift frequency does not exactly measure the velocity through a particular vessel, it reflects the velocity.

In spectrum analysis, the vertical axis denotes the velocity and the horizontal axis the time. Doppler waveforms or the spectrum depends on the resistance offered to blood in the particular vessel sampled. The frequency shift can be measured at any point along the cardiac cycle. Low resistance circulation is denoted by good flow in diastole. When there is high resistance circulation, the flow is either reduced or becomes nil. Doppler study is useful for studying the blood flow within the heart particularly in pathological states such as incompetence of valves and presence of shunts. Clinical approach of Doppler velocimetry is mainly used for measuring through downstream resistance to the flow of blood (Figure 8.1). This is based on the concept that the mean flow is proportional to the mean pressure and inversely proportional to the mean downstream resistance ($QM = P_m/R_m$).

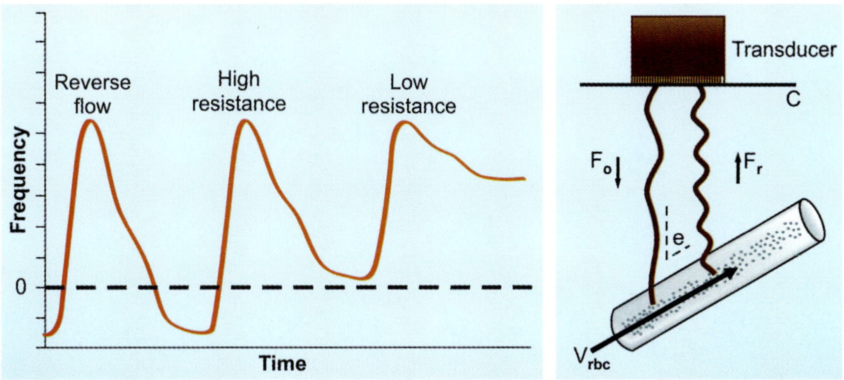

Figure 8.1 Basic biophysical understanding of the Doppler

This concept however, only applies to steady nonpulsatile flow conditions. In a medical setting, where flow is pulsatile, vascular impedance rather than vascular resistance describes opposition to blood flow. Downstream resistance is just one component of vascular impedance which is also dependent on the pulse frequency, blood inertia, dispensability of the vessel wall and wave reflection. In present scenario controversy still occurs because of our inability to measure vascular impedance in clinical settings.

Doppler indices correlate well with impedance to pulsatile flow, pressure pulsality and vascular resistance. Doppler, therefore has useful application in detection of emergency conditions such as fetal distress.

FETAL CARDIOVASCULAR PHYSIOLOGY

Anatomically, the fetal circulation (Figure 8.2) is quite different from that of an adult and both the ventricles are operating in parallel rather than in series. Lungs are bypassed with help of foramen ovale and ductus arteriosus in fetus allows blood to flow from the right to left circulation. Though the majority of the blood from the right ventricle gets entry into ductus arteriosus and then flow into thoracic aorta, still some small amount of blood gets entry into the lungs via both the pulmonary arteries. From thoracic aorta, blood returns to the placenta via umbilical artery and gets oxygen form mother. Then this highly oxygenated blood returns to fetus via umbilical vein.

Ductus venosus takes half of the oxygenated blood from the umbilical vein and other half of blood enters into the portal system and hepatic veins. Blood from the ductus venosus and left hepatic vein gets entry into the right atrium. From there, the foramen ovale makes it possible to get access directly into the left atrium. During each ventricular diastole blood is ejected from left atrium into left ventricle.

So the almighty has given beautiful mechanism of shunting by which cardiac muscles and brain receive blood, which is very high in oxygen content. Right ventricular volume flow exceeds the left ventricle volume flow in the fetus by ratio of 1.3:1. The combined ventricular output flow in the fetus at term is approximately

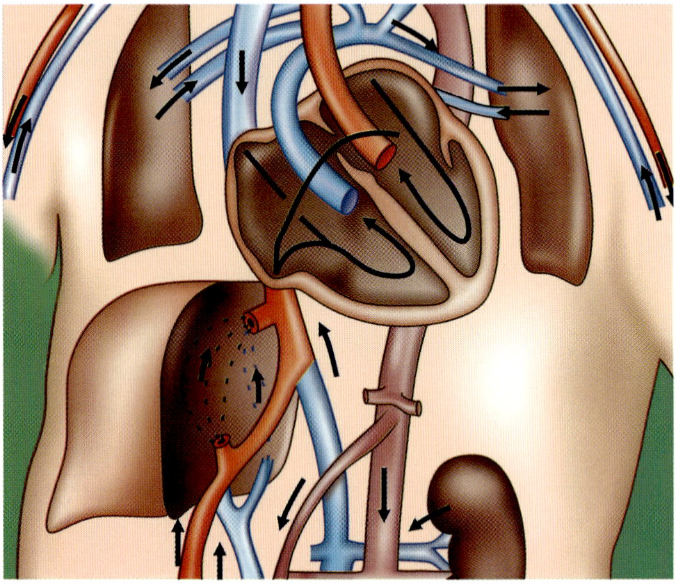

Figure 8.2 Normal circulation through the fetal heart

1,735 mL/min, whereas flow indicated for estimated fetal weight is constant at mean value of 553 ± 153 mL/min/kg. Stroke volume increases exponentially with advancing gestation. It measures from 0.7 mL at 20 weeks to 7.6 mL at term for the right ventricle and 0.7 mL at 20 weeks to 5. 2 mL at term for the left ventricle.

DOPPLER WAVEFORM QUANTIFICATION

Understanding the Terms RI, PI and SD (Figure 8.3)

Doppler indices are ratio of frequency shifts obtained from the same cardiac cycle and thus independent of the angle of insonation:

- Pulsatility index (PI) = SD/M
- Resistivity index (RI) = SD/S
- SD ratio = S/D
- Peak velocity = The maximum velocity on the Doppler spectrum (cm/sec)
- Time to peak velocity (TPV) = The time from onset to peak velocity (msec), also referred to as acceleration time
- Deceleration time = The time from the peak of waveforms to the intersection of the descending slope with the baseline (msec)
- Time-velocity integral (TVI) = The measurement of the area under the Doppler waveform over one cardiac cycle (cm)
- Time-averaged velocity (TAV) = This is equal to TVI divided by the time period (cm/sec)
- E/A ratio = A measurement used to quantify Doppler waveforms across the atrioventricular valves. E represents peak velocity during early ventricular filling and A represents peak velocity during the atrial contraction

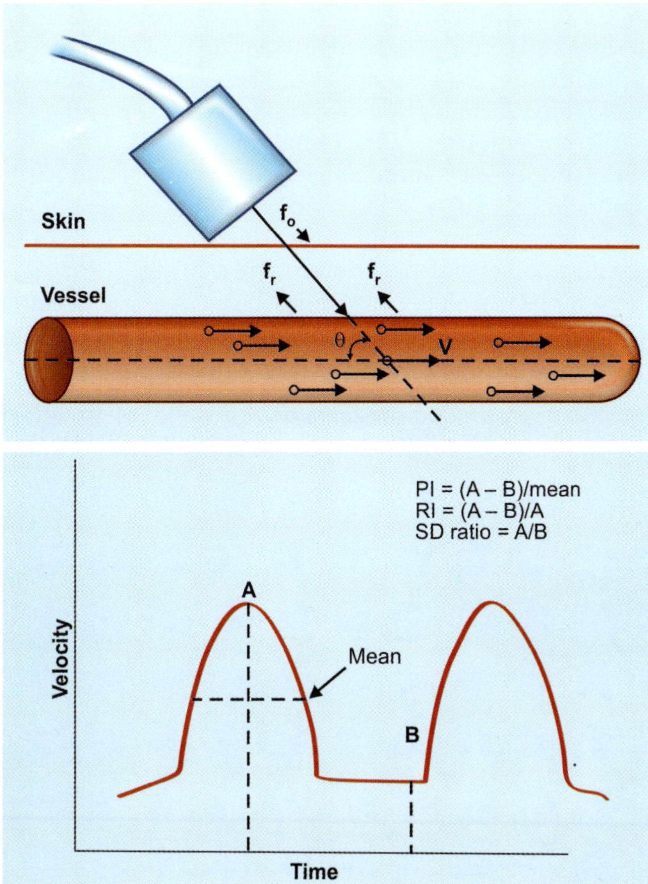

Figure 8.3 Biophysics and a graphical representation for understanding of the terms PI, RI, SD

- Filling time = The diastolic time of cardiac cycle (msec)
- Ejection time = The systolic time of cardiac cycle (msec)
- Percent reverse flow = A measurement used to quantify Doppler waveforms in the inferior vena cava. It represents the TVI of the reverse flow segment (arterial contraction) divided by the TVI of the total forward flow multiplied by 100.
- S/A= A measurement used to quantify Doppler waveforms in the ductus venosus. S represents maximum systolic velocity and A represents the atrial nadir.

ATRIOVENTRICULAR VALVES

As routine we have to take good basal apical four chamber view and we have to be sure that angle of insonation should be less than 20° from the direction of blood flow across the atrioventricular valves. We have to place the Doppler sample volume within the ventricle and on the apical side of the mitral or tricuspid valves.

Just look at the fantastic normal waveform of AV valve Doppler (Figures 8.4A and B). They show or correspond to ventricular filling during diastole and are biphasic. The first phase of the waveform is known as E wave; it corresponds to the early ventricular filling. Second phase of waveform is known as the A wave and it corresponds to active ventricular filling (atrial contraction).

As we know that there is continuity between the mitral and aortic valves so we can see aortic flow during systolic component, but we do not see same for pulmonary valve across the tricuspid valve. The E/A ratio is used for Doppler waveform quantification across the atrioventricular valves.

Doppler waveforms across the atrioventricular valves are dependent on the compliance of the ventricular muscle, preload and afterload. If we want to measure

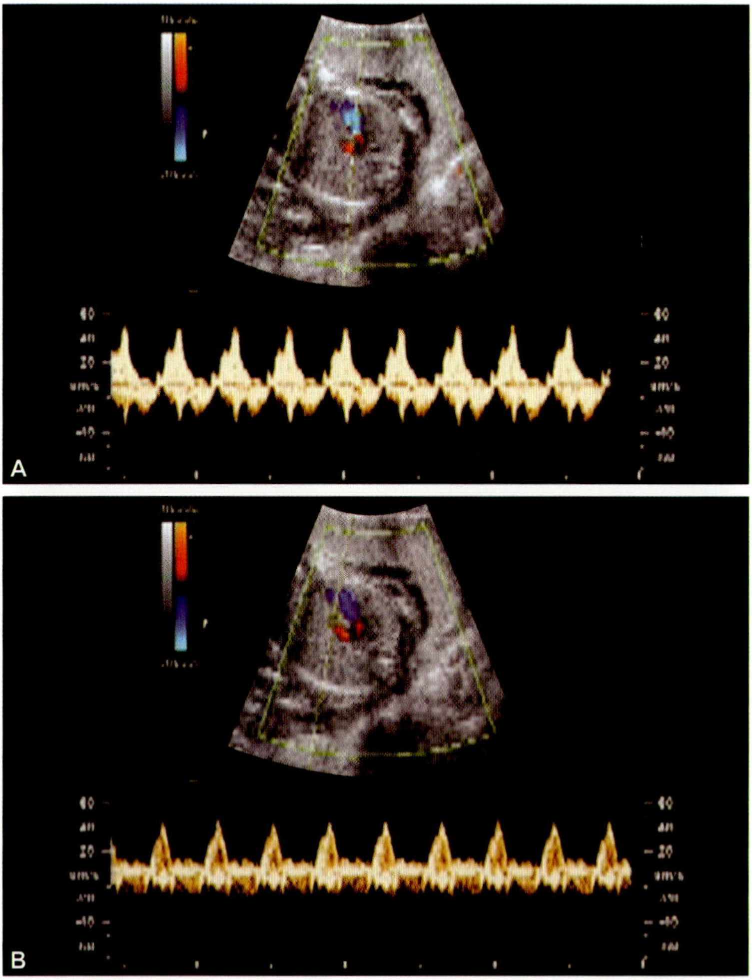

Figures 8.4A and B Use of Doppler across atrioventricular valves

the diastolic function of the ventricle, E/A ratio is an ideal index. The peak of A wave is higher in the fetus because of the increased cardiac muscle stiffness during the fetal life.

NUTSHELL

1. Doppler shift is the difference in frequency of transmitted sound and the reflected sound echoes.
2. In spectrum vertical axis denotes the velocity and horizontal axis is the time. The frequency shift can be measured at any point along the cardiac cycle.
3. Fetal circulation is based on three shunts:
   A. Foramen ovale, B. Ductus venosus. C. Ductus arteriosus.
4. All indices has its own importance and thanks to higher end machine which will give us readymade calculation by just pressing one button, i.e. auto-calculation.
5. Doppler waves across the valve are dependence of the ventricular muscle, preload and after load.
6. Tricuspid regurgitation has got association with chromosomal abnormality, i.e. trisomy 21 (Down syndrome).

9

Fetal Arrhythmias

In order to diagnose fetal arrhythmias, we must know and understand the electrophysiology of the arrhythmias and gain knowledge regarding the fetomaternal pharmacology and the pharmacokinetics of the antiarrhythmic drugs.

We must know that all antiarrhythmic drugs may cause great amount of toxicity to both the mother as well as the baby. So, we must take into consideration, the risk versus benefits ratio before the implementation of treatment. Fetal ECG is ideal clinical tool for analysis. It is very difficult to do fetal ECG except while using a scalp electrode.

With advent of ultrasound and new modalities of M-mode, pulse Doppler and Doppler color flow, it has become very easy to understand arrhythmias. Diagnostic tracing of M-mode is indicative of arrhythmias, but first we must learn to put M-mode sampling line or cursor line correctly.

We have to put a line across the atria and ventricles simultaneously, so it can cut both in same line and give us very good visualization of the rate of atrioventricular contraction.

Now we have to understand fetal behavior as it is not a constant subject. The fetus moves with the beat and may change position depending on its own wishes. Therefore correct M-mode placement is not an easy job. However, now with the use of new modality such as pulsed wave Doppler, it has become easier for us to analyze fetal cardiac arrhythmias, because pulse Doppler records intravascular or intracardiac blood flow against time.

We know that in fetal life, fetal heart is more dependent upon active atrial contraction for adequate ventricular filling so what we actually get in form of Doppler flow would be either transmitral or transtricuspid flow (Figure 9.1).

If we cannot look for fetal cardiac rhythm at the time of assessment, we must put a cursor at the junction of ventricular inflow and outflow tract at left ventricle in aortic outflow (LVOT). So here we can see both ventricles filling as well as emptying opposite to the baseline on either side. Other areas of placement of sample volume are at the level of:

- Overlapping of the pulmonary venous and arterial flow
- Overlapping of the ascending aorta and superior vena cava

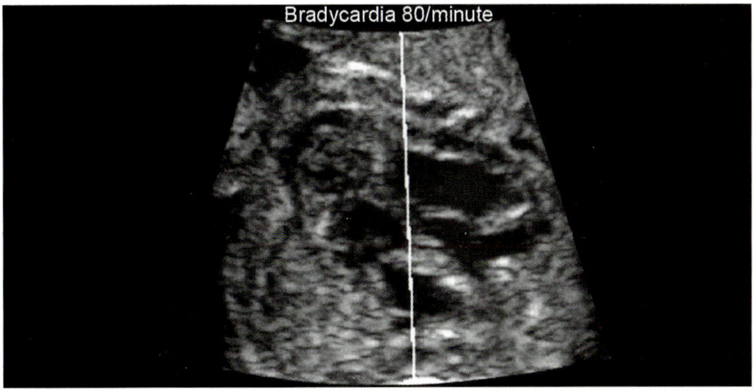

Figure 9.1 Color Doppler image of the tricuspid regurgitation

So, now we should be convinced that M-mode ECG is more helpful for detection of arrhythmias in comparison to the pulse Doppler tracing for rhythm analysis.

Doppler is best tool for analysis of physiological impact of fetal arrhythmias on the fetal cardiovascular system.

We can easily pick-up rhythm abnormalities when we hear irregular heartbeats, but we must remember that variable heart rate decelerations can commonly occur in second trimester and when the mother is in supine position. The most common irregularity in fetal heart is in form of some pause or extrabeat.

We all know how to feel the rhythm of heart and love to hear its sound during the systole and diastole. Rhythm is just last S... of PASS...S. If the squeeze is normal, usually rhythm is also normal.

Though the incidence of fetal arrhythmias is very low, only about 1–2%, it may account for almost 10% cases of neonatal morbidity and mortality.

In set-up of neonatal cardiologist, referrals for arrhythmias usually account for 15% of the OPD cases.

If we observe the development of fetal heart, pulsations can be visualized from 35–37 days of gestation. Primitive atrial muscle acts as a pacemaker. Specialized conducting system of the heart develops as the pregnancy advances. Connective tissue separates atria from ventricles. Heart rate may vary between 100-160-160-170-140-150 bpm. Sometimes, we may observe the fetal heart rate to fall below 90 bpm; this is known as embryonic bradycardia.

CONDUCTION SYSTEM

The conduction system of the heart comprises of the following (Figure 9.2):

- *SA node*: Present near the superior vena caval opening
- *AV node*: Located at triangle of Koch
- *Bundle of His*: Located in ventricular septum and passes through both the ventricular walls
- *Purkinje's system*: Located at the base of ventricles

Maturity of conducting system progresses throughout fetal life to postnatal life.

ASSESSMENT OF FETAL RHYTHM

- Assessment of the fetal rhythm can be done with the help of following:
  - *Fetal ECG*: In literature, this is an old method for diagnosing fetal rhythm, but we all know that fetus is in constant motion and therefore this method is not very useful nowadays.
  - *Fetal heart—M-mode ultrasound*: With invention of real time M-mode ultrasound, it is now easy to use ultrasound at level of atria and ventricles.
  - *Doppler*: This modality helps in giving real time images easily and fast.
- Arrhythmias must be suspected when at the time of antenatal check-up, any of the following findings are detected:
  - Maternal connective tissue disorder
  - Family/sibling history of structural heart defects
  - Maternal/fetal thyrotoxicosis
  - Maternal ingestion of drugs such as digoxin, isoprenaline, etc.
  - Familial syndromes such as WPW syndrome and long QT syndrome.
- Fetal arrhythmia assessment involves assessment of the following parameters: Cardiac wall motion for rhythm, cardiac structure, cardiac function and fetal well-being.

ARRHYTHMIA

We must suspect arrhythmias if irregularity of fetal cardiac rhythm occurs at irregular intervals, with a pattern suggestive of a pause or an extrabeat.

A supraventricular extrasystole happening very early in the diastole may occur during the atrioventricular conduction system's refractory period and therefore may not be conducted into the ventricles in order to initiate a ventricular response.

The atrial pace maker is reset, resulting in a longer pause between ventricular ejections than normal. The absence of ejection into the fetal arteries results in a

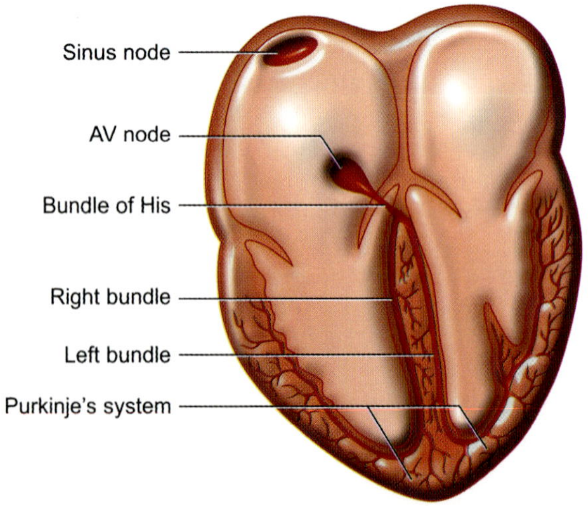

Figure 9.2 Normal conductive system of the heart

skipped beat, which may be heard, even though the underlying electrophysiology actually is that of an extrabeat. The abnormalities in the rhythm of fetal heart could be described as follows:

- Bradycardia < 90 bpm
- Tachycardia > 200 bpm
- Irregular rhythm.

Irregular Rhythm

This could be in the following forms:

- Atrial extrasystole
- Ventricular extrasystole
- Blocked atrial ectopic
- Bigeminal.

Irregular rhythm is the most common occurrence in the fetal life and most of the times, it is self-limiting. Close follow-up is required and sometimes the second degree AV block can progress to a complete heart block. It is advisable to counsel mothers for avoiding caffeine and smoking during pregnancy as this may sometimes cause irregular rhythm in the babies.

Bradycardia

Sinus bradycardia (Figure 9.3) is usually seen in fetus while performing fetal echo. This may be due to the pressure on fetal heart and it usually subsides within fraction of a second as pressure is relieved from the baby. If sinus bradycardia persists for long, it may cause complete heart block and may even sometimes lead to 2nd degree heart block.

Complete Heart Block (CHB)

This is usually seen in cases of AV dissociation. In these cases, the atrial rate is 120–130 bpm and in comparison to that ventricular rate may be 50–90 bpm. In this type of situation, we have to look for the presence of some congenital anomaly

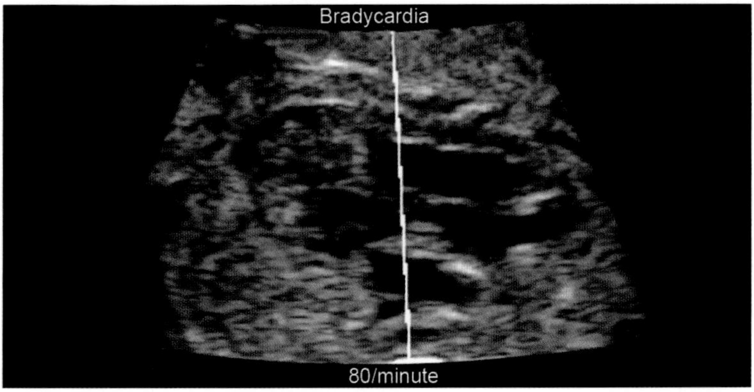

Figure 9.3 Bradycardia

such as structural malformation (AVSD) or corrected TGV or maybe some tumor like rhabdomyoma.

Isolated CHB

Clinical examination of mother is necessary and sometimes we may encounter maternal rheumatism and upon investigation may find positive serology suggestive of Ro (SSA) and LA (SSB). These antibodies may transfer from mother to fetus > 18 weeks.

CHB Monitoring

We have take close look in this situation and monitor parameters such as fetal growth, BPP and signs of fetal heart failure.

Fetal therapy for CHB

- In cases of CHB with CHD, the prognosis is poor.
- In cases of isolated CHB, prognosis is good. We may offer fetal pacing as a part of fetal therapy and sometimes administration of drugs like prednisone to mother may help in achieving wonders in this type of situation.
- In cases of CHB, we may allow lady to deliver vaginally, but we have to be more cautious because vagal stimulation at time of delivery may reduce heart rate. In order to detect fetal distress, we have to monitor fetal scalp pH and internal fetal lead to monitor atrial rate.

TACHYARRHYTHMIAS

Tachyarrhythmias can be defined as disturbances in the heart rhythm associated with an abnormal increase in the heart rate. Various abnormalities of fetal rhythm which could be associated with an increased heart rate are as follows:

- Atrial tachycardia (Figure 9.4)
- Atrial flutter
- Atrial fibrillation

Sometimes, when the fetus is performing fast movements, the heart rate may show an abnormal increase. The sonologist must also look for the presence of following structural defects:

- Aneurysm of foramen ovale flap
- Ebstein anomaly
- Tumors like rhabdomyoma.

Atrial Tachycardia

In atrial tachycardia, the heart rate varies between 200–300 bpm, with a 1:1 conduction. The sonologist must assess whether it is persistent or intermittent and also look for the signs of cardiac failure.

Atrial Flutter/Fibrillation

Atrial flutter results form a circular re-entrant movement of electrical energy within the atrium, with the heart rate varying between 300–400 bpm/min.

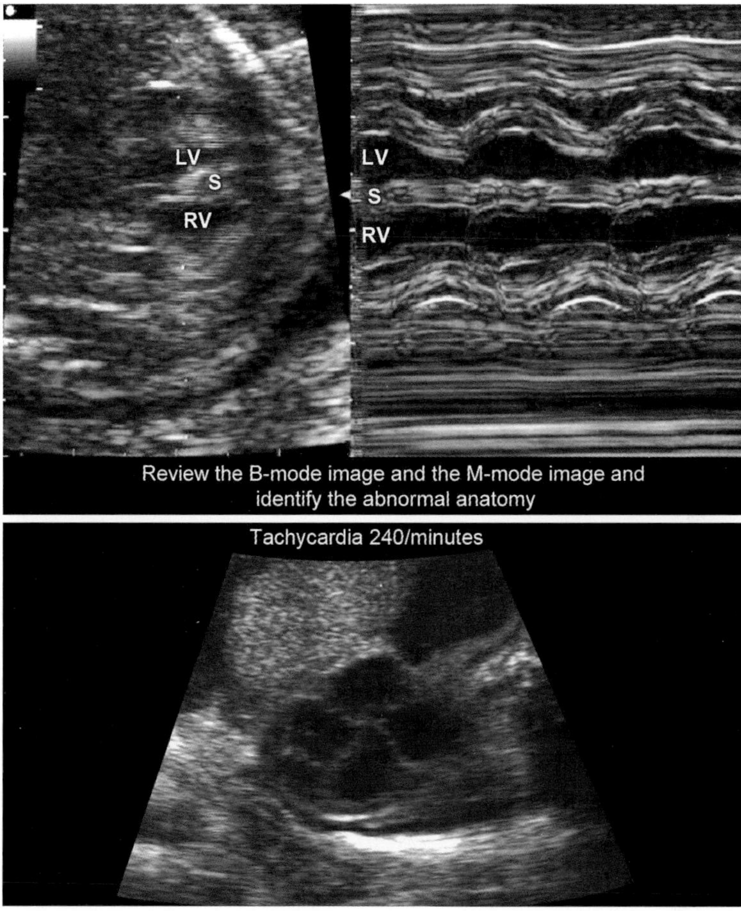

Figure 9.4 Tachycardia with heart rate of 240/min

Varying degree of atrioventricular block is present, resulting in varying ventricular response rates, which may be fixed and unresponsive to fetal activity.

The presence of atrioventricular block is a further evidence that atrioventricular re-entry via the atrioventricular node is not the underlying electrophysiological mechanism behind atrial flutter.

In flutter, regular atrial contractions occur, while in cases of fibrillation, there are irregular atrial contractions. A 3:1 or 2:1 AV block occurs in order to save the ventricles.

Atrial tachycardia is very common and spontaneous resolution usually occurs, but we must first rule out conditions such as hydrops fetalis. If it is not there, we must simply adopt a "wait and watch policy".

We know that the normal fetal ventricular function depends upon an effective atrial pump, so failure to control atrial flutter, may result in elevated atrial pressures with dilatation of the failing atrial pump leading to further increases in systemic venous pressure and all this together adds up, making the fetus even more hydrotic.

So our mission is to restore normal function, i.e. 1:1 atrioventricular contraction in sequence. For this, we have to give medicaments to the mother. The traditionally used drug, digoxin, acts as "old is gold" and helps in controlling the ventricular rate. To this we can add drugs such as procainamide or flecainide.

After giving dioxin, we must monitor maternal digoxin levels. This may be difficult in a country like India because of the high costs involved. However, we can also monitor by ECG, using corrected QT intervals.

Sometimes, we might have to give drugs directly into the umbilical vein, particularly in cases of fetal hydrops. Believe me, with the advent of fetal interventions like cordocentesis with help of color Doppler, this is not so difficult and may bypass maternal circulation and very minimal dose may be required. This may help in curing the disease fast. Moreover, in cases of hydrops, we are also treating anemia and at the same time, we can give drugs to the baby.

We have to institute treatment for babies with persistent tachycardia or very premature fetuses *in utero* in whom signs of hydrops are evident. In these cases, we must go for planned cesarean section before 36 weeks and hand the baby over to the neonatologist for further management.

We must counsel parents before hand for risk as well as benefits of fetal therapy. We usually put a 12 lead ECG on the mother for monitoring and carefully watch the response of therapy because we are not sure for fetal response. Sometimes cardioversion may fail to occur with treatment. It may remain transient and if we are lucky, it may sometimes remain sustained as well.

Postnatal follow-up is very crucial. For this, a 12 lead ECG with ECHO may be necessary and if the tachycardia is persistent, it may require treatment.

Ventricular Tachycardia

It is very rare, but known entity and usually coexists with some kind of ventricular tumors or ventricular dysfunction. B-mode and M-mode images of both the ventricular chambers with interventricular septum have been shown in Figures 9.5 and 9.6.

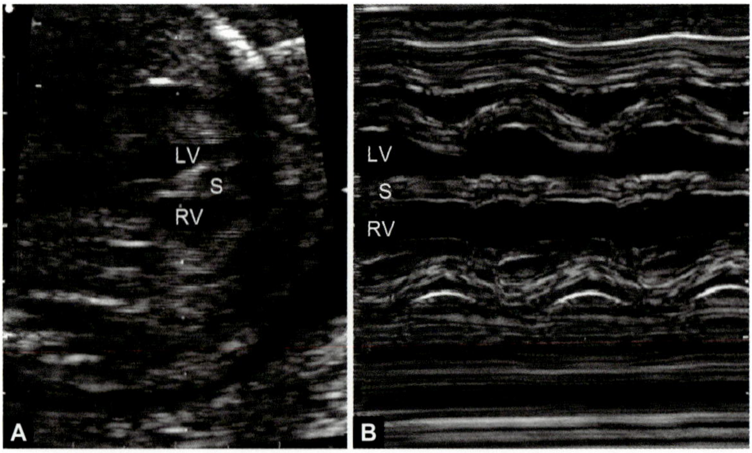

Figures 9.5A and B (A) B-mode and (B) M-mode image of the both the ventricular chambers with interventricular septum

In this type of ventricular tachycardia, ventricular activity is usually unrelated to atrial events. This may be because of retrograde conduction and supraventricular tachycardia. Sometimes, this may be also associated with long QT intervals.

Supraventricular tachyarrhythmias with 1:1 conduction may land up in congestive cardiac failure and we have to give transumbilical digoxin to baby along with maternal oral digoxin treatment. With this combination, postnatal outcomes will usually be good. So we can conclude that in structurally normal heart without signs of failure, close follow-up is mandatory. Sometimes, cases of infrequent ectopics may be innocuous. If we detect persistent tachycardia with failing heart, we must plan for fetal therapy.

Now, let us see how Doppler is helpful in cases of arrhythmias.

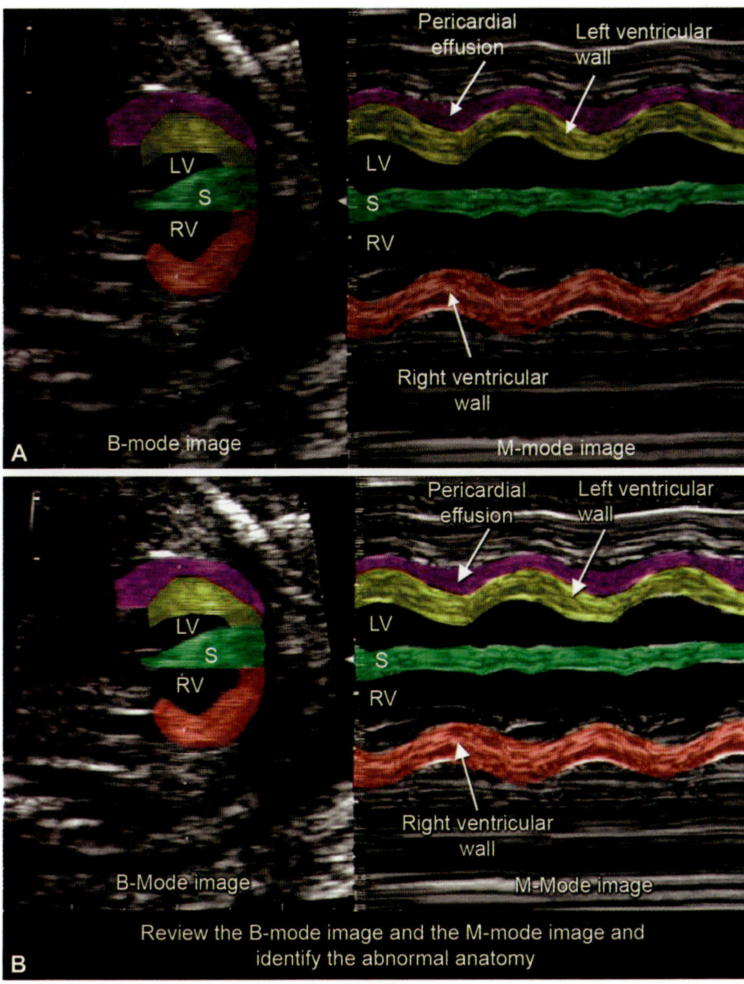

Figures 9.6A and B Labeled images of the B-mode and M-mode of both the normal ventricular chambers with septum

As Doppler is an essential tool for diagnosis of fetal anemia and AV malformations, we usually see high velocity in MCA Doppler and a typical saw toothed pattern in umbilical artery. Sometimes pulsatile umbilical vein is also there, which is corresponding to an increased reverse flow in IVC. Moreover, the flow in the ductus venosus also gets reversed.

Now we can describe this condition in three categories as follows:

1. *Mild*: The condition is described as mild, if at the gestational age of 36–37 weeks, there is mild cardiac failure along with mild pulsatile flow in the umbilical vein.
2. *Moderate:* The condition is described as moderate, if at the gestational age of 34–35 weeks, the sonologist observes placental insufficiency, hypoxic status, cardiac failure and pulsatility in umbilical and portal veins and ductus venosus.
3. *Severe*: The condition is described as severe, if at the gestational age of 17–18 weeks, we see signs of nonimmune hydrops, cardiac anomaly with heart failure and severe pulsatile flow in umbilical and portal vein and IVC.

NUTSHELL

1. Fetal arrhythmias can be diagnosed by getting good M-mode tracing for that fetus must be co-operative and cardiac examination friendly.
2. It is very difficult to take fetal ECG for diagnosis of arrhythmias but it can be done with use of fetal scalp electrode.
3. All anti-arrhythmic drugs can cause side effect to mother so we have to see risk v/s benefit ration before starting.
4. With advent of new modalities like M-mode and Pulse Doppler it is very easy to understand fetal arrhythmias.
5. Fetus is constantly moving subjet so it will be very difficult to put M-mode cursor perfectly.
6. Ideal placement for Doppler is at the junction of ventricular inflow and out flow tract at LVOT so we can see both ventricular filling as well as emptying to the base line on either side, other 2 area are... Overlapping of the pulmonary venous and arterial flow and overlapping of the ascending aorta and superior vena cava.
7. In PASS...S, if last S means squeeze is good means rhythm is good.
8. The conduction system made up of SA node, AV node, Bundle of His, Purkinje's system and it is progressing throughout fetal life to post natal life.
9. Fetal heart arrhythmias are of irregular rhythm, bradycardia, complete heart block, and tachyarrhythmias—such as atrial tachycardia, atrial flutter and fibrillation, ventricular tachycardia.

10

Outflow Tract Abnormalities

After having sufficient knowledge of normal tract LVOT and RVOT, we have to think and describe normal as normal and abnormal as abnormal.

If we are able to detect normal cardiovascular tract (Figure 10.1), it would be easy to look for abnormal or outflow tract abnormalities. From the discussion in previous chapters, we feel that by using a normal four-chamber view, we would be able to detect only 50–60% of major cardiac abnormalities.

According to the guidelines of ISUOG, if we also include outflow tract in imaging techniques, rest of abnormalities of heart disease would also be picked up, with the detection rate of 75%. This is also known as extended basic examination of fetal heart.

Prenatal detection of outflow anomalies like transposition of the great vessels (TGV) is important because it is a surgically corrected anomaly, having very good prognosis for fetus. Thus, we can guide parents accordingly and advise them to deliver the baby at a place where surgical facilities are available.

The next question we need to answer is "when should we have suspicion of having outflow tract abnormalities on basic fetal examination?"

To find the answer, let us go to basic PASS....S:

- *Position*: Normal or abnormal
- *Axis*: Usually the cardiac axis is increased

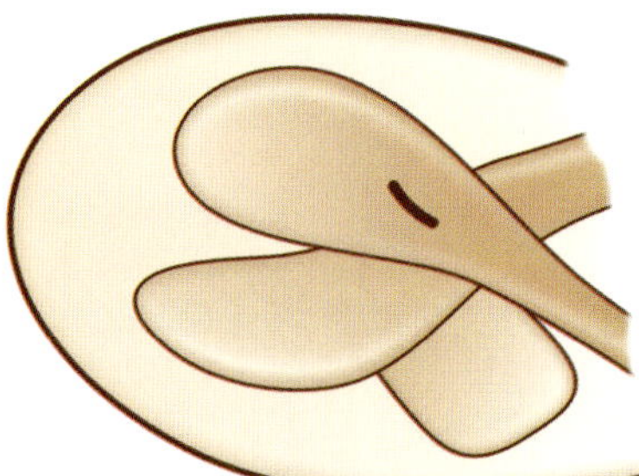

Figure 10.1 Normal tract

- *Size*: Sometimes we may observe ventricles which are unequal in size
- *Symmetry* may be lost because of:
  - Narrow or dilated outflow tracts
  - Abnormal semilunar valves
  - Parallel placed outflow tracts.

OUTFLOW TRACT ABNORMALITIES

Outflow tract abnormalities (Figure 10.2) are mainly as follows:
- Double outlet right ventricle (DORV)
- Transposition of great arteries (TGA)
- Tetralogy of Fallot (TOF)

Double Outlet Right Ventricle

- In this anomaly, both aorta and pulmonary artery arise from right ventricle and mostly they occupy 50% of right ventricle each.
- We can see malaligned ventricular septal defect (VSD) in form of subaortic, subpulmonary, doubly committed or a noncommitted defect. We can see the double outlet right ventricle in Figures 10.3A and B.
- This is basically an outflow tract anomaly and subaortic VSD. Therefore, the circulation is usually similar to TOF.
- If DORV has subpulmonic VSD, then the hemodynamics are similar to that of complete TGA.
- Association of trisomy 18 is increased with DORV.
- Since it is not easy to see DORV, we must think what it should look like on ultrasound examination (Figures 10.3 to 10.5):
  - Both aorta and PA arise from RV
  - Two types of aorta—PA relationships are possible: Aorta may be posterior and to the right of the pulmonary artery or aorta may be parallel to the pulmonary artery with aorta being anterior and to the right.

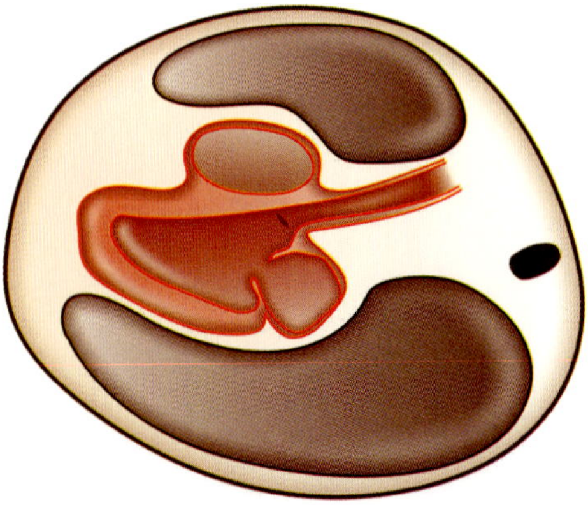

Figure 10.2 Tract abnormalities

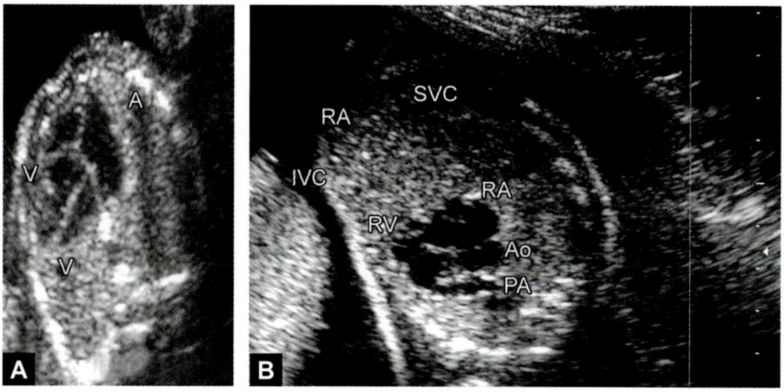

Figures 10.3A and B Ultrasound image of double outlet right ventricle (DORV)

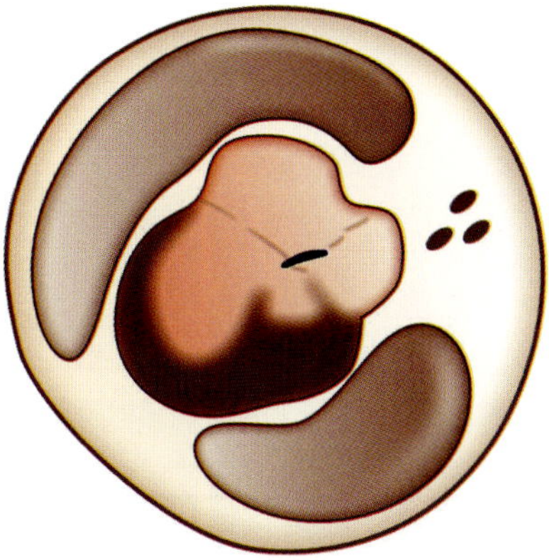

Figure 10.4 Diagrammatic representation of double outlet right ventricle

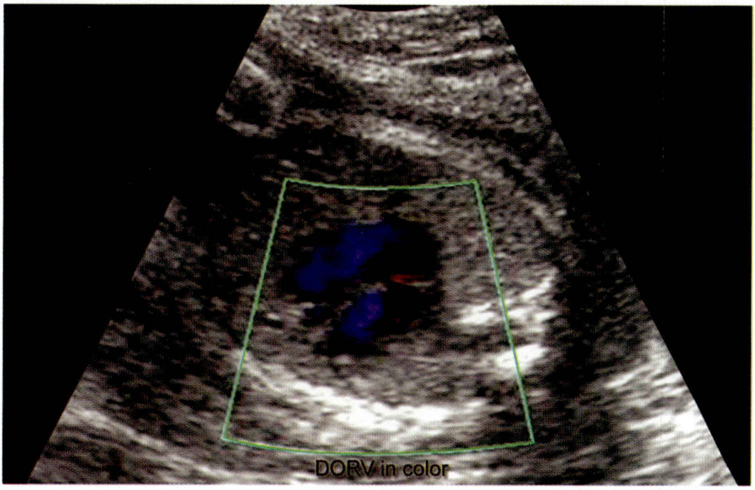

Figure 10.5 Doppler image of double outlet right ventricle

- When we see one abnormality, it is mandatory to search for presence of some other abnormalities also. Lets see and watch ...... What the picture displays?

Treatment

- DORV is a correctable anomaly and very good 10-year-survival rates may be seen in up to 97% cases after surgery.
- Type of surgery totally depends upon the location and size of VSD and relation and position of aorta and pulmonary vessel.

Tetralogy of Fallot (TOF) (Figures 10.6A to E)

- It comprises of the following components:
  - Over-riding of the aorta
  - Ventricular septal defect (Figure 10.7)

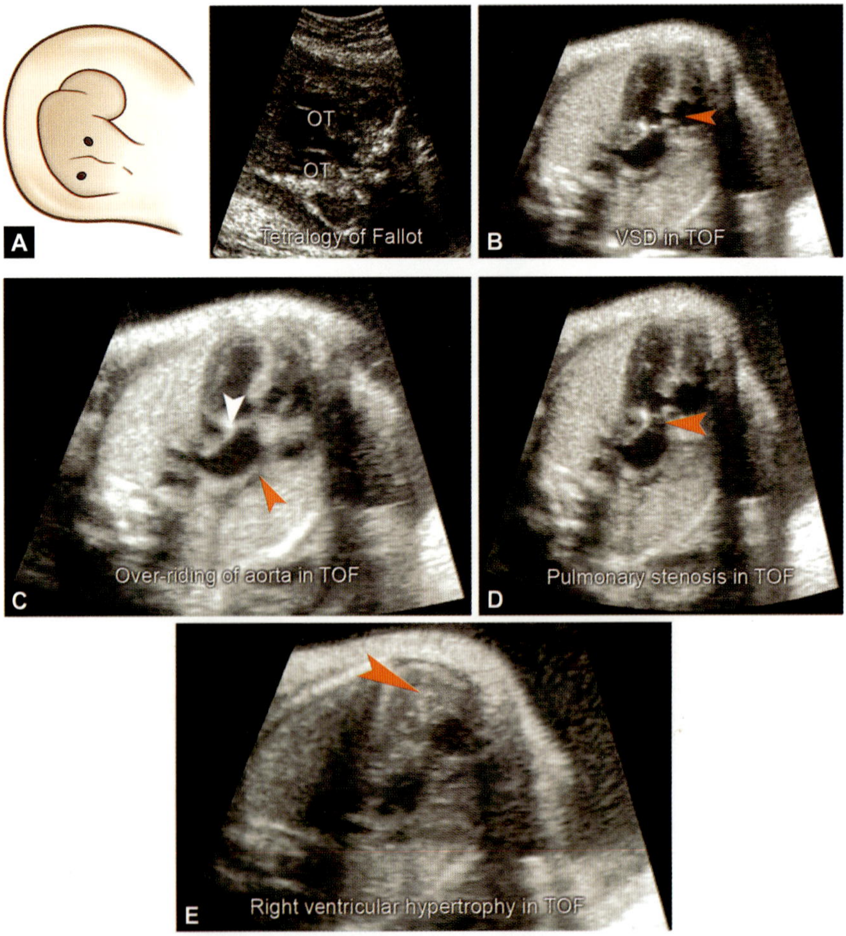

Figures 10.6A to E (A) Tetralogy of Fallot; (B) VSD in tetralogy of Fallot; (C) Over-riding of aorta in tetralogy of Fallot; (D) Pulmonary stenosis in tetralogy of Fallot; (E) Right ventricular hypertrophy in tetralogy of Fallot

  - Subvalvular stenosis, pulmonary hypertension (RV outflow tract obstruction) (Figure 10.8)
  - RV hypertrophy.
- Presence of all these four components is essential to establish a diagnosis of tetralogy of Fallot. However, we may not always be able to appreciate right ventricular function in utero. We may also sometimes see pulmonary valve obstruction in only 20% of the patients.

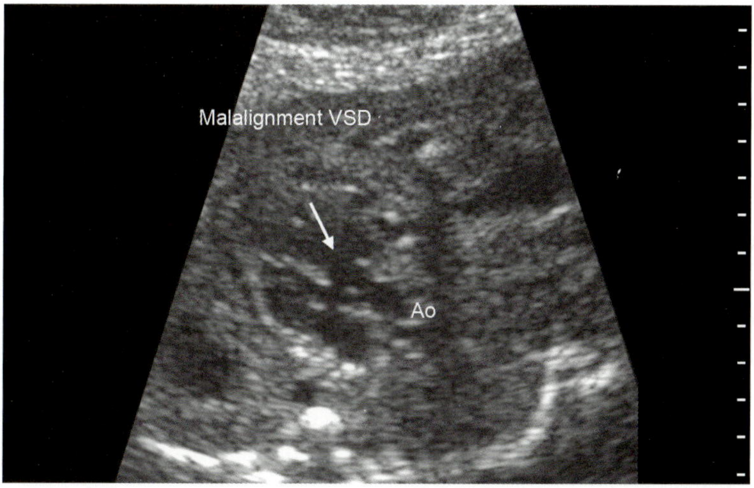

Figure 10.7 Ventricular septal defect

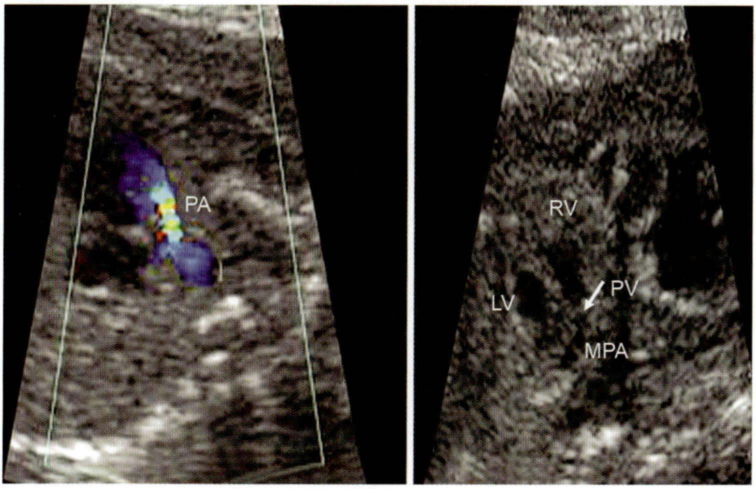

Figure 10.8 Pulmonary hypertension

Abbreviations: AV, atrioventricular; LV, left ventricle; MPA, main pulmonary artery; PA, pulmonary artery; PV, pulmonary vein

- Atrial septal defect (ASD), ventricular septal defect (VSD) and patent ductus arteriosus (PDA) may also be seen.
- Tetralogy of Fallot may also be associated with extracardiac anomalies in approximately 20–30% babies.

Ultrasound

Ultrasound diagnosis of TOF is based on the following parameters:

- Over-riding of dilated aorta can be easily identified
- Malalignment of VSD extending to perimembranous position.

Doppler Examination

Doppler examination is based on the following parameters:

- Aorta receives blood from both the ventricles
- RVOT obstruction can be easily made out
- 25% cases are associated with right aortic arch
- PA is dilated with absent valves
- Other cardiac abnormalities are also present.

Management

- This is the most common cyanotic heart disease which is diagnosed after 1 year of age
- As the age advances, cyanotic spells worsen the prognosis. So, if we are able to diagnose TOF prenatally, we can guide the parents accordingly, because surgical outcome is usually fine with this type of anomaly
- Size of pulmonary artery determines the surgical outcome
- Cardiothoracic surgeon usually perform total correction in all patients either in single or double sitting, if size of pulmonary artery is favorable
- If on neonatal Doppler, we find size of pulmonary artery to be hypoplastic, we can offer palliative shunts to the diseased one
- Surgery has fantastic outcome of up to 85% of cure with very good survival rates.

Transposition of Great Arteries (TGA)

In these cases, the God has designed the outlets from different ventricles in comparison to the normal. Normally, left ventricle gives rise to aorta and right ventricle gives rise to the pulmonary artery. However, in cases of TGA, the aorta arises from right ventricle and pulmonary artery arises from left ventricle (Figures 10.9A and B). Since two independent circulations are operating at both the systemic as well as pulmonary levels, shunts are a must for survival of fetus in form of ASD/VSD/PDA.

Ultrasound Diagnosis

The following features can be observed on ultrasound examination:

- Parallel orientation of the outflow tracts
- Aorta arises from the right ventricle

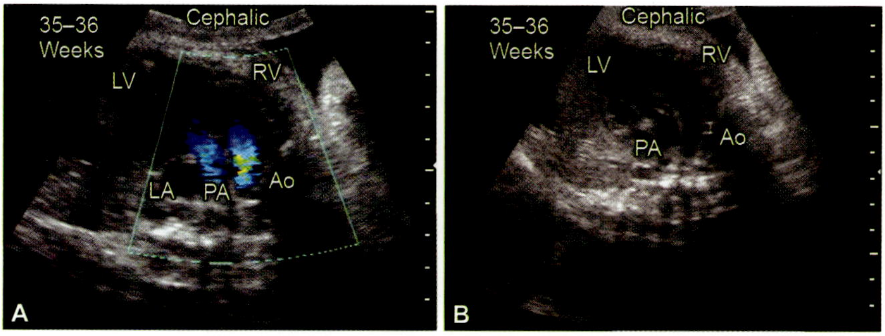

Figures 10.9A and B Transposition of great vessels

- Pulmonary artery arises from the left ventricle
- Aorta arises anterior to pulmonary arteries
- One must look for the presence of VSD.

Usually, we can see both great vessels crossing each other at 90°, so we can see criss-cross here. If this does not occur, we can see both vessels parallel to each other.

Management

- At birth, fetus is cyanosed and it is in distress
- We have to see that the ductal arch must remain open so we may have to give prostaglandin E1 (PGE1) infusion to the neonate
- Sometimes palliative procedure such as atrial septostomy (Rashkind) is carried out
- Main goal is to opt for cardiac surgical procedures such as:
  - Jatene's arterial switch operation
  - Mustard or senning atrial switch procedures.

Result of surgery is good after arterial and atrial switch surgery.

CRUX ABNORMALITY (FIGURES 10.10 AND 10.11)

Dysplastic Heart Valves

- Could be associated with trisomy 18.
- This could manifest in form of aortic or pulmonary stenosis (Figures 10.12 to 10.16).

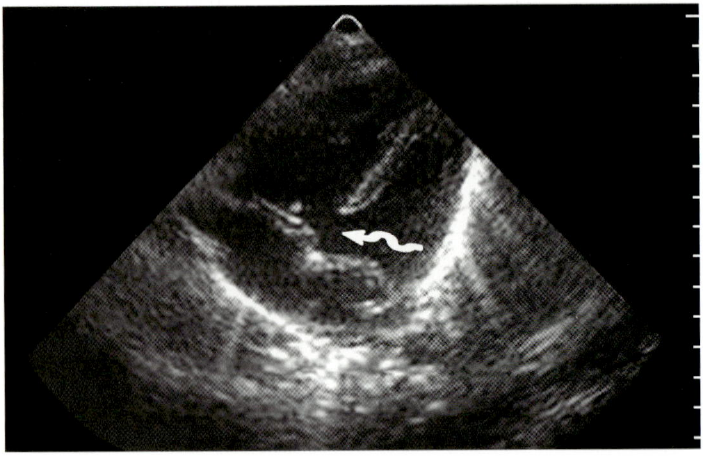

Figure 10.10 Crux abnormality

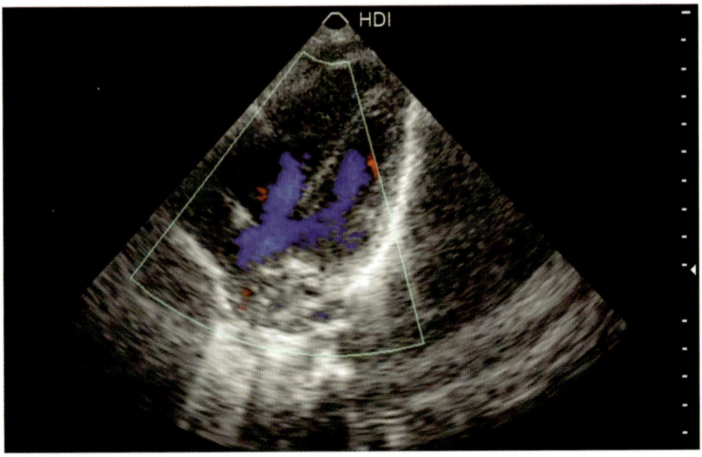

Figure 10.11 Color flow at crux

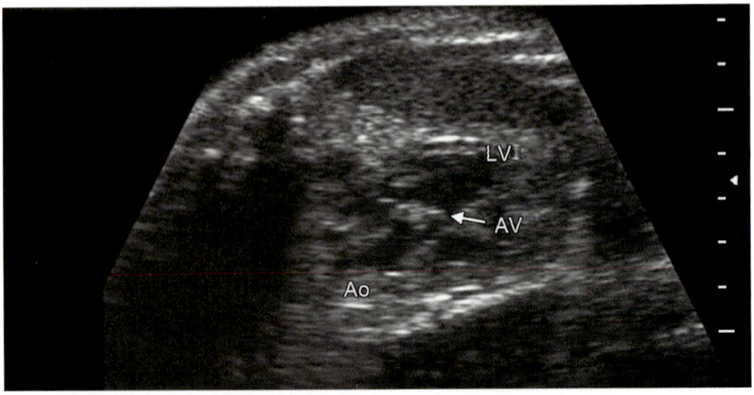

Figure 10.12 Dysplastic aortic valve

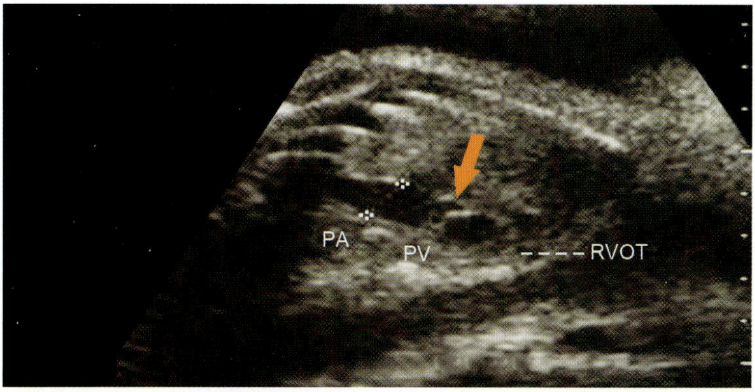

Figure 10.13 Pulmonary valve

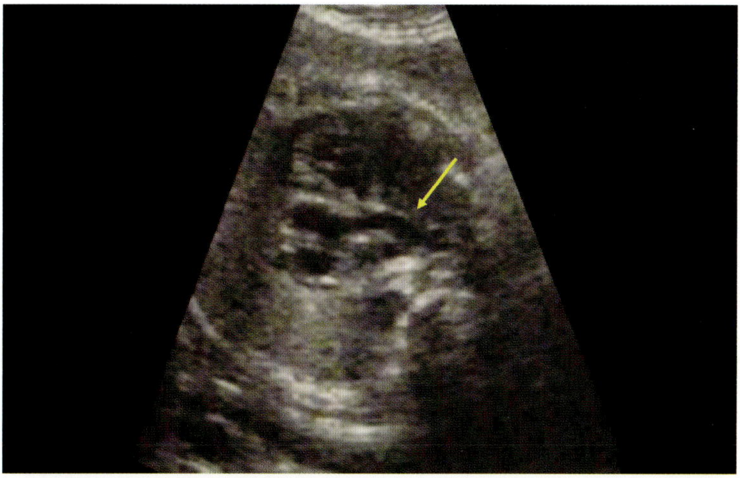

Figure 10.14 Aortic stenosis

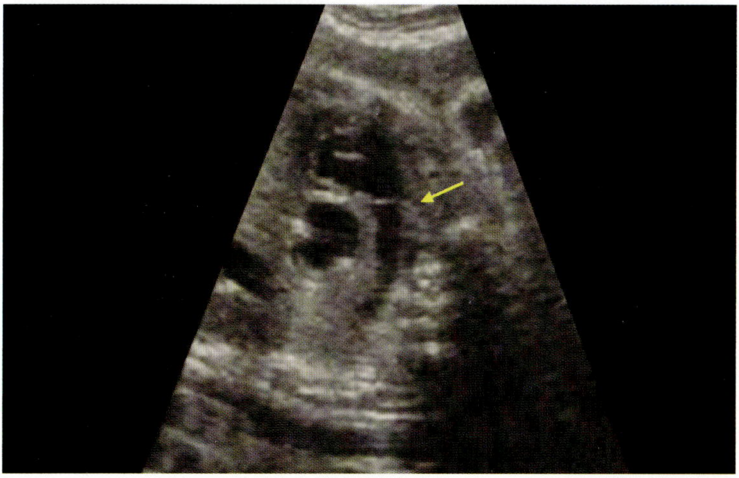

Figure 10.15 Aorta

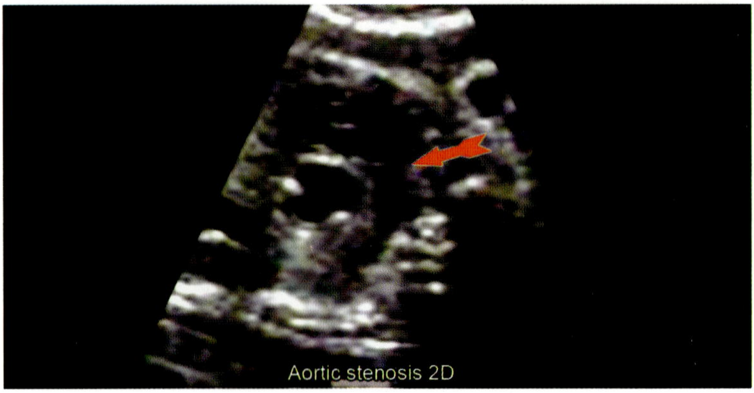

Figure 10.16 Color aliasing in the aorta

NUTSHELL

1. As given in ISUOG guideline, outflow tract should be imagine as extended basic program and so many heart abnormality missed by four-chamber view, will be easily diagnosed and discussed with parent for plan of delivery.
2. Again go to PASS...S and here, if outflow tract abnormality is there will be symmetry loss.
3. DORV, TGA and TOF are three main and discussed in detail.

11

Fetal Dissection

Nowadays in busy practice we might forget all the basic fundamentals taught by our teachers during first day of our admission in first MBBS class during the Anatomy lecture at the time of dissection.

Back to basics, I believe that the principle to learn any new thing in life is to define what is normal, then it becomes very easy to define what is abnormal.

So in this atlas of fetal echo, let us start our first step towards learning the basic style of dissection (Figures 11.1 to 11.21):

- As per the rule, we have to follow the curvature of vascular flow for the dissection and on that basis we have to identify all vessels, chambers and the tracts
- Before dissection of the heart, we have to follow the basic standard protocol for autopsy

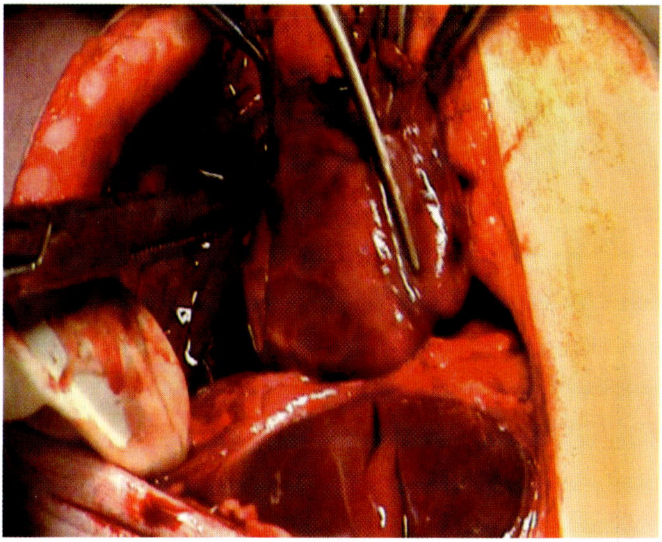

Figure 11.1 The anterior surface of the heart with dissected neck

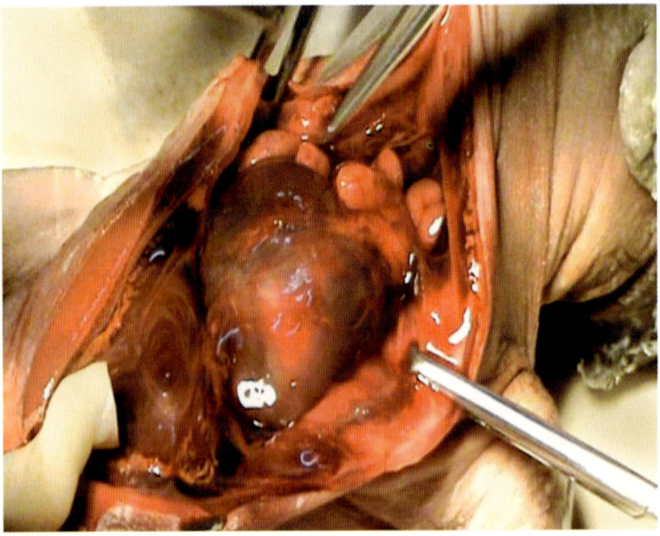

Figure 11.2 The opened pericardium with anterior surface of the heart

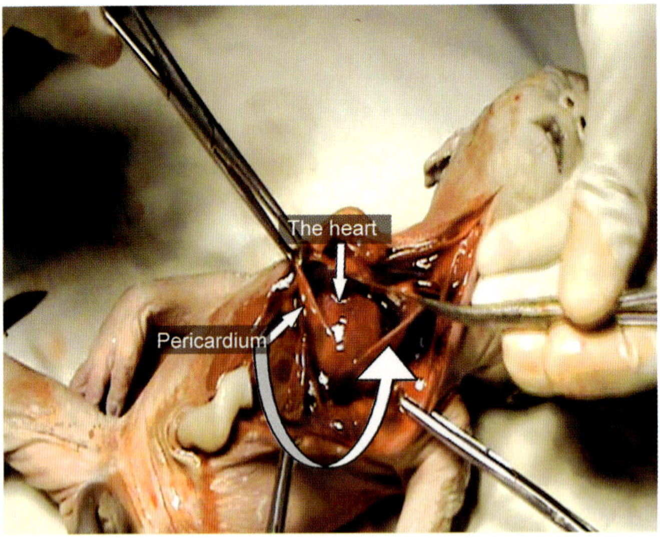

Figure 11.3 The opened pericardium with anterior surface of the heart

- First we look at the external appearance of fetus and then look for any gross fetal malformations
- Just like in ultrasound biometry, there are protocols for measurement in the fetus as well
- Firstly, we have to measure the total length of fetus, then head to rump length (CRL) and lastly the leg length and foot length.

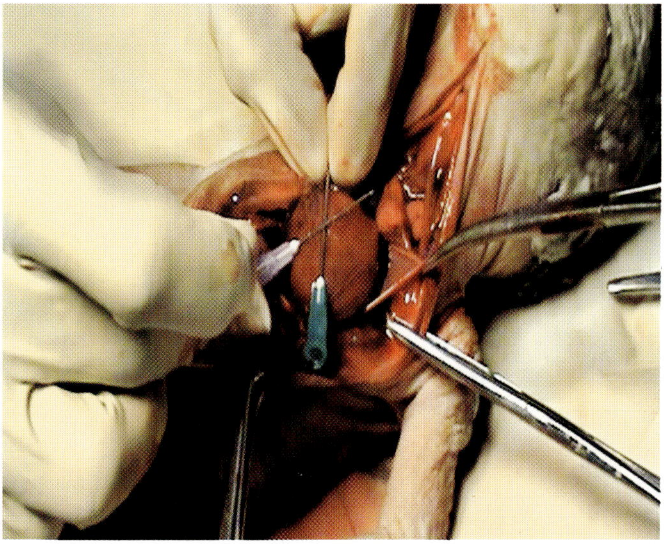

Figure 11.4 Axis of the heart

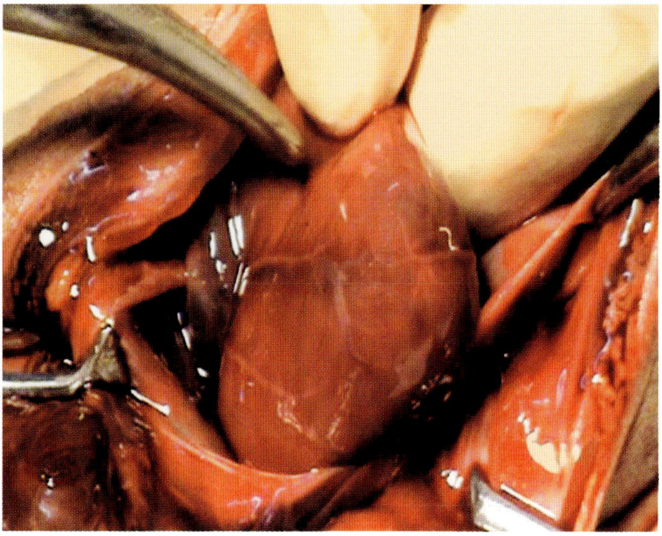

Figure 11.5 Anterolateral surface of the heart with right auricle

- Secondly, we have to measure the head circumference.
- Next, we have to look for the alignment of nose and the mandible. They should be in same line for symmetry and we must be able to diagnose micrognathia
- There are nomograms available on the basis of which we can assign the exact age of the fetus depending on the fetal biometry and the exact developmental defect.

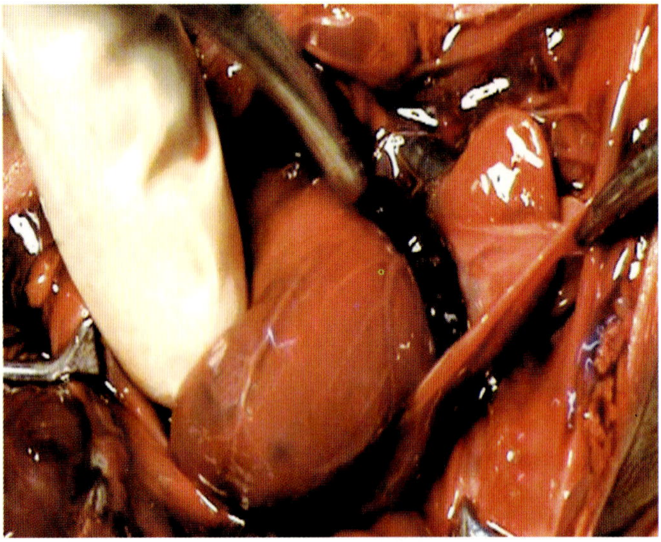

Figure 11.6 Left auricle, anterior interventricular groove, pericardium

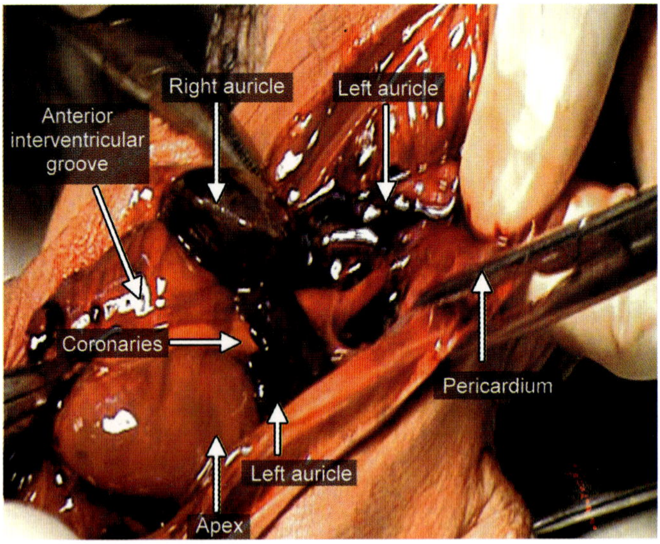

Figure 11.7 Labeled showing left auricle, anterior interventricular groove, pericardium

- The anus must be probed in order to confirm patency
- After external examination and measurement, we have to make a cut extending from the neck to the symphysis, taking care not to injure the structures below, especially in cases where the gestational age is very less.
- After cutting sternum we can see beneath, what is lying in the pericardium. The thinness may vary according to the gestational age of fetus.

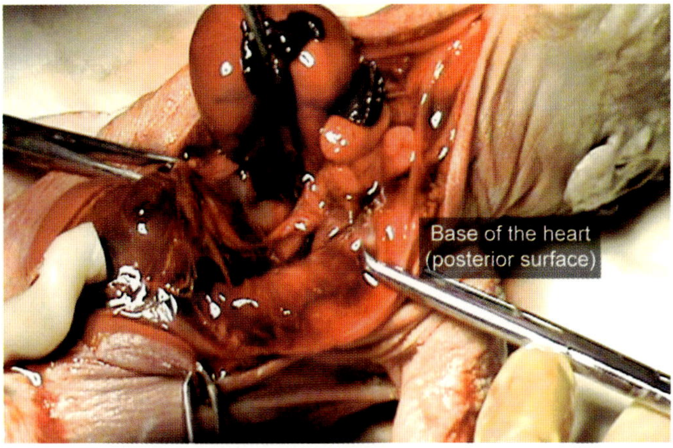

Figure 11.8 The posterior surface of the heart

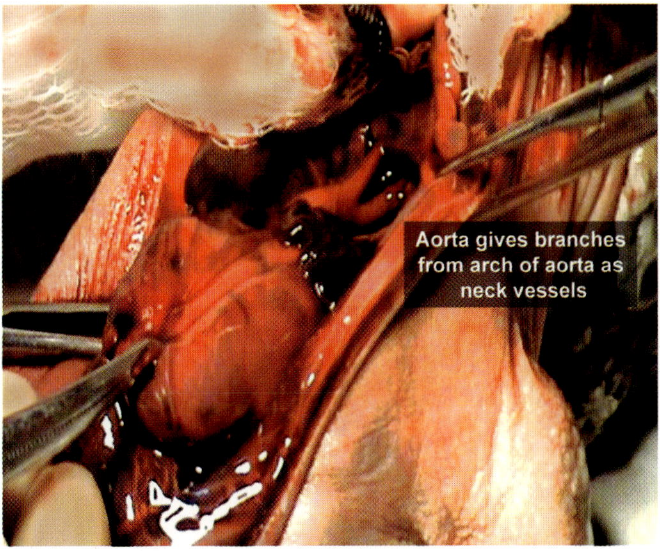

Figure 11.9 Aortic arch with two main branches

- After opening the pericardium, we must assess whether the pericardiac fluid is present or not and if present we must estimate its amount
- Just above the heart, a large thymus is usually visualized because in neonatal life thymus is very big and sometimes may cover whole of the front of the heart.
- We just need to reflect the thymus to see front of the heart, which shows right and left atrial appendages, out of which the right atrial appendage is a little larger than the left.

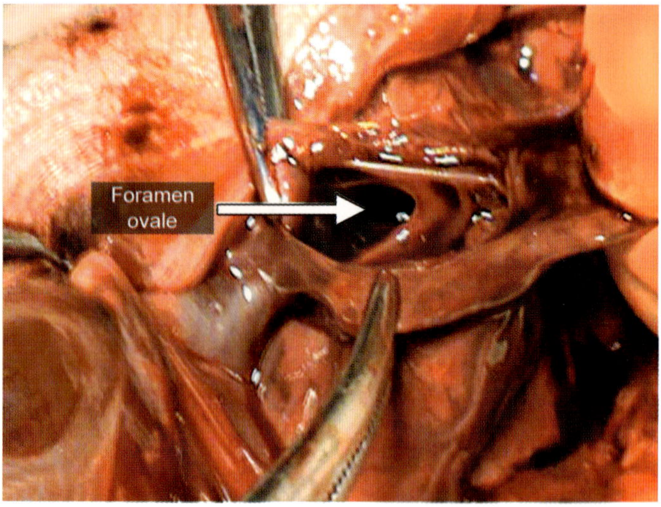

Figure 11.10 Foramen ovale opening from RA to LA

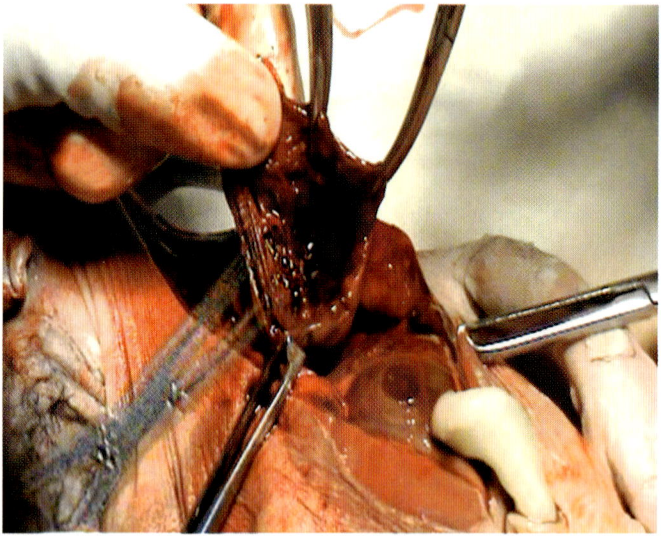

Figure 11.11 Opened right auricle

- Now its time to look for interventricular groove, which on the inner side shows IVS, i.e. the interventricular septum
- Look at the external features of the heart, including the chamber position, symmetry and association of all outflow tracts from their origin to insertion
- We have to look for external features of the outflow at aorta and three vessels branching, i.e. the innominate artery, common carotid and subclavian artery
- Whole specimen should be cut out with both lungs, stomach with liver and intact diaphragm from below and esophagus with trachea from above

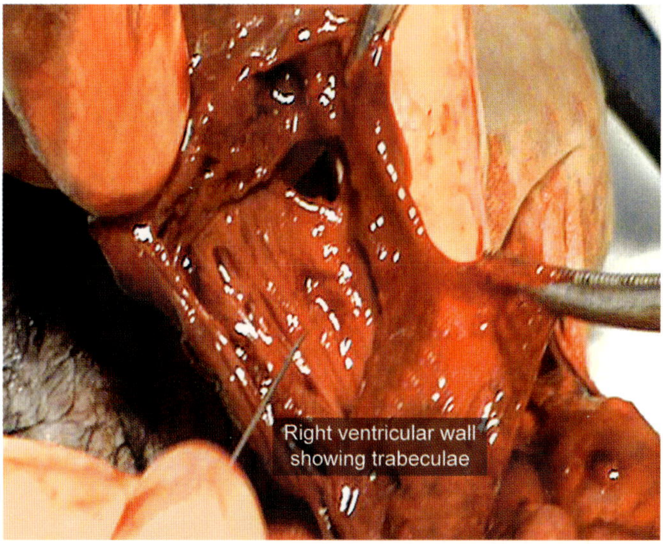

Figure 11.12 Opened right ventricle (dirty chamber)

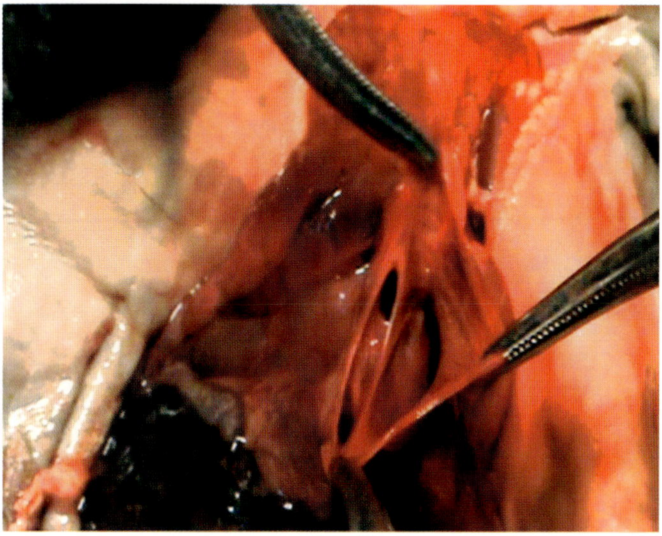

Figure 11.13 Opened aortic and pulmonary valves

- *Let us start with venous connection:* Both SVC and IVC are draining into the right atrium, so we just need to put a guide probe into it and cut along the vascular line. Now we are in right atrium which drains both vena cava and has the right appendicular appendage, which is on the anterior surface of the heart.
- Right atrium opens into right ventricle via tricuspid valve, so now we have to cut along with the vascular connection of tricuspid valve and enter onto the right ventricle having moderator band as an identification mark on ultrasound

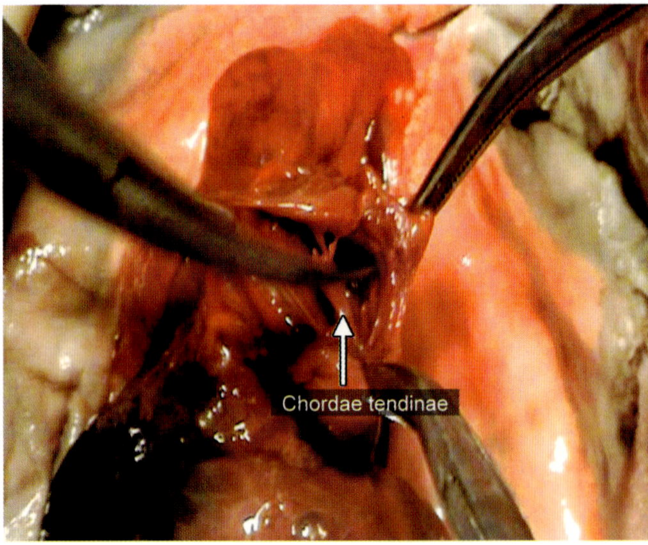

Figure 11.14 Opened ventricle and chordae tendinae

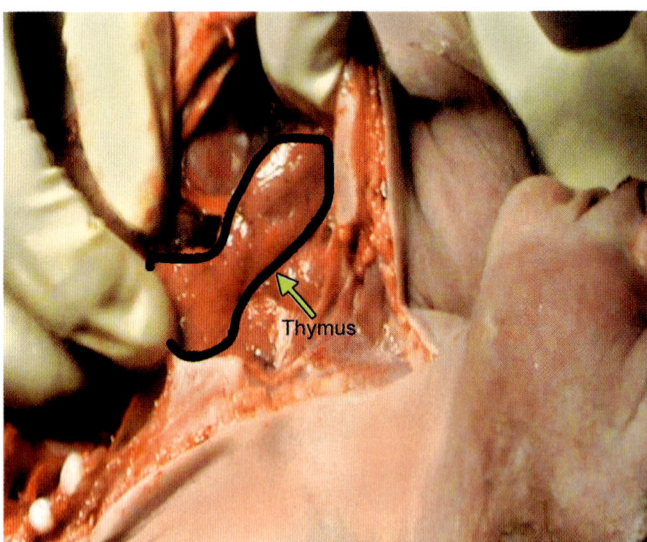

Figure 11.15 Thymus

as well as *in situ*. Tricuspid valve, as the name suggests has three cusps, namely anterior, posterior and septal. Tricuspid valve inserts more apically into the interventricular septum in comparison to the mitral valve. The anterior leaflet is larger than the other two leaflets.

- Right ventricular outflow tract (RVOT) mainly comprises of the pulmonary arteries. From right ventricle, the blood drains into lungs via the pulmonary arteries so we must cut open the vessels entering into the lungs.

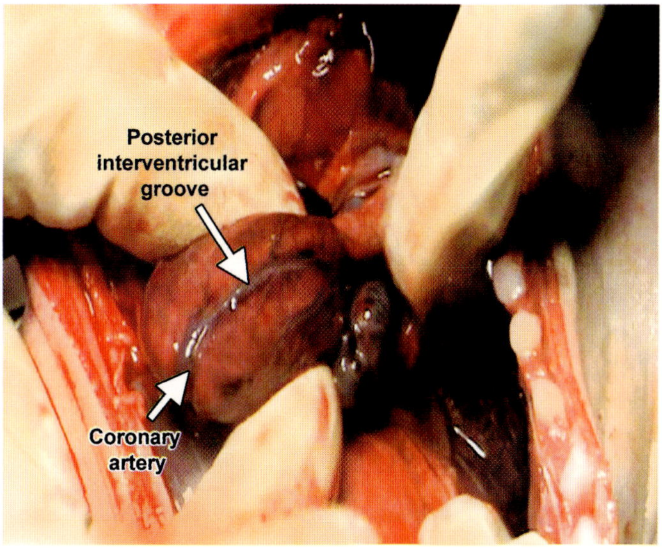

Figure 11.16 Posterior interventricular groove with coronary artery

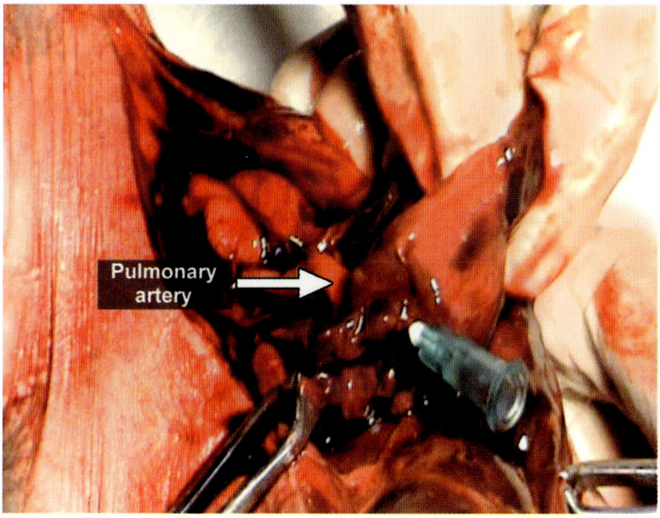

Figure 11.17 Origin of the pulmonary artery from the right ventricle

- Now if we look at the back of heart, we would be able to see the posterior part of left atrium and both pulmonary veins entering into the left atrium from the posterior side. So again following the rule of thumb, we must cut according to the vessels, so that by cutting open the veins, we are in the left atrium and opening this would enable us to visualize the left atrial appendages.

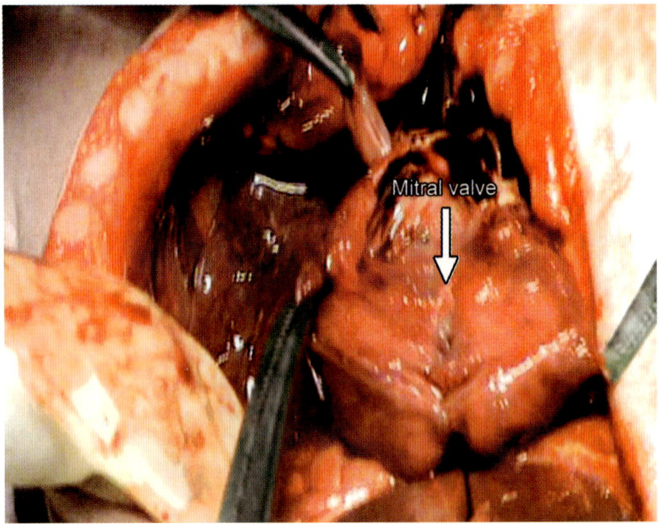

Figure 11.18 The open mitral valve and left ventricular chamber

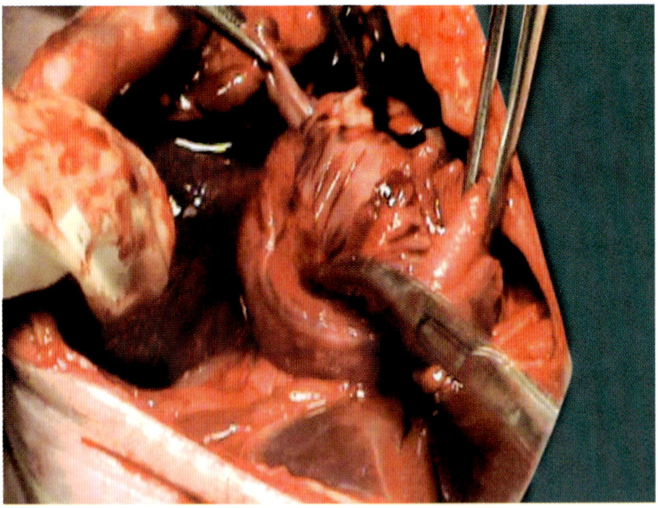

Figure 11.19 Opened right ventricle

- We can see foramen ovale flap opening onto the left atrium and can also visualize septum primum and septum secundum.
- Now we have to cut again along the vascular margins so we have to open from LA into LV via mitral valve which has two cusps as the name suggests. We can also see the normal offset between the two valves. The tricuspid valve is normally placed more apically in comparison to the mitral valve

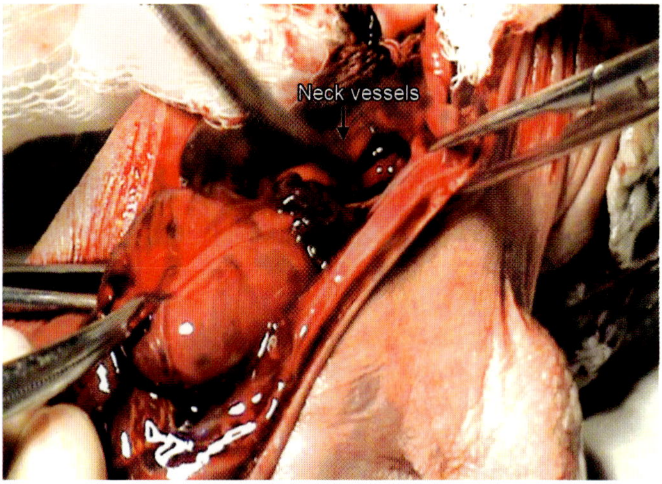

Figure 11.20 Dissected neck vessels

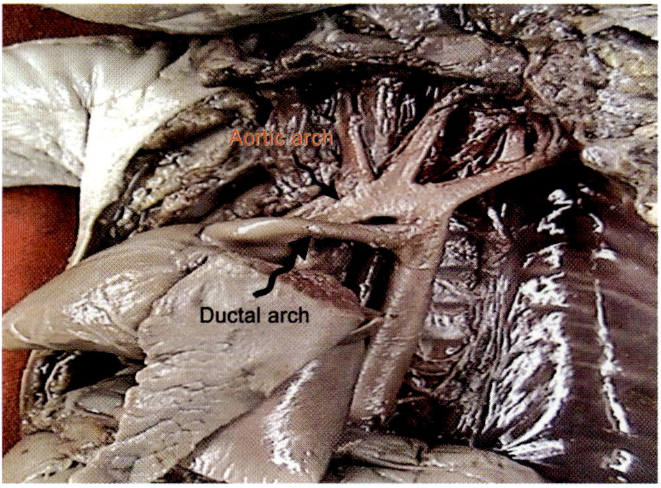

Figure 11.21 The ductal arch

- Left ventricle is little bit more clearer than the right ventricle, which is more occupied with chordae tendi. So in comparison, the left ventricle has a much clearer chamber than the right ventricle.
- *Mitral leaflets have two cusps:* Anterior and posterior. Anterior leaflet is larger than posterior leaflet. The leaflets of the valve are attached to their respective ventricular walls through the chordae tendi and papillary muscles.
- The crux of the heart is formed by the atrioventricular valves, membranous portion of the IVS and septum primum

- Left ventricle gives out LVOT which is narrow and is known as the aortic isthmus. The LVOT and aorta are posterior to the RVOT and pulmonary artery. The anterior mitral leaflets are continuous with the posterior aortic wall and interventricular septum is continuous with the anterior aortic wall.
- Left ventricular outflow tract (LVOT) is truly an aortic tract and we can see by opening of semilunar valve at the level of left ventricle that we are in the aorta.
- The aortic arch is usually left sided and gives rise to the brachiocephalic, left common carotid and left subclavian arteries.
- The ductus arteriosus is present only in fetal life and is the conduit between the left pulmonary artery and the descending thoracic aorta just beyond the origin of the left subclavian artery.
- The pulmonary artery, ductus arteriosus and descending aorta together form the ductal arch and aortic arch is also separate one. While doing dissection we are able to observe the difference in both, including their origin and difference in shape like hockey stick and drum stick shape at the region where the ductal arch joins the arch of aorta.
- The ductal arch joins the aortic arch by a connection known as ductia arteries. This is a very high flow connection named as aortic fundal flow and we can have wave pattern of it with gradation. We can predict outcome of baby's brain status as this vessel diverts bold flow from heart to the vessel of the brain via three arteries.

NUTSHELL

1. For internal examination put incision—chin to pubis or inverted "y".
2. Systematically examine thoracic cavity and abdominal organ and take note of it.
3. Dissection of heart can be done *in situ* or remove enblock with lungs and liver.
4. For external examination see for size, situs and axis, interventricular groves, arterial appendages, superior and inferior vena cava, pulmonary veins, aorta and pulmonary artery.
5. Heart dissection → follow the flow of blood beginning on right side, → cut through the systemic inflow tracts (SVC & IVC), → cut through the superior venacava to open right atrium → next cut across the tricuspid valve to open into the right ventricle → insert probe into the right ventricle out flow tract and cut across → cut through the pulmonary vein to open left atrium → next cut to open mitral valve to open into left ventricle → insert probe into left ventricular outflow tract and cut across.

12

Images of Fetal ECHO Tract and Dissection

IMAGES OF FETAL ECHO (FIGURES 12.1 TO 12.6)

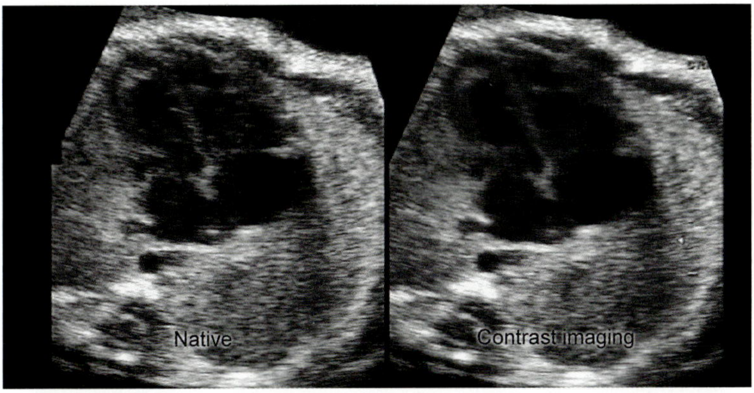

Figure 12.1 Contrast imaging

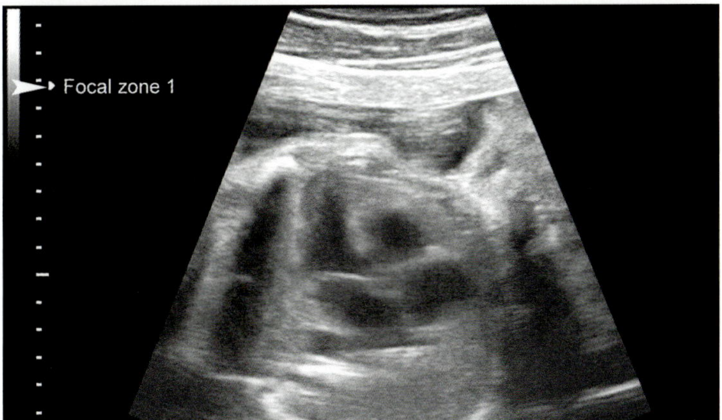

Figure 12.2A

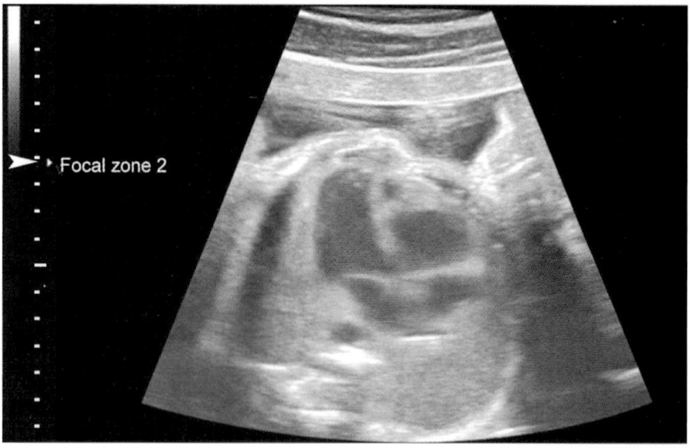

Figure 12.2B

Figures 12.2A and B Focal zone imaging showing zone 1 and zone 2

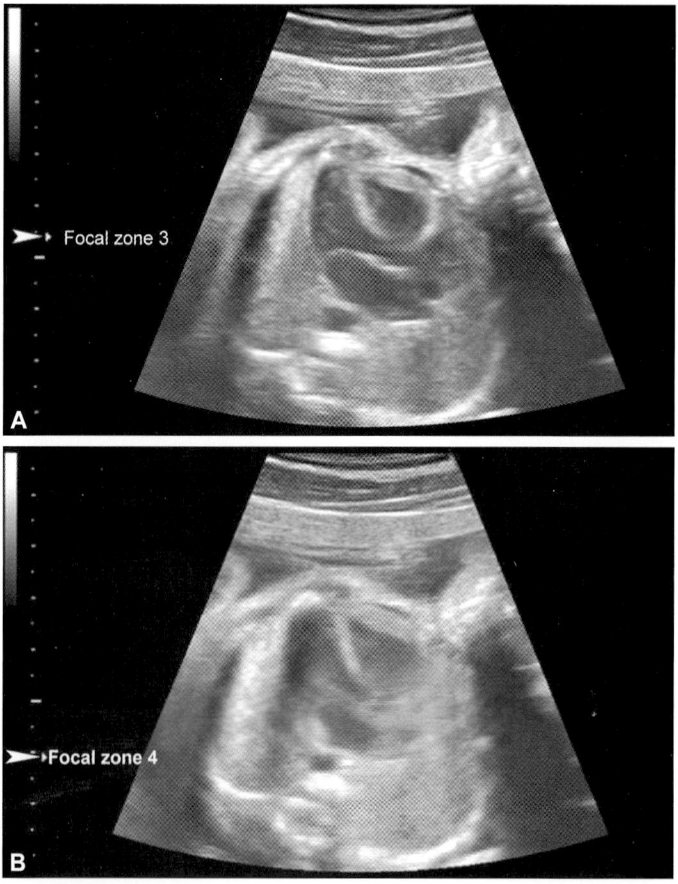

Figures 12.3A and B Focal zone imaging showing zone 3 and 4

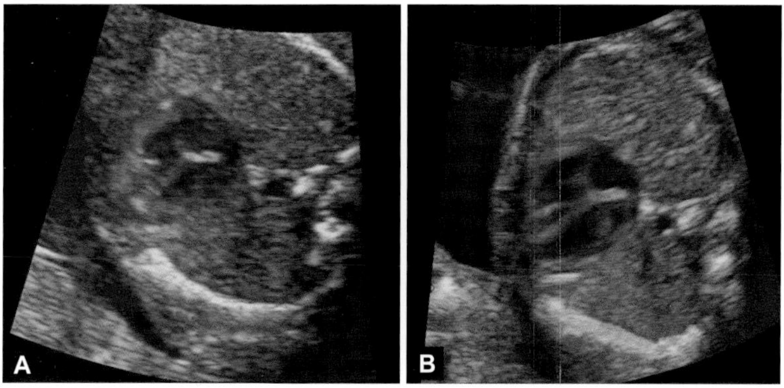

Figures 12.4A and B Difference between (A) Low; and (B) High frequency transducer

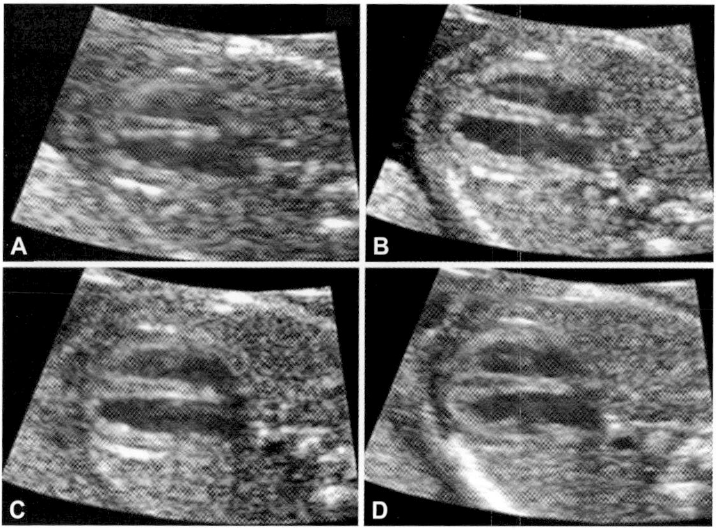

Figures 12.5A to D Difference between native image and various harmonics

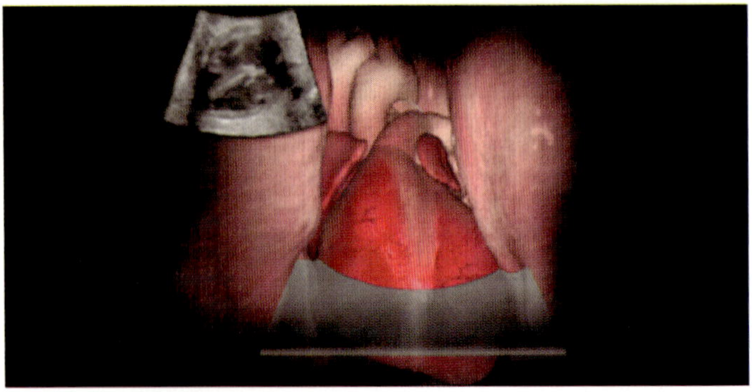

Figure 12.6 Four-chamber view of fetal heart

■ ASSESSMENT OF FETAL CARDIAC AXIS (FIGURES 12.7 TO 12.10)

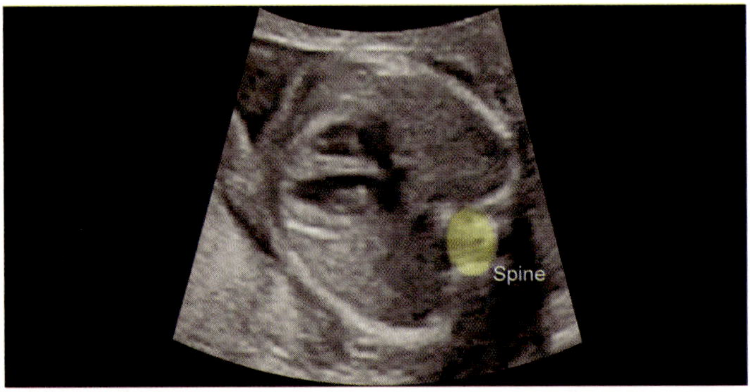

Figure 12.7 *Step 1:* Identification of fetal spine

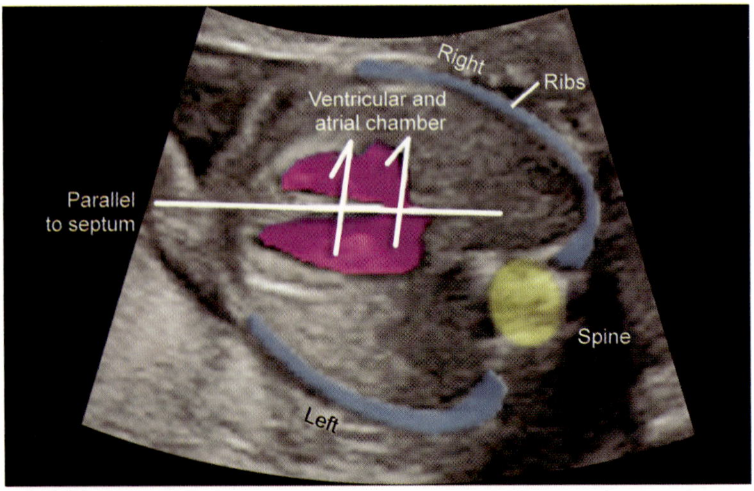

Figure 12.8: *Step 2:* A line which runs parallel to the interventricular septum

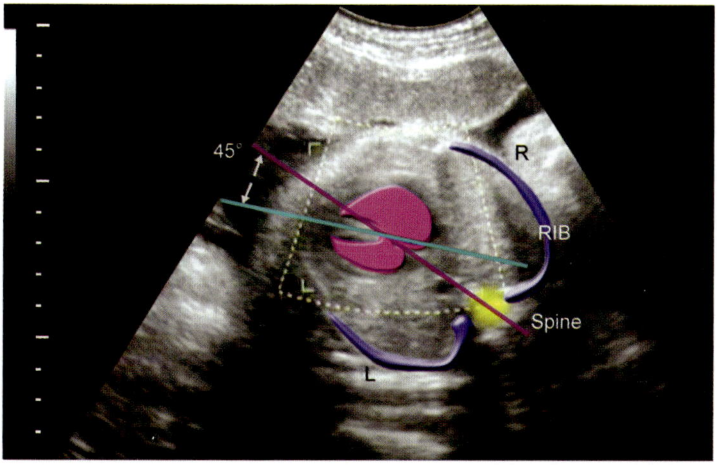

Figure 12.9 *Step 3:* The angle between the line from the spine to the anterior chest wall intersects the line parallel to the septum at a 45° angle (± 20°)

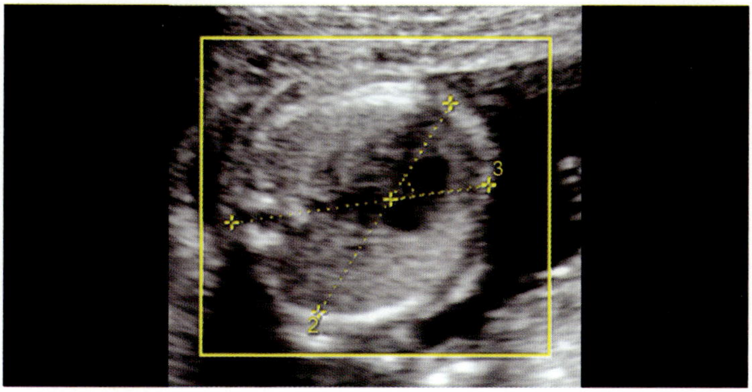

Figure 12.10 Panoramic view of the heart

■ ASSESSMENT OF FETAL SITUS (FIGURES 12.11 TO 12.17)

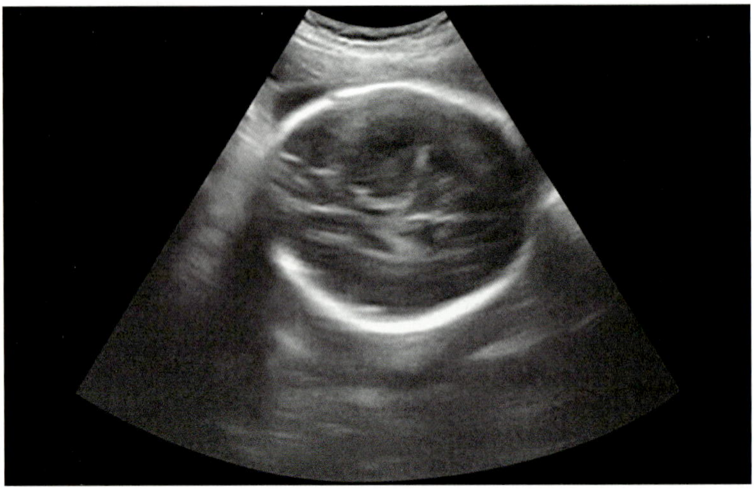

Figure 12.11 *Step 1:* The transducer is placed transversely at the level of the fetal head; in this example the head is in the vertex position

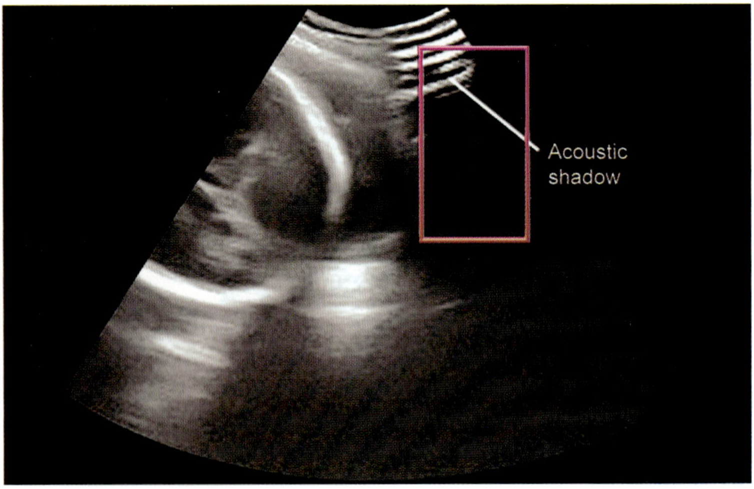

Figure 12.12 *Step 2:* As the examiner faces the transducer, the right edge of the transducer is lifted from the maternal abdomen and the corresponding acoustic shadow is identified

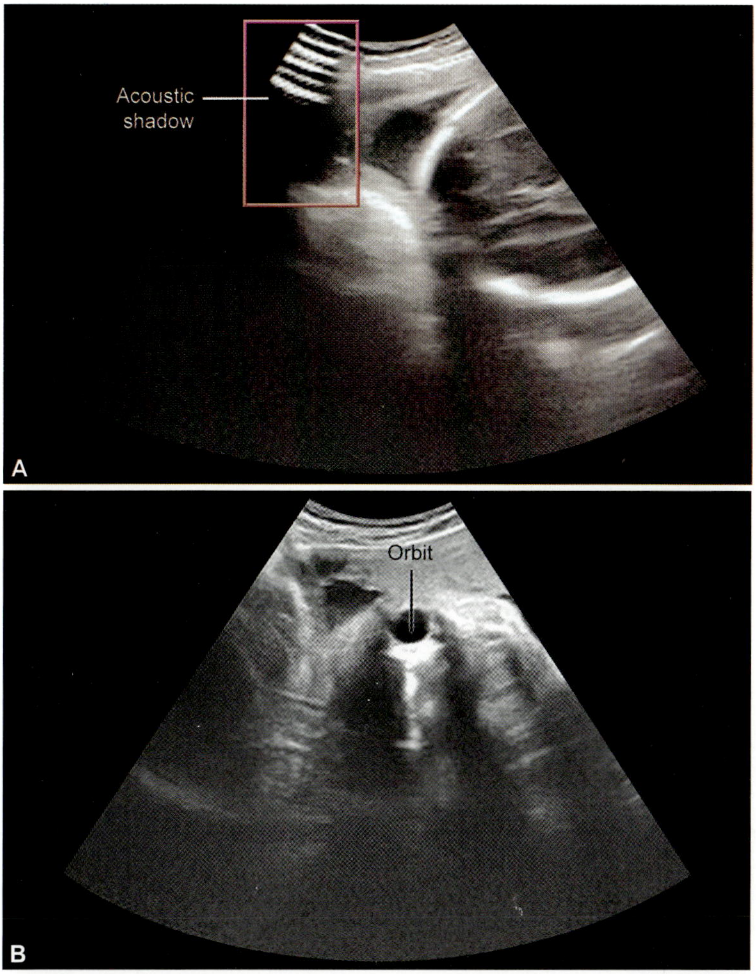

Figures 12.13A and B *Step 3:* If the shadow is on the same side as the edge of the lifted transducer, then there is synchrony between the two. If the examiner faces the transducer, then right edge of the transducer is lifted from the maternal abdomen, and the acoustic shadow identified is on the other side of the screen, then the examiner needs to rotate the transducer by 180° so that there is synchrony between the transducer position and the ultrasound image

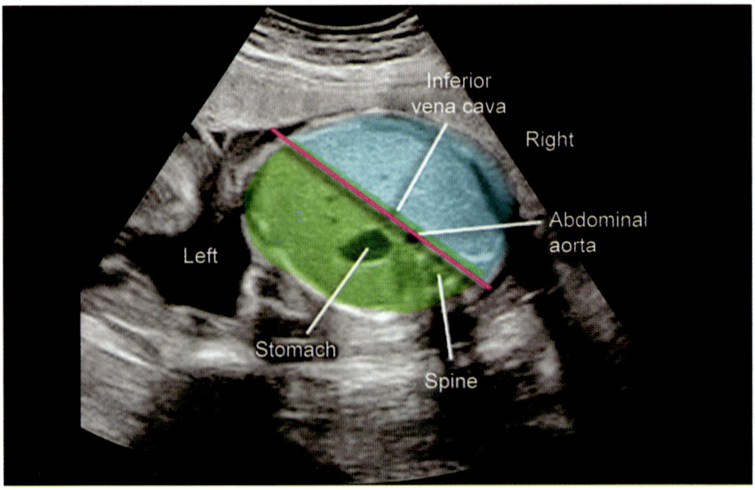

Figure 12.14 *Step 4:* Obtaining a transverse view of fetal abdomen by rotating the transducer by 90° from the sagittal view. The fetal stomach is located on the left side of the fetal abdomen

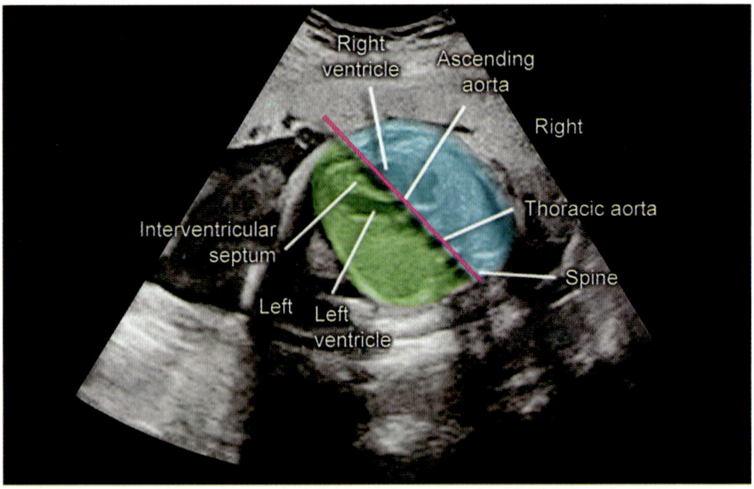

Figure 12.15 *Step 5:* Given the position of the fetal head, the transducer is directed at the level of the four-chamber view. The heart is located in the left side of the chest

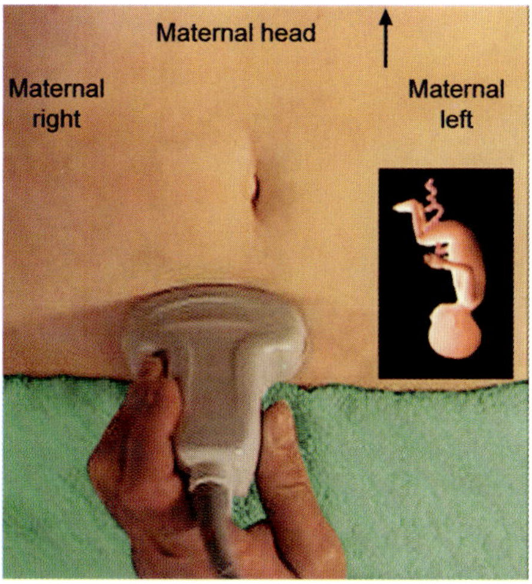

Figure 12.16 Transducer locates for maternal right and maternal left in vertex position

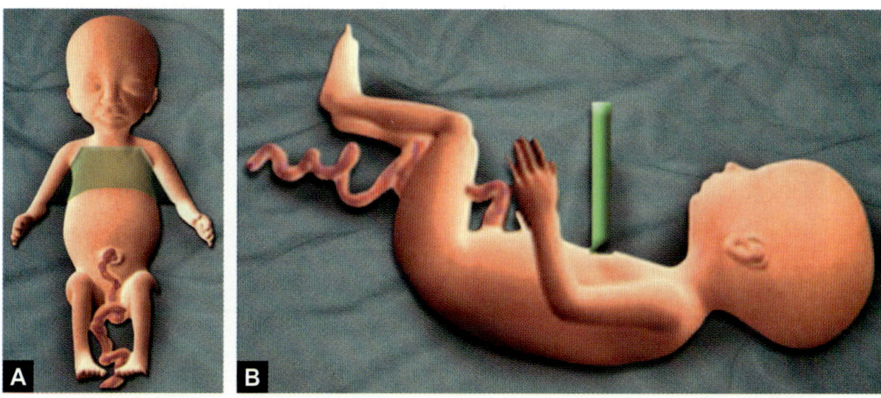

Figures 12.17A and B Level of the heart for the normal four-chamber view

FOUR-CHAMBER VIEW OF NORMAL HEART (FIGURES 12.18 TO 12.35)

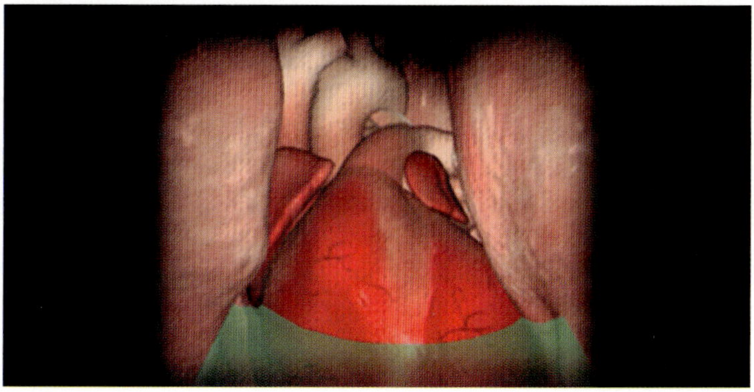

Figure 12.18 Four-chamber view of normal heart

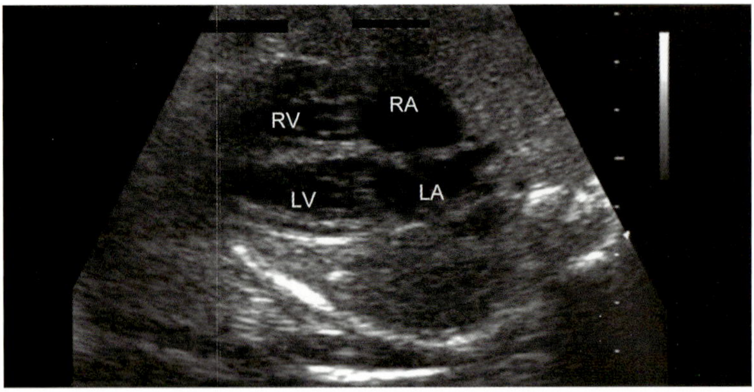

Figure 12.19 Two-dimensional image of normal four-chamber of the heart

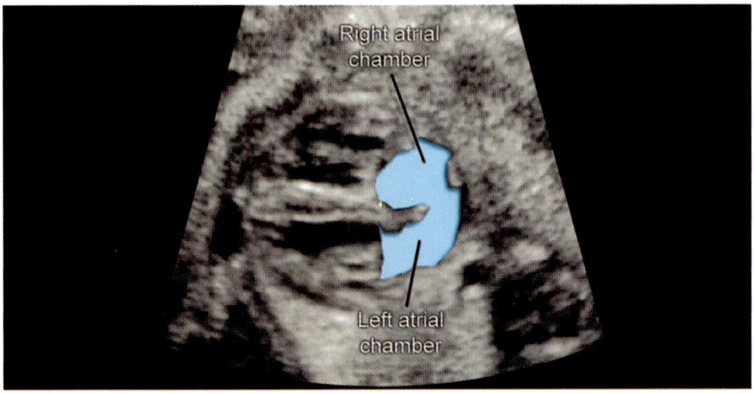

Figure 12.20 Both the atrial chambers of the heart

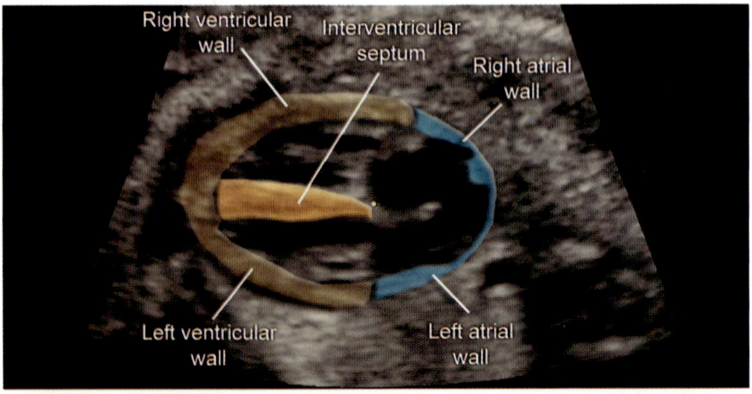

Figure 12.21 Ventricular and atrial walls with interventricular septum

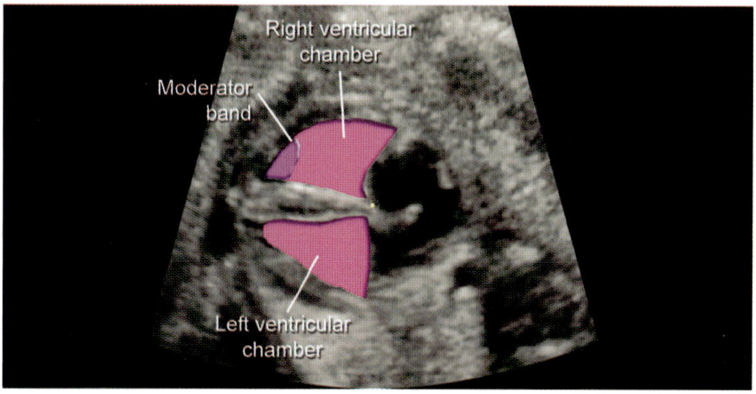

Figure 12.22 Ventricular chamber with moderator band in right ventricle

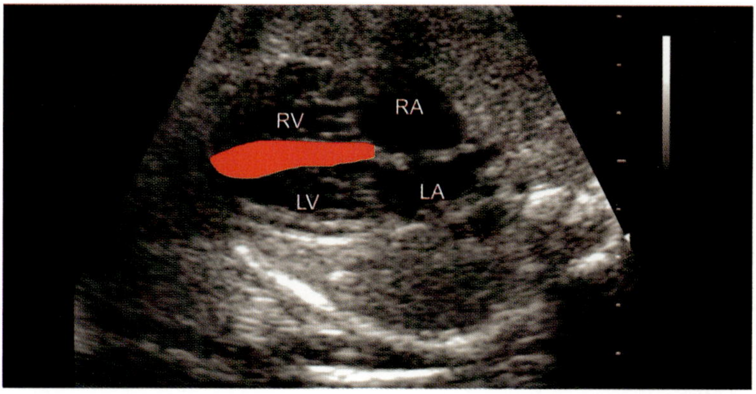

Figure 12.23 Ventricular septum

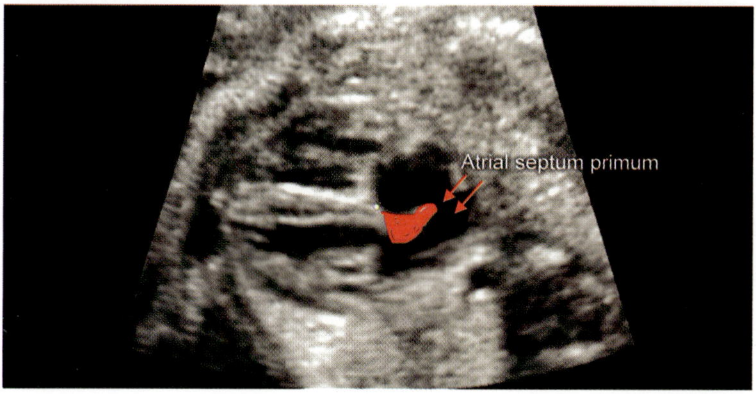

Figure 12.24 Atrial septum primum

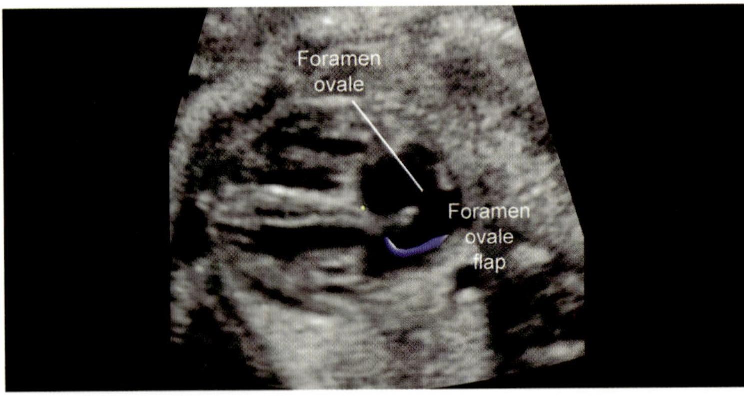

Figure 12.25 Foramen ovale

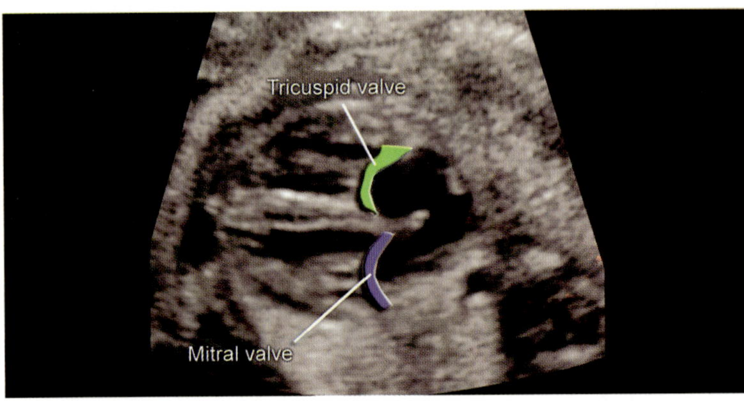

Figure 12.26 Atrioventricular valves

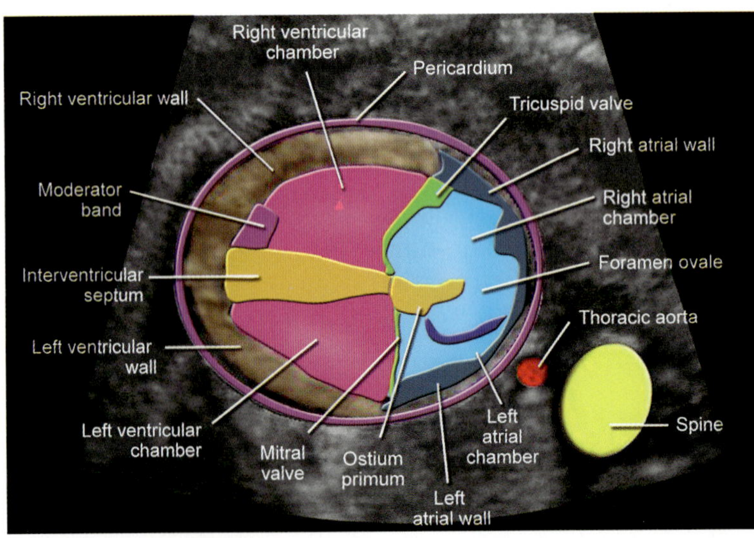

Figure 12.27 Labeled image of the normal heart showing all the important structures

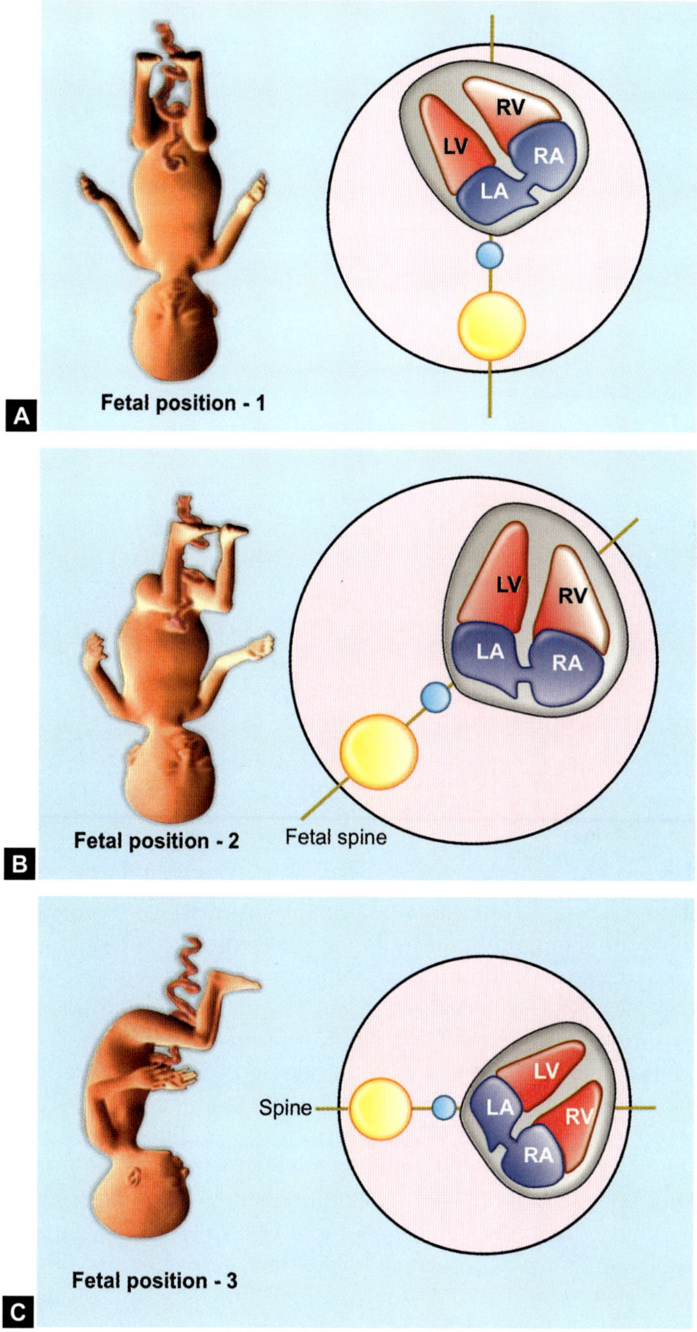

Figures 12.28A to C

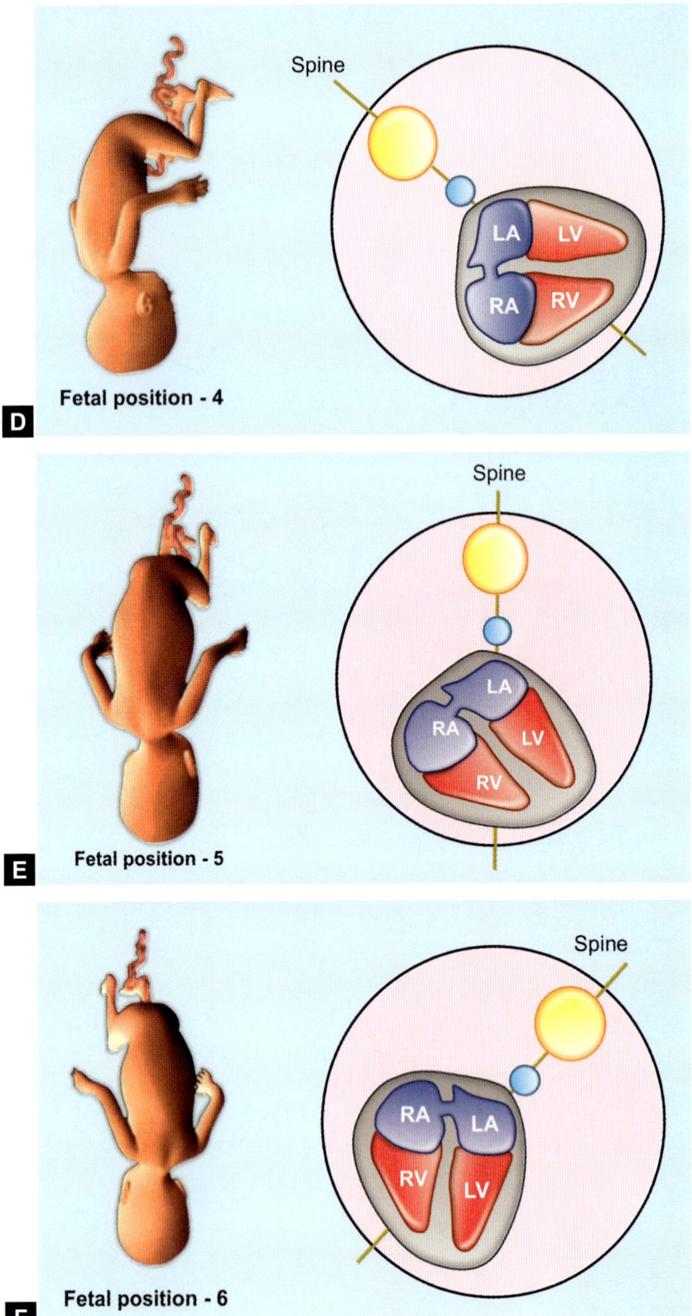

Figures 12.28D to F

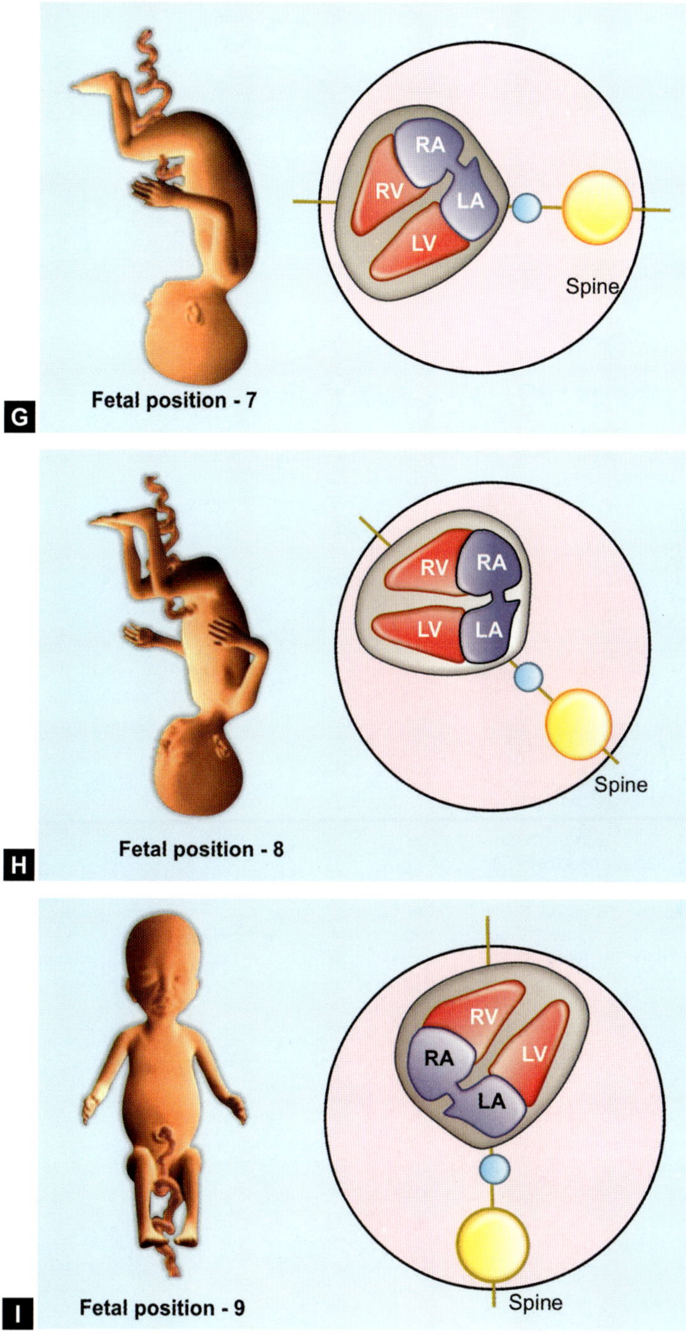

Figures 12.28G to I

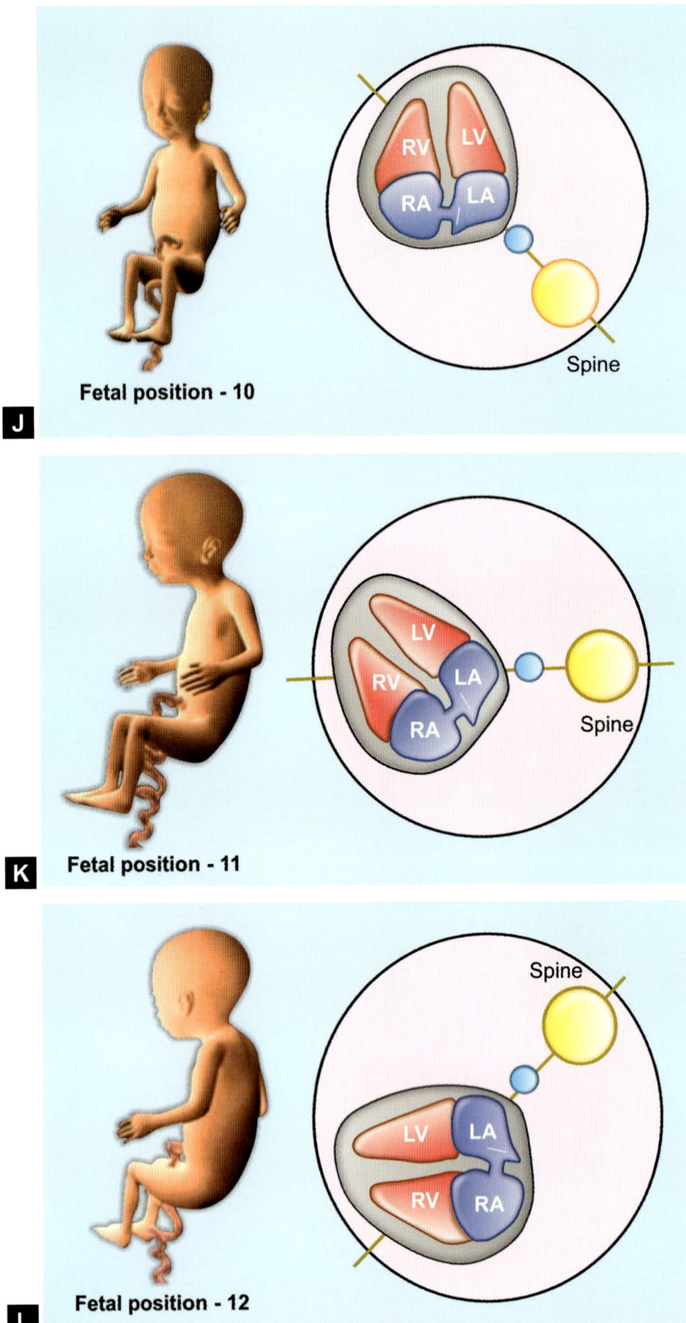

Figures 12.28J to L

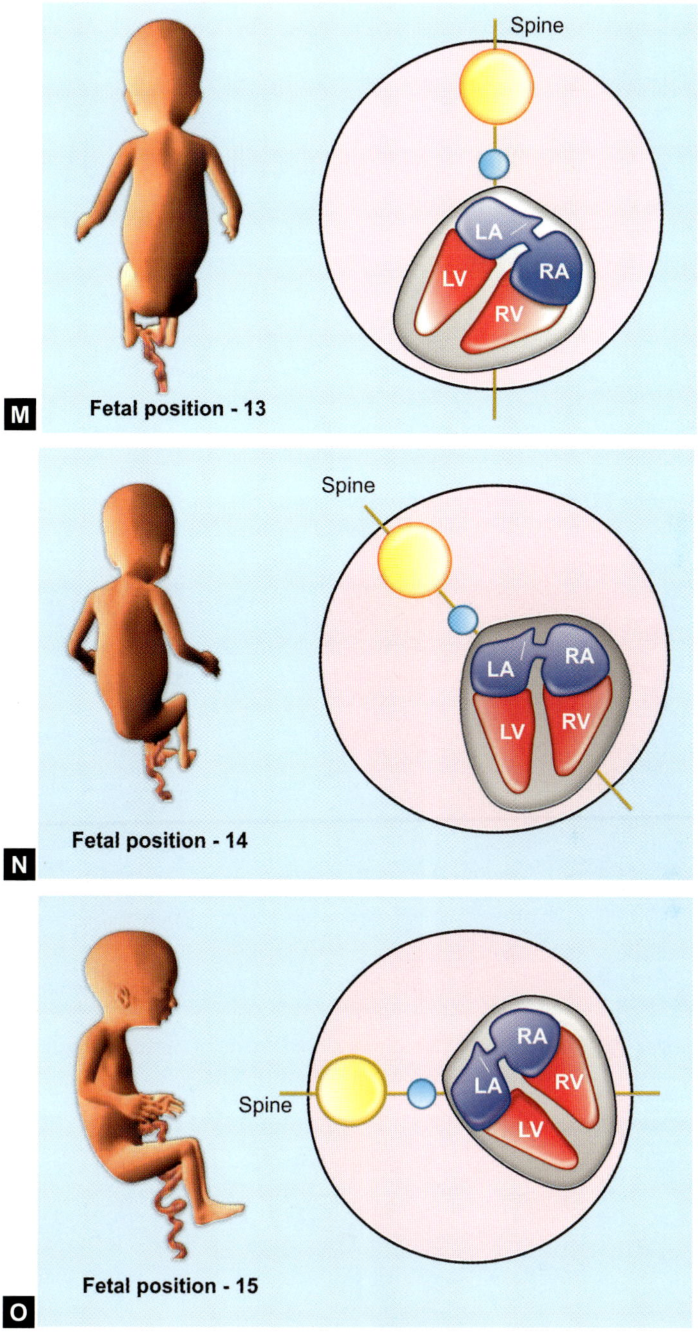

Figures 12.28M to O

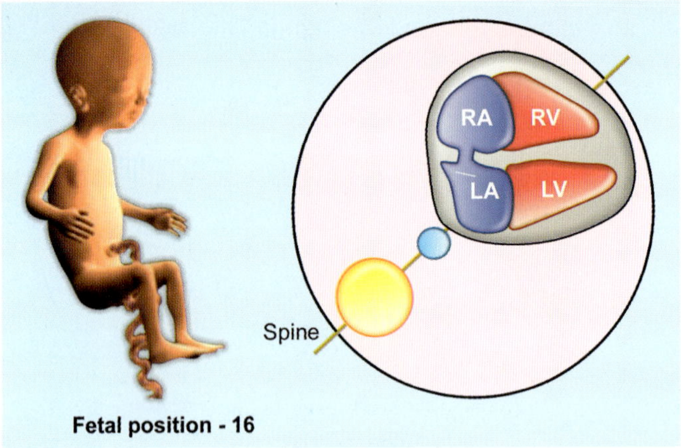

Figure 12.28P

Figures 12.28A to P Comparison of various baby positions for four-chamber view with schematic heart positions

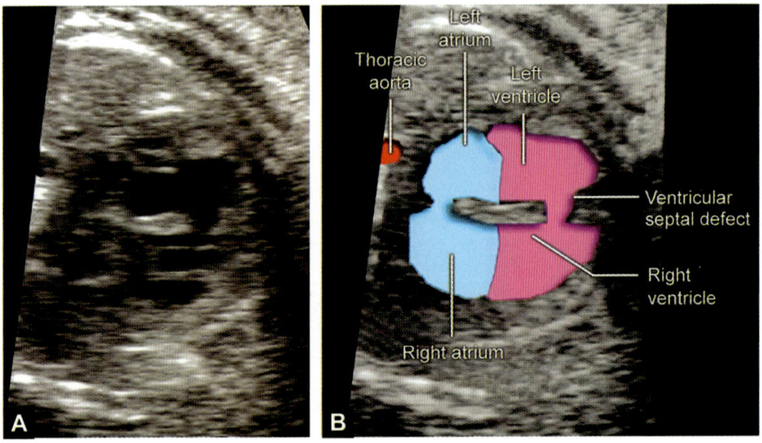

Figures 12.29A and B (A) Two-dimensional image of ventricular septal defect; (B) Labeled image of VSD

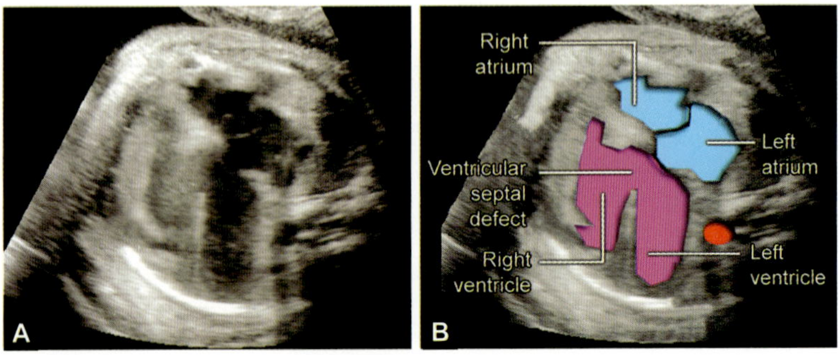

Figures 12.30A and B (A) Large ventricular septal defect; (B) Labeled image of VSD

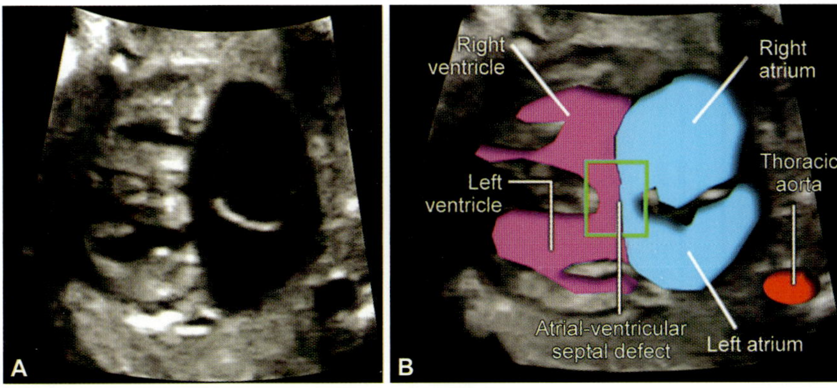

Figures 12.31A and B (A) Atrioventricular septal defect; (B) Labeled image showing atrioventricular septal defect

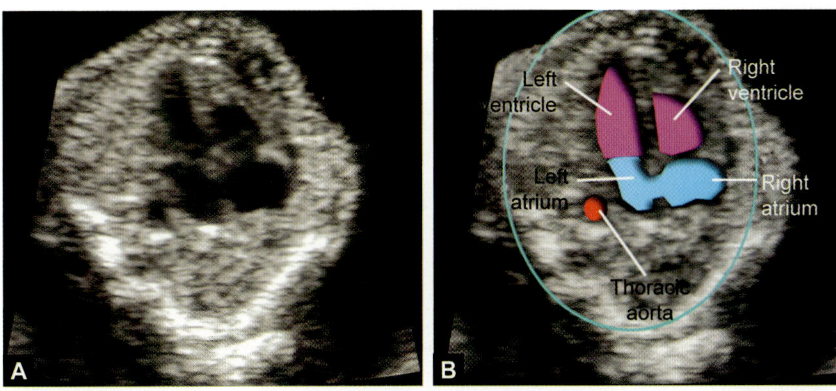

Figures 12.32A and B (A) Left axis deviation; (B) Labeled image showing left axis deviation

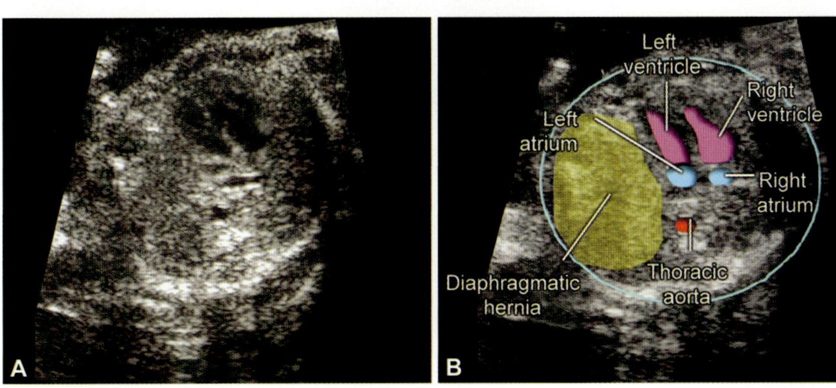

Figures 12.33A and B (A) Diaphragmatic hernia; (B) Labeled image

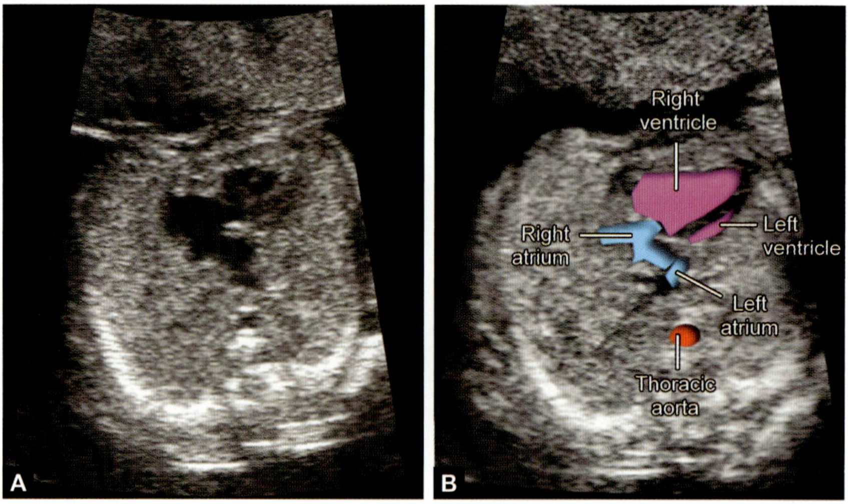

Figures 12.34A and B (A) Hypoplastic left ventricle; (B) Labeled image

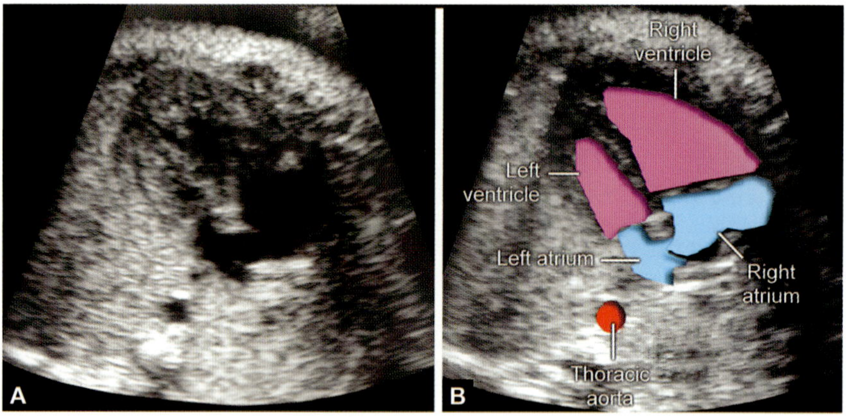

Figures 12.35A and B (A) Enlarged right chambers; (B) Labeled image

LEFT VENTRICULAR OUTFLOW TRACT (LVOT) (FIGURES 12.36 TO 12.50)

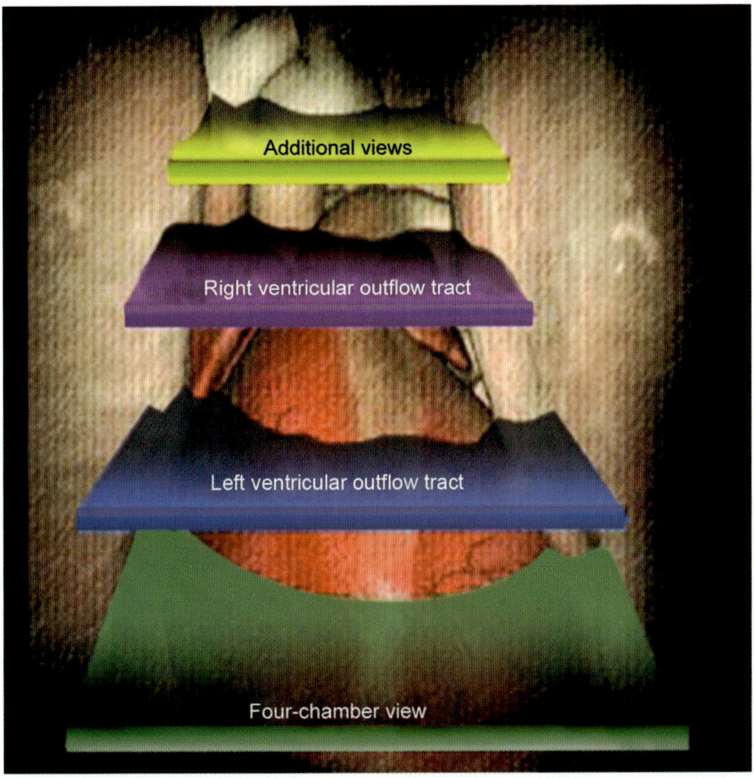

Figure 12.36 Stepwise examination of heart starting from the four chambers and then cephalad to it

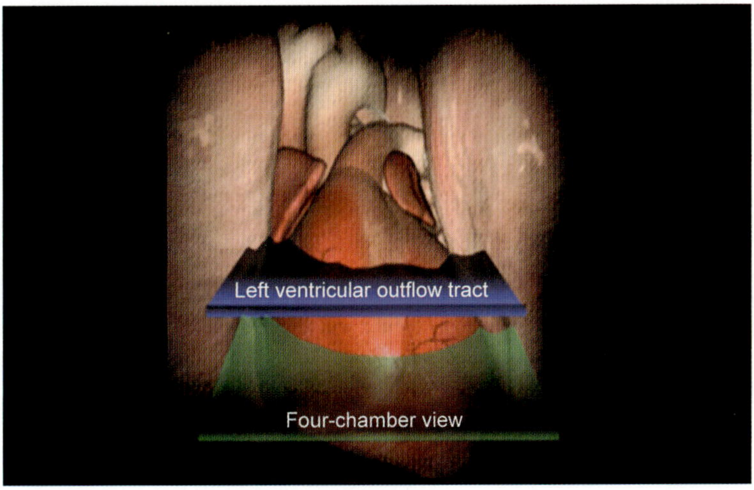

Figure 12.37 Left ventricular outflow tract

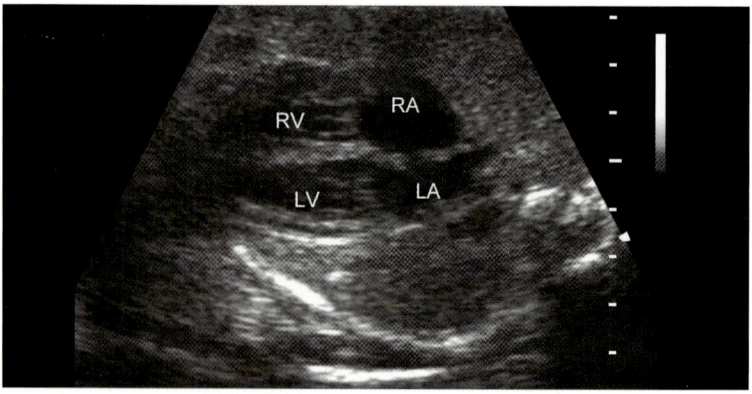

Figure 12.38 Two-dimensional four-chamber view of normal heart

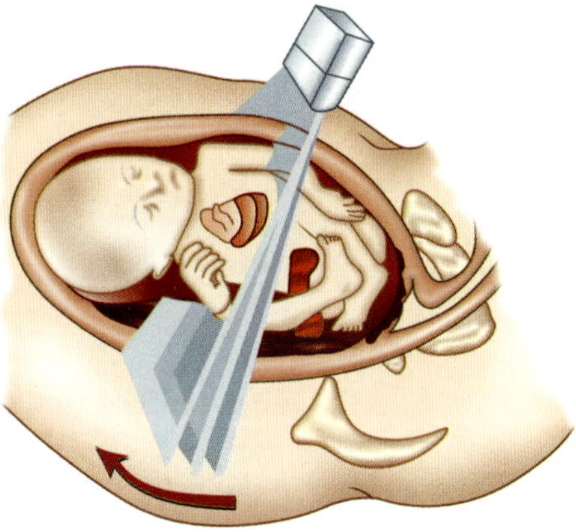

Figure 12.39 The LVOT is imaged by directing the ultrasound beam cephalad from the four-chamber view

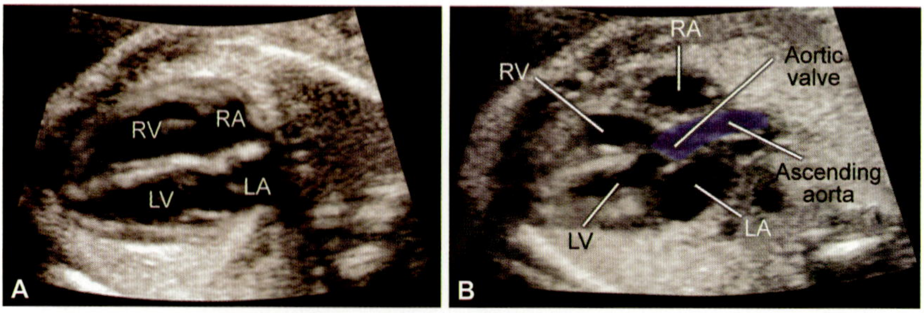

Figures 12.40A and B (A) Four-chamber view of the normal heart; (B) View of left ventricular outflow tract

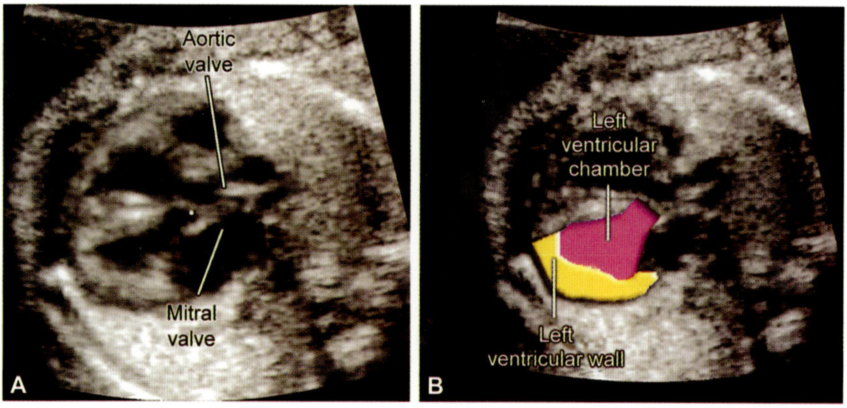

Figures 12.41A and B (A) Two-dimensional view of left ventricular wall and left ventricular chamber; (B) Labeled view

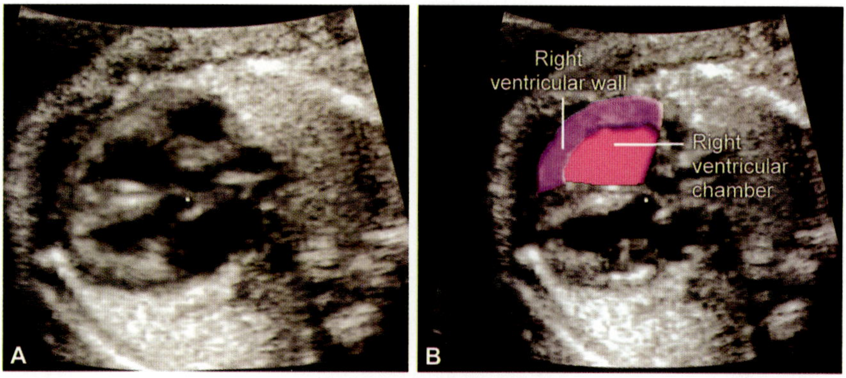

Figures 12.42 A and B (A) Two-dimensional view of right ventricular wall and right ventricular chamber; (B) Labeled view

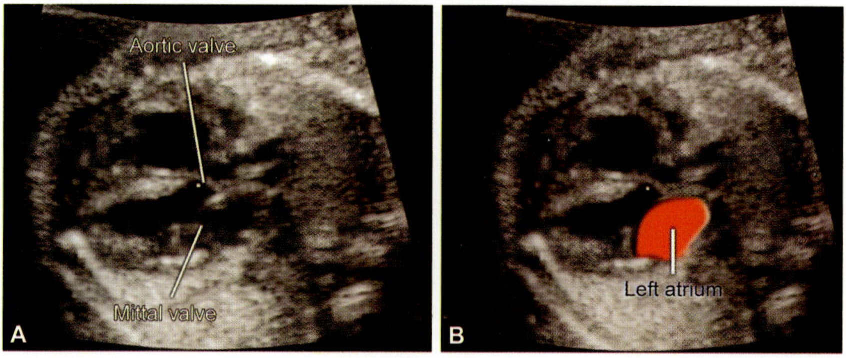

Figures 12.43A and B (A) Two-dimensional view showing left atrium in LVOT; (B) Labeled image

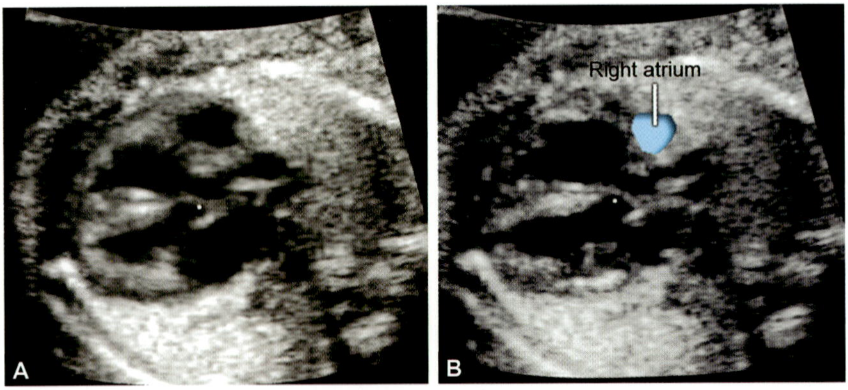

Figures 12.44A and B (A) Two-dimensional view showing right atrium position in LVOT; (B) Labeled image

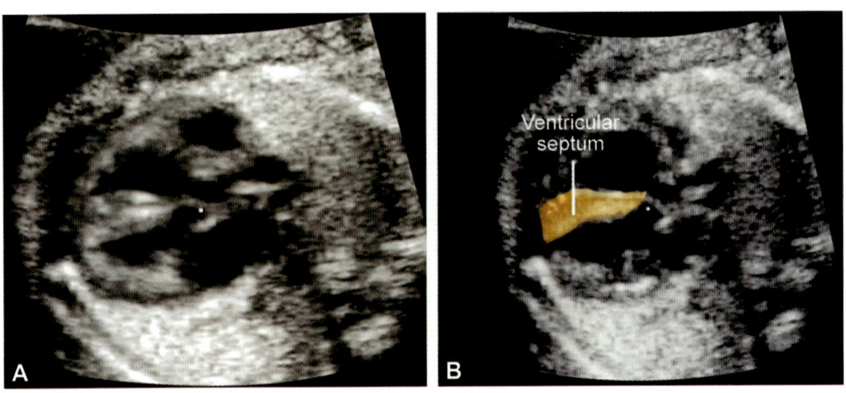

Figures 12.45A and B (A) Two-dimensional image showing ventricular septum in LVOT; (B) Labeled image

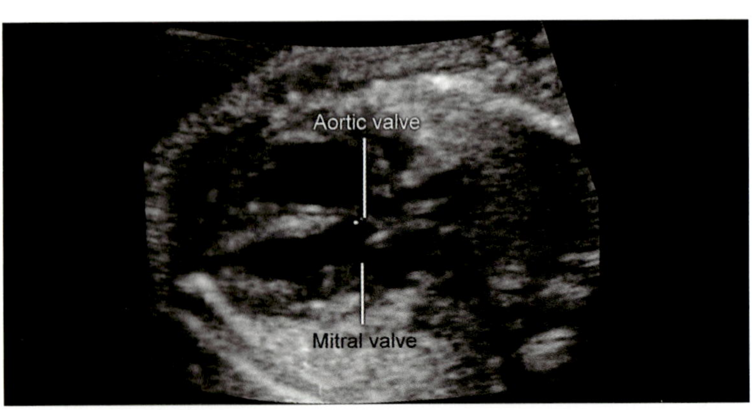

Figure 12.46 Aortic and mitral valve in LVOT; ventricular wall and aortic valve are in continuity (aortoseptal continuity)

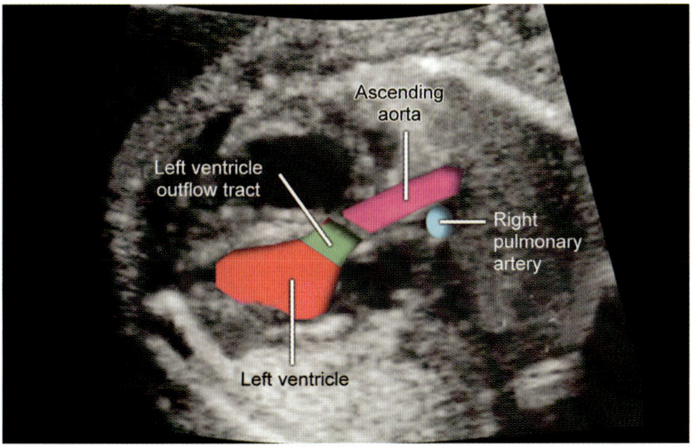

Figure 12.47 Left ventricle outflow tract labeled

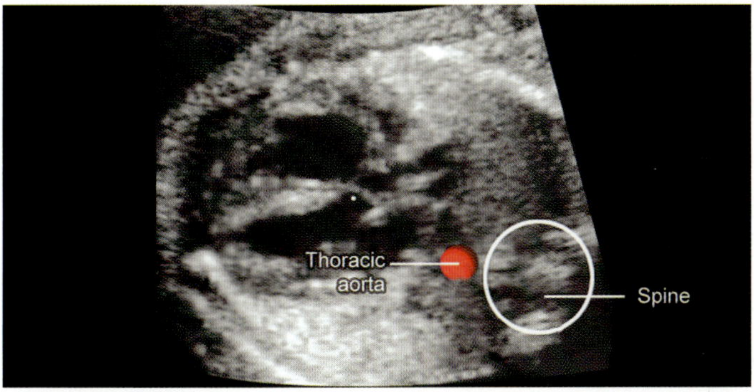

Figure 12.48 Thoracic aorta and spine in LVOT

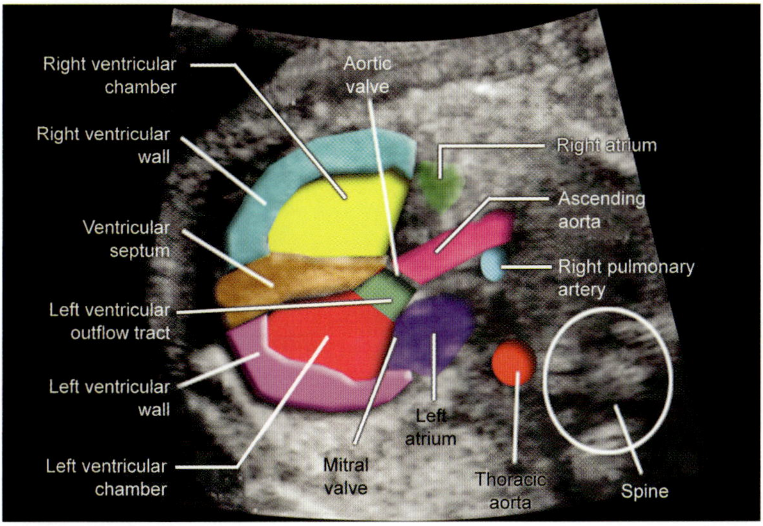

Figure 12.49 Complete graphical representation of LVOT

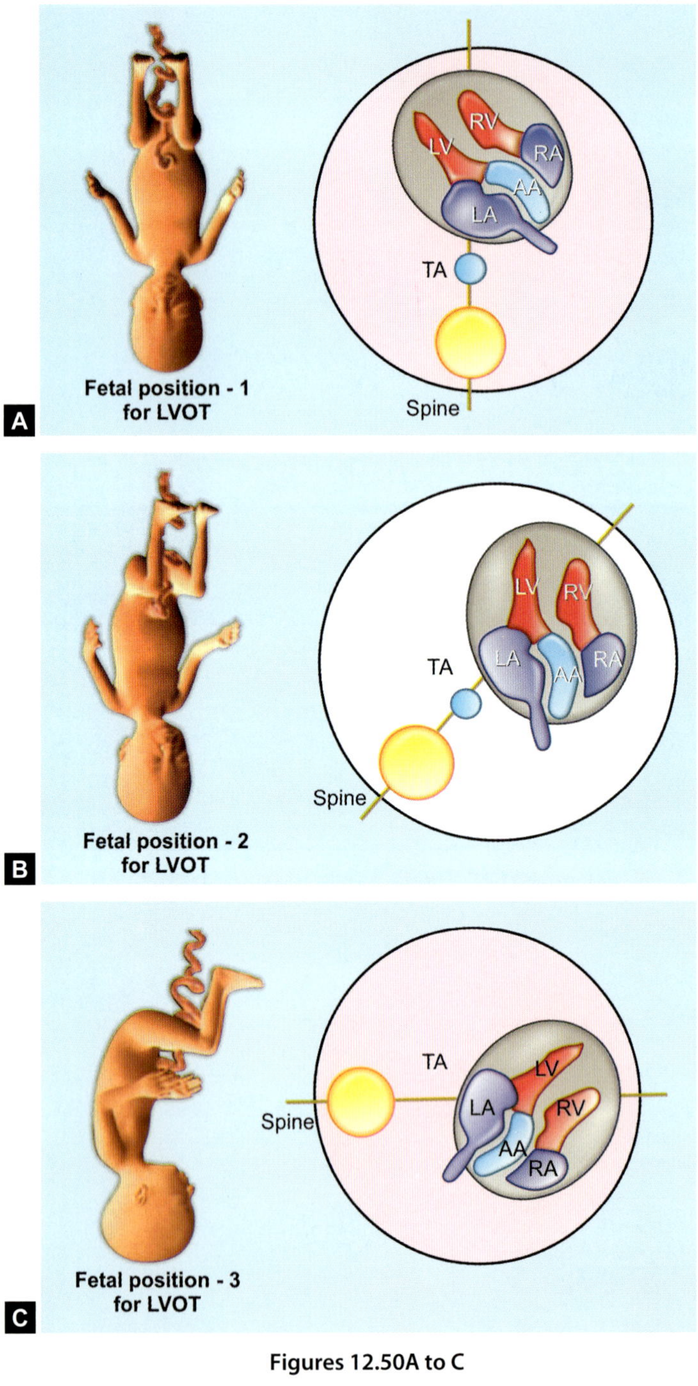

Figures 12.50A to C

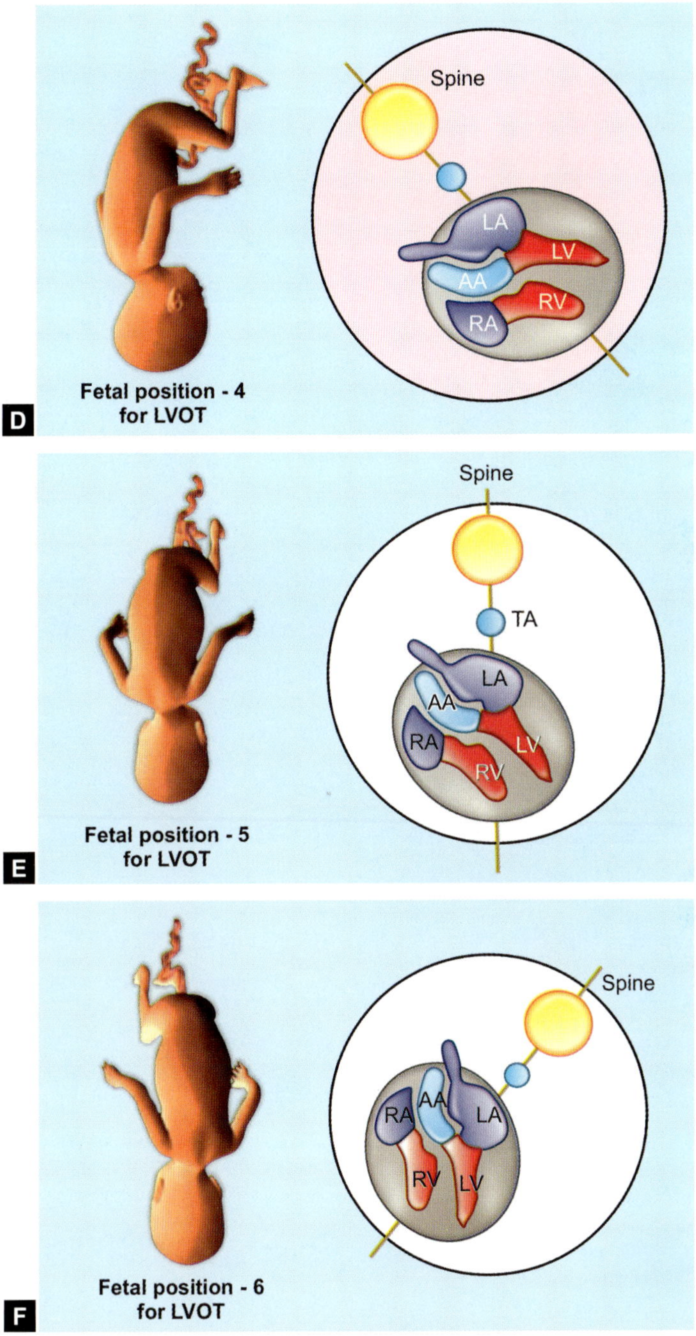

Figures 12.50D to F

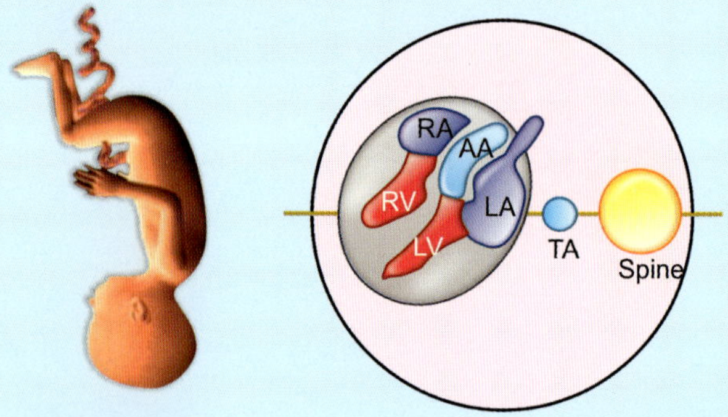

Fetal position - 7
for LVOT

G

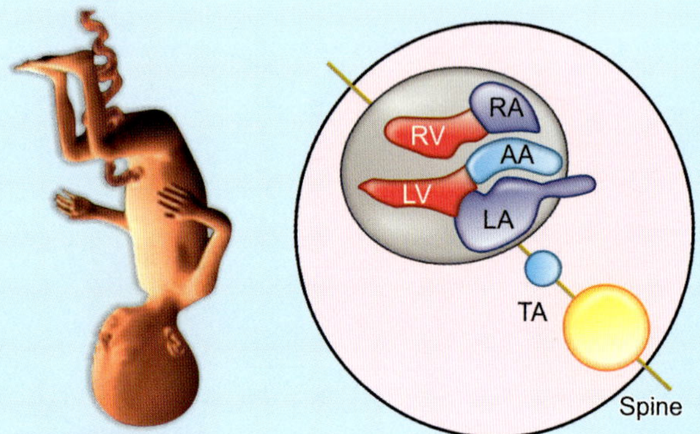

Fetal position - 8
for LVOT

H

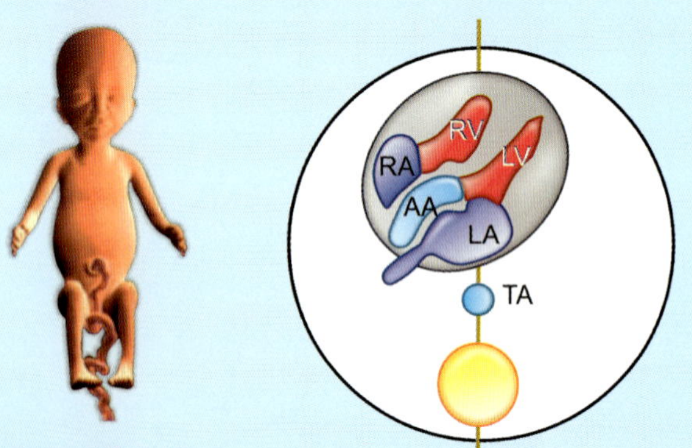

Fetal position - 9
for LVOT

I

Figures 12.50G to I

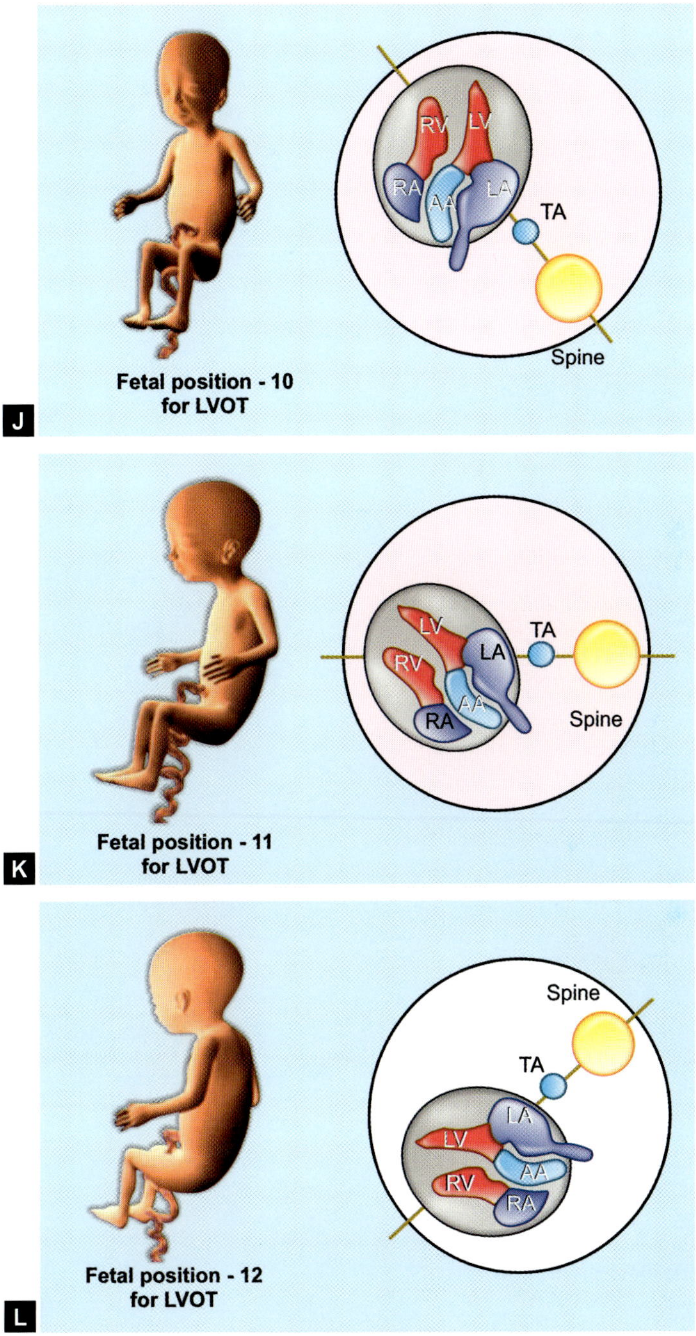

Figures 12.50J to L

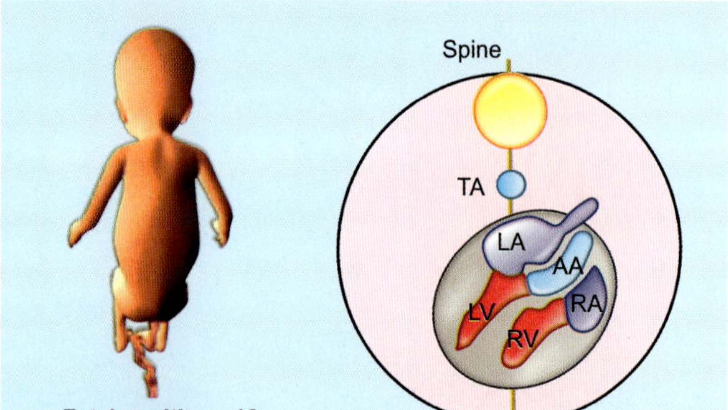

Fetal position - 13 for LVOT

M

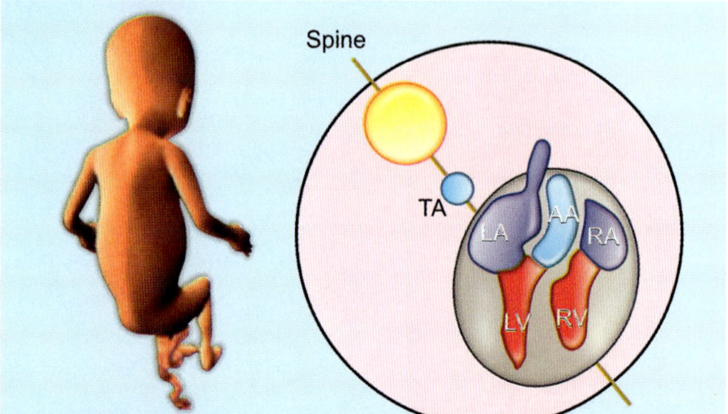

Fetal position - 14 for LVOT

N

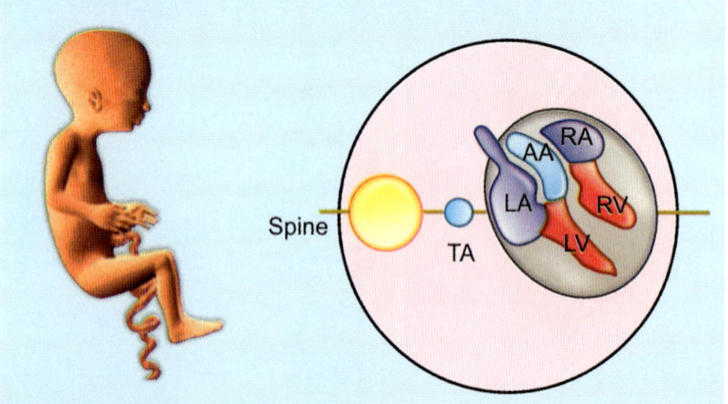

Fetal position - 15 for LVOT

O

Figures 12.50M to O

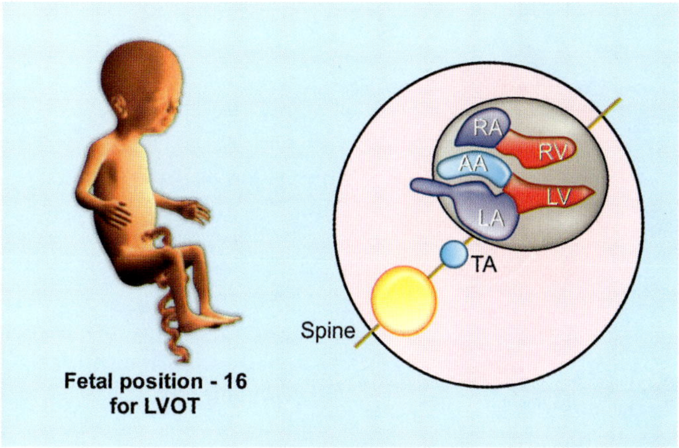

Figure 12.50P

Figures 12.50A to P Left ventricular outflow tract with various fetal positions

RIGHT VENTRICULAR OUTFLOW TRACT (RVOT) (FIGURES 12.51 TO 12.61)

As a routine, first we have to take four-chamber view. Then we just need to angulate the transducer cephalad to have LVOT and another slight angulation in the further cephalad direction gives us RVOT.

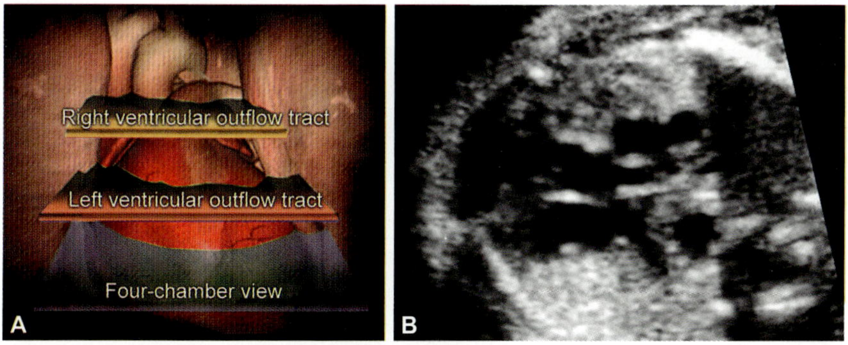

Figures 12.51A and B Right ventricular outflow tract (RVOT)

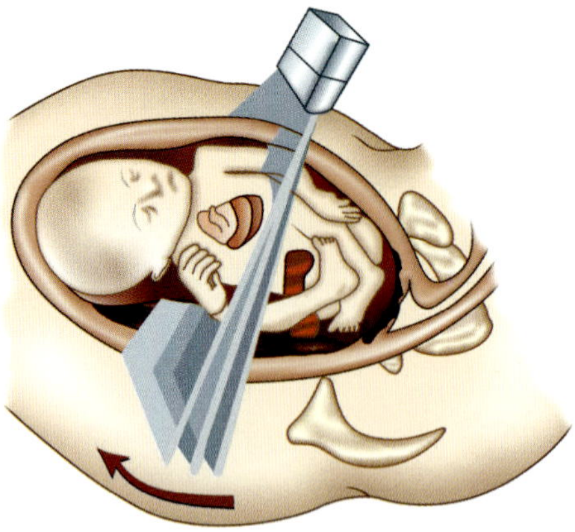

Figure 12.52 The RVOT is viewed by slight cephalad angulation of the transducer from LVOT plane

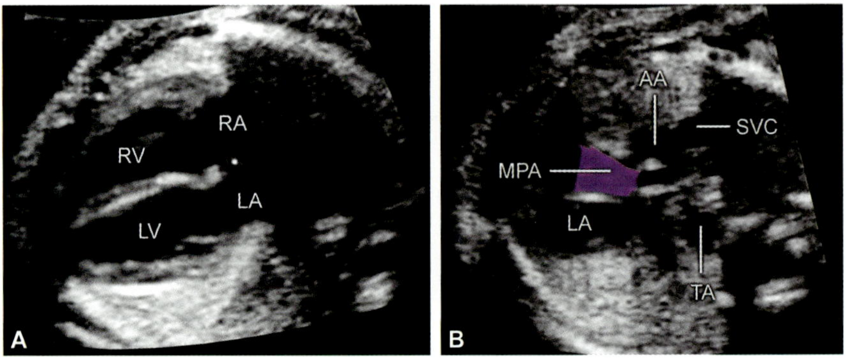

Figures 12.53A and B (A) Two-dimensional image showing four-chamber view of heart with RVOT; (B) Labeled image

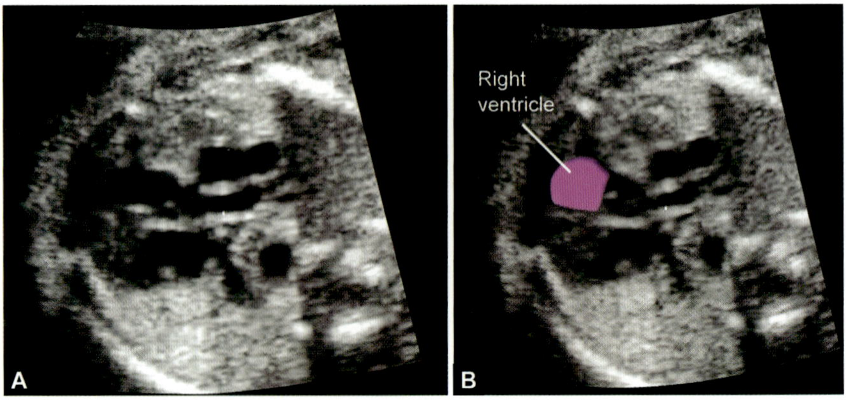

Figures 12.54A and B (A) Right ventricle in RVOT; (B) Labeled image

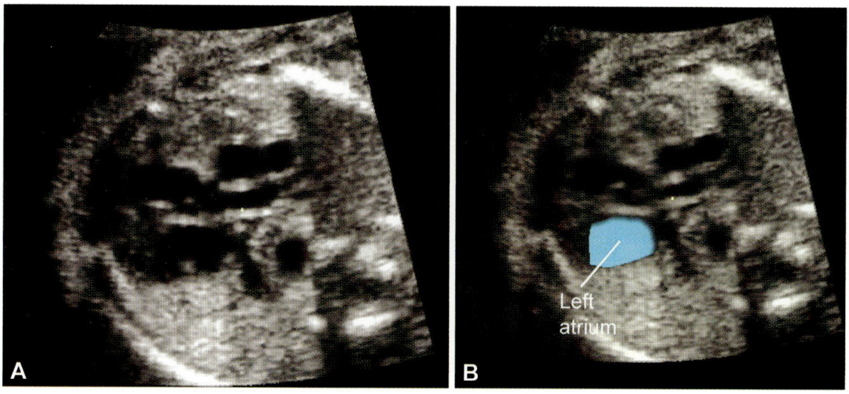

Figures 12.55A and B (A) Two-dimensional image showing left atrium in RVOT; (B) Labeled image

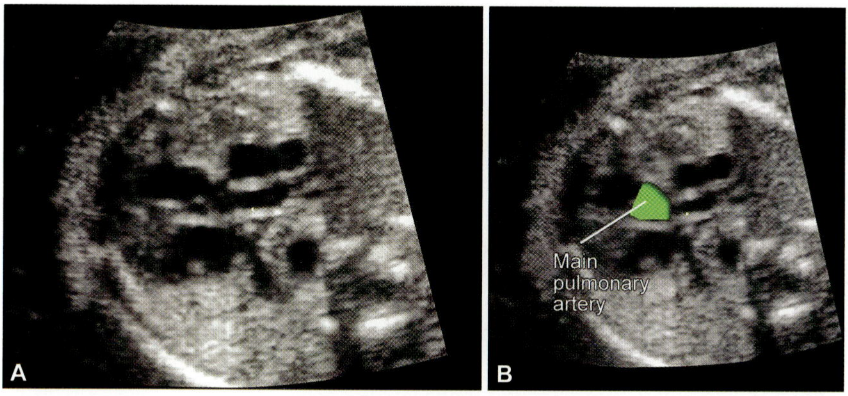

Figures 12.56A and B (A) Two-dimensional image showing main pulmonary artery in RVOT; (B) Labeled image

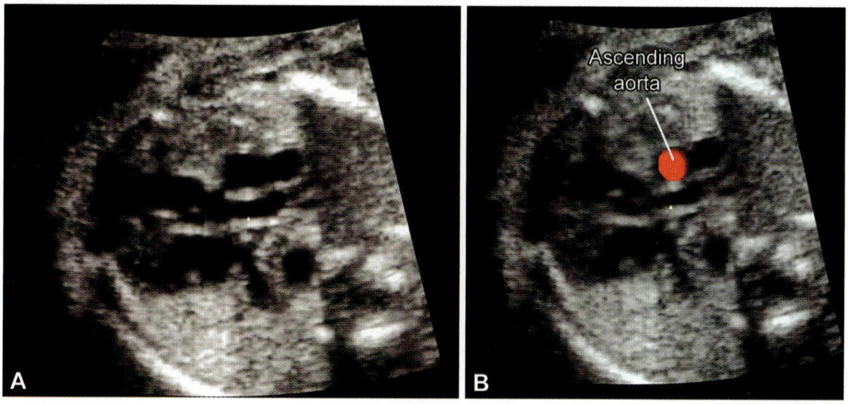

Figures 12.57A and B (A) Two-dimensional image showing ascending aorta in RVOT; (B) Labeled image

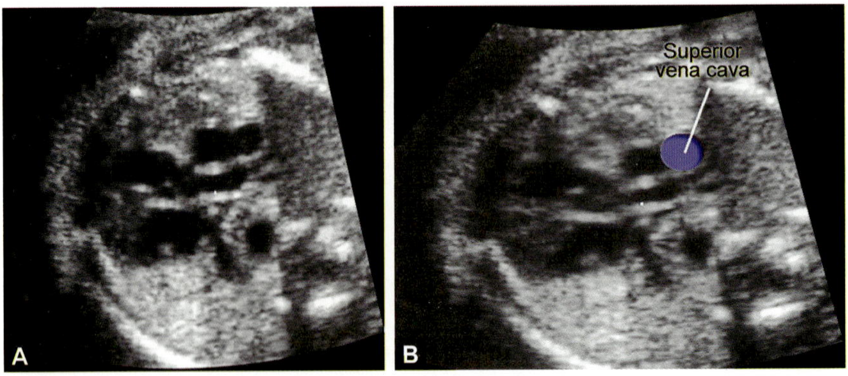

Figures 12.58A and B (A) Two-dimensional image showing superior vena cava in RVOT; (B) Labeled view

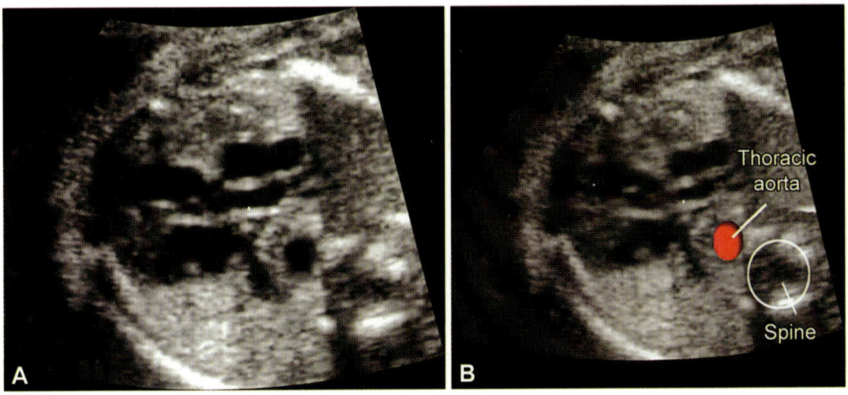

Figures 12.59A and B (A) Two-dimensional image showing thoracic aorta and spine in RVOT; (B) Labeled image

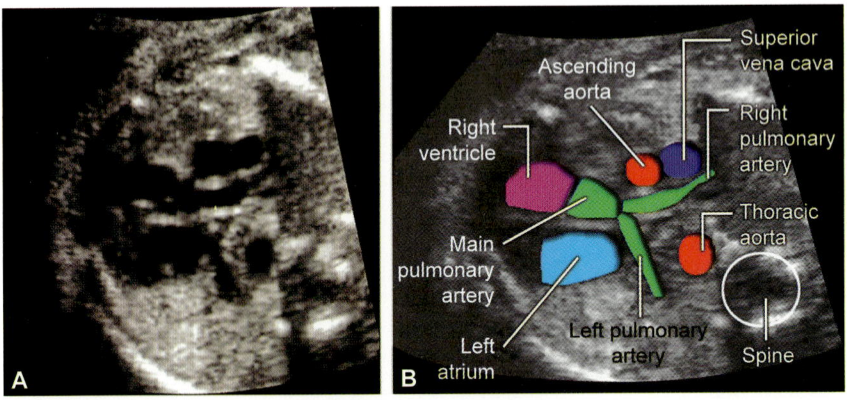

Figures 12.60A and B (A) Two-dimensional image of the structures associated with RVOT; (B) Labeled image

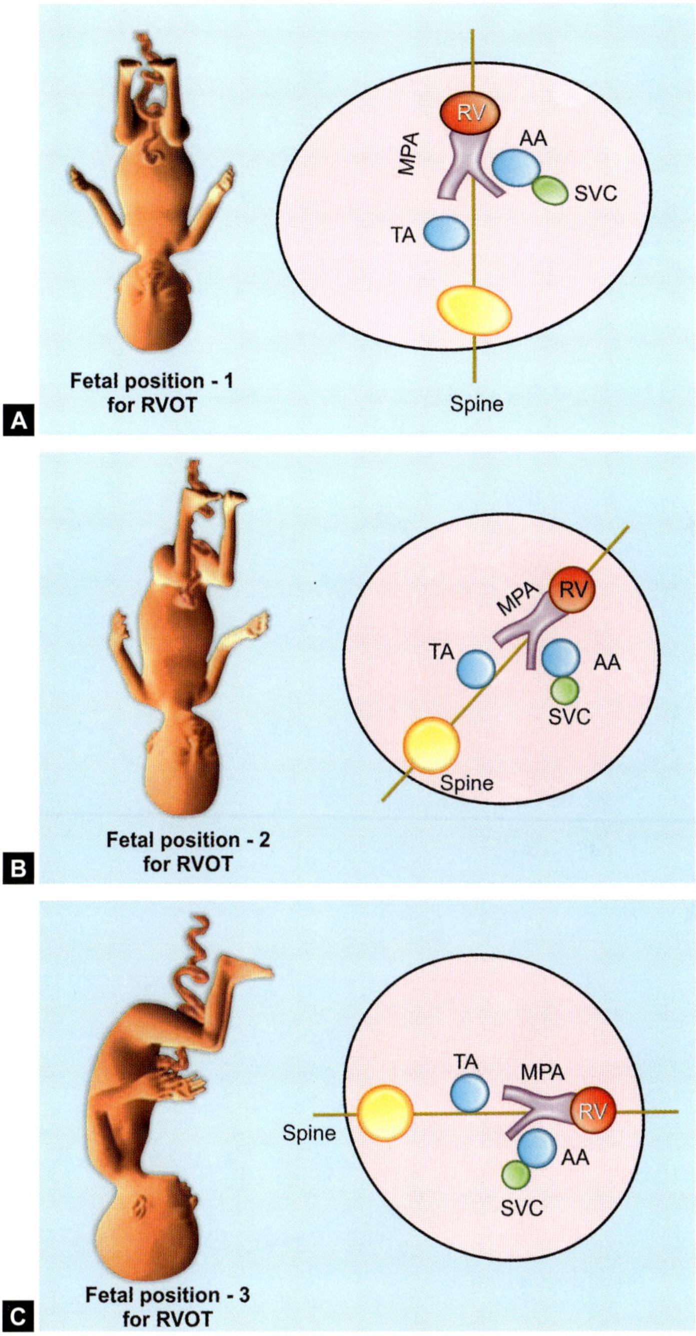

Figures 12.61A to C

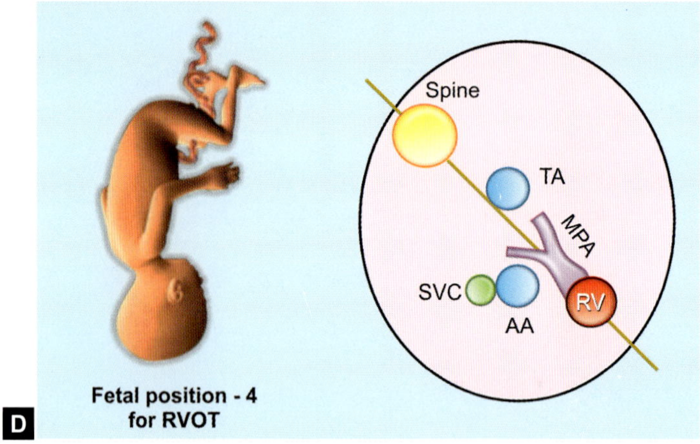

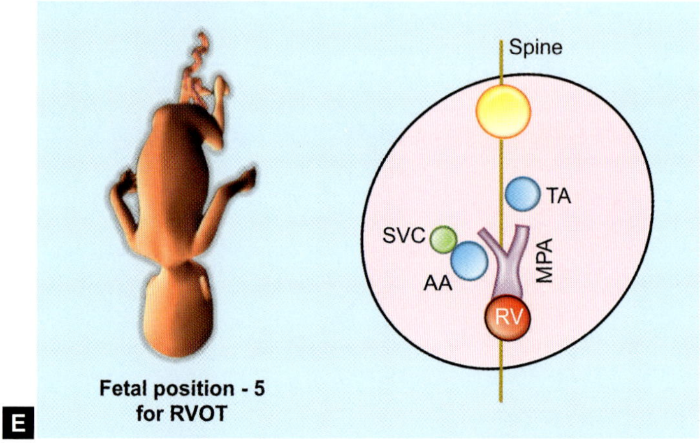

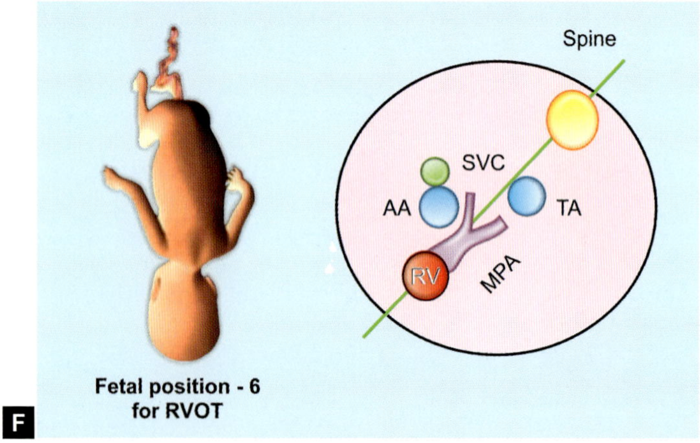

Figures 12.61D to F

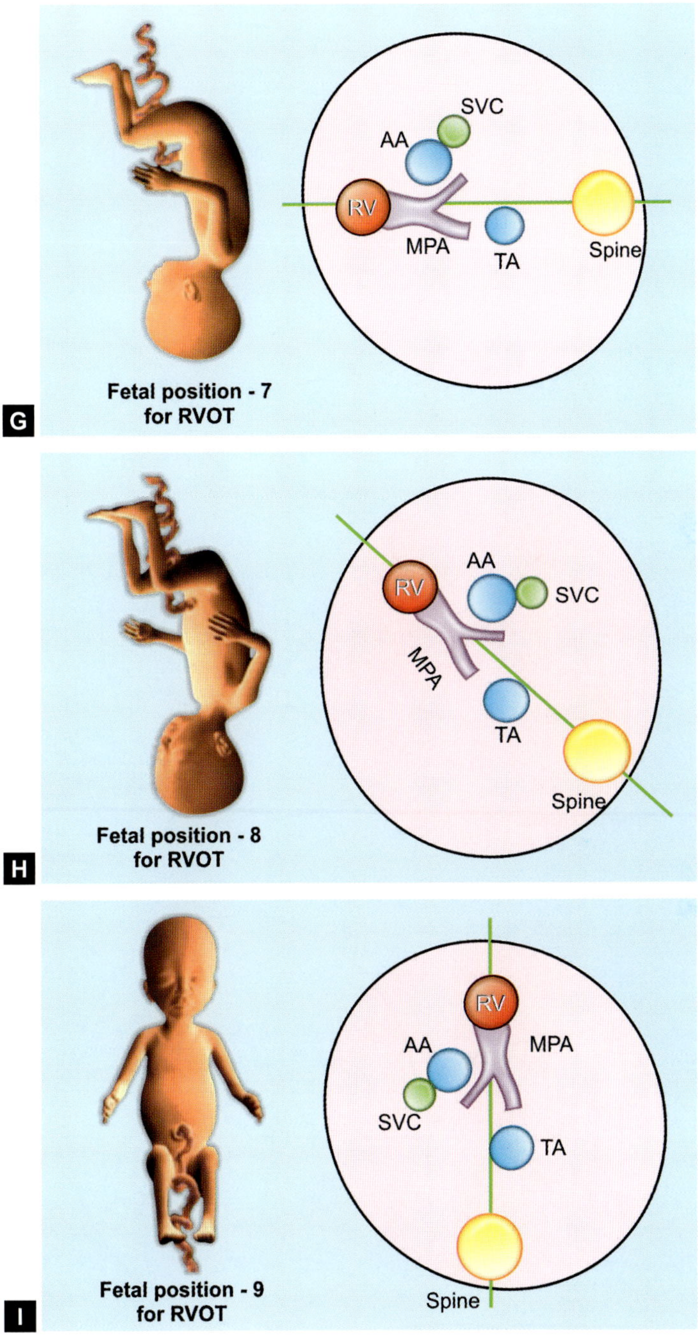

Figures 12.61G to I

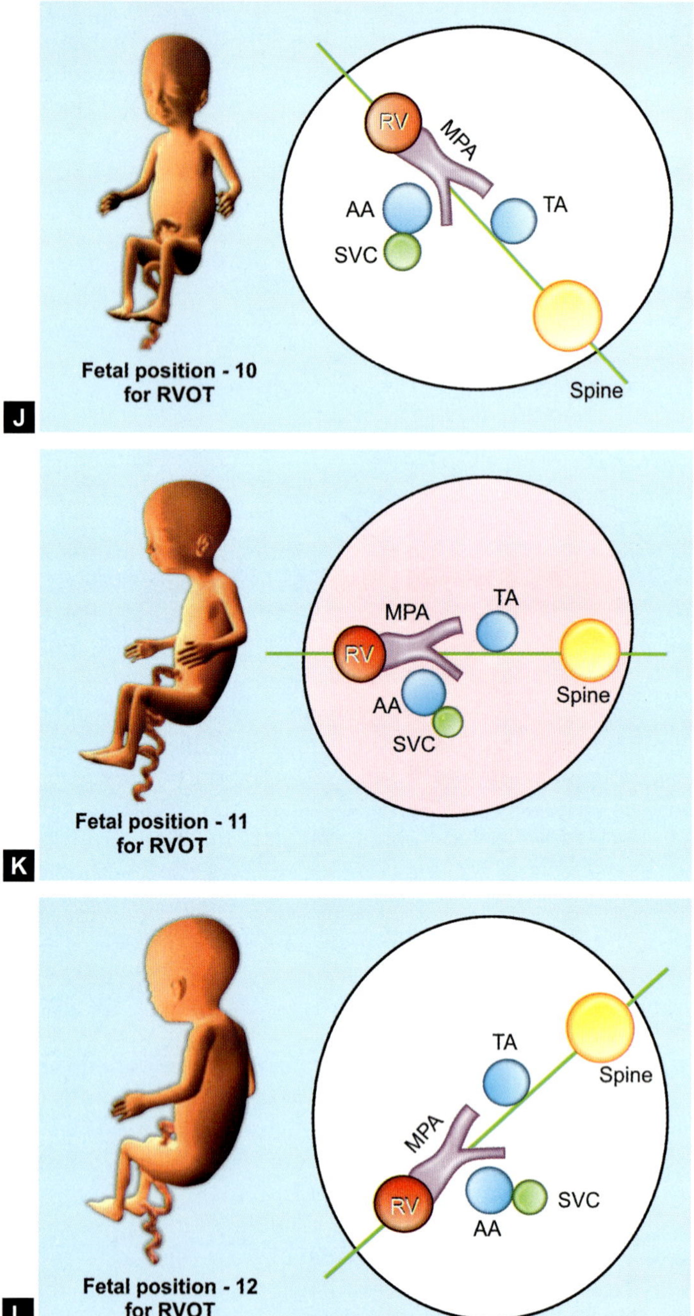

Figures 12.61J to L

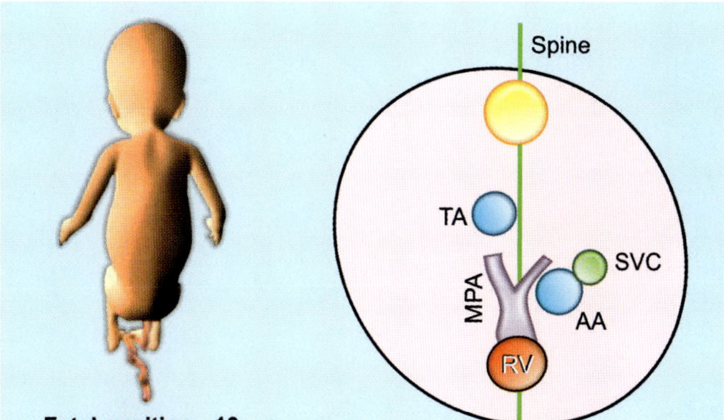

Fetal position - 13
for RVOT

M

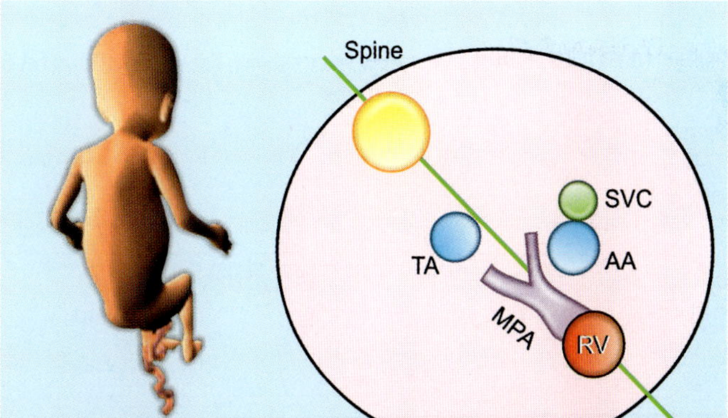

Fetal position - 14
for RVOT

N

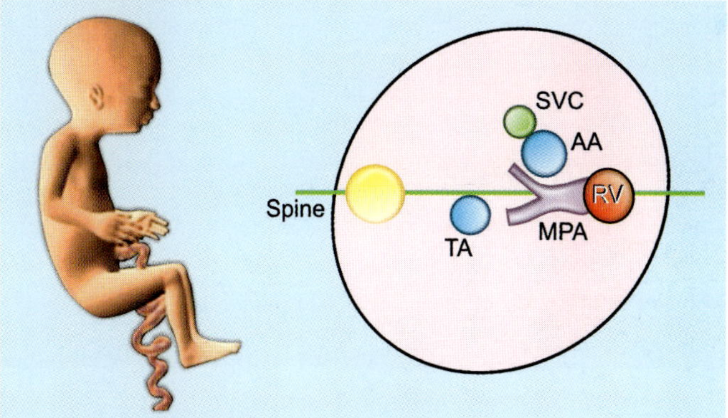

Fetal position - 15
for RVOT

O

Figures 12.61M to O

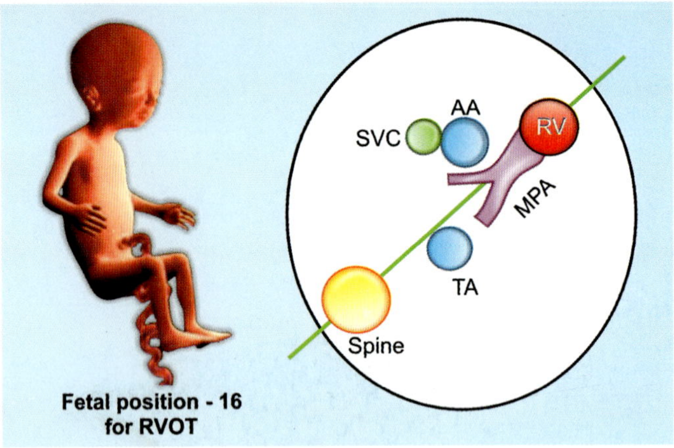

Figure 12.61P

Figures 12.61A to P Right ventricular outflow tract with various fetal positions

TRACHEAL AND ARCH VIEWS OF THE HEART (FIGURES 12.62 TO 12.70)

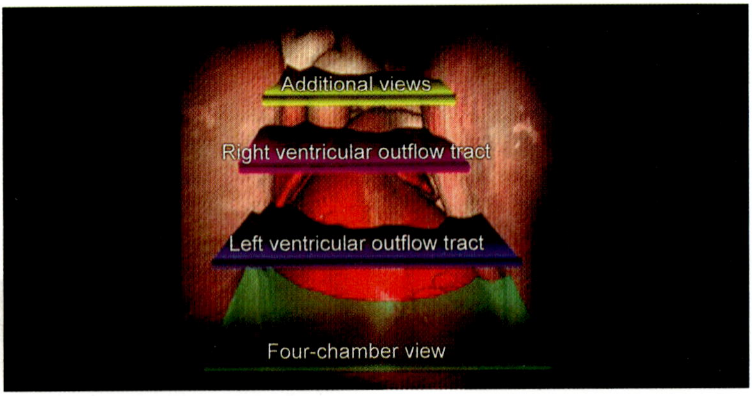

Figure 12.62 Additional views of the heart

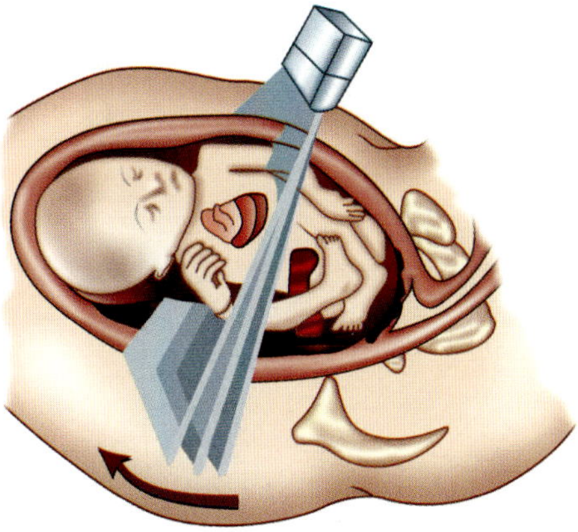

Figure 12.63 The arch views are imaged by directing the ultrasound beam cephalad from the four-chamber view

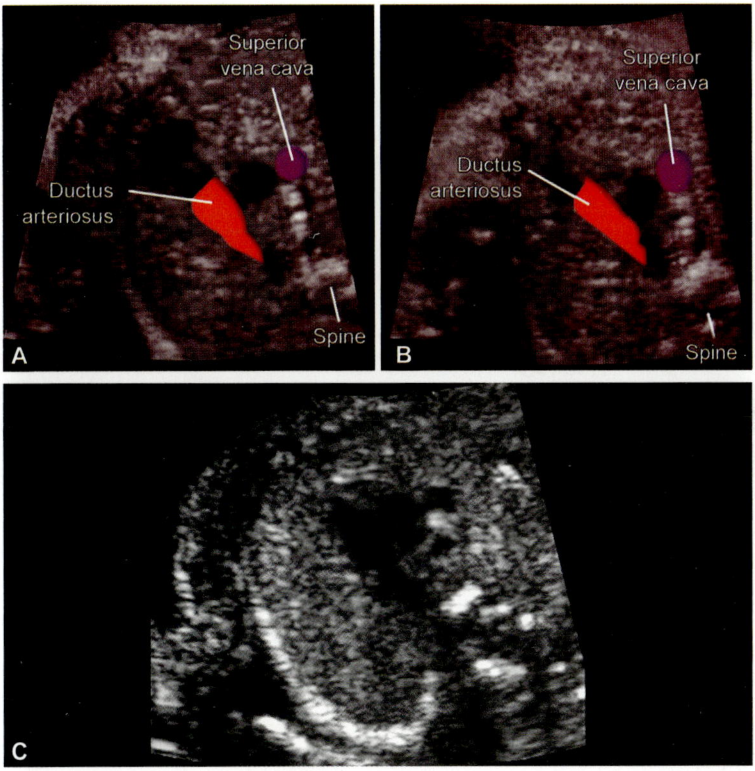

Figures 12.64A to C (A and B) Labeled images showing ductus arteriosus and superior vena cava in an arch view; (C) Two-dimensional view

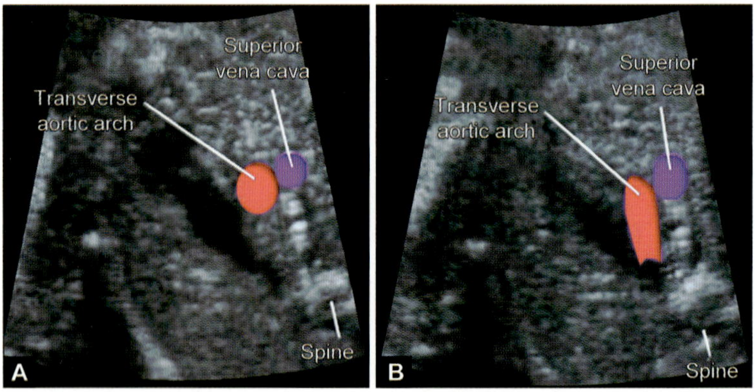

Figures 12.65A and B Labeled images showing superior vena cava and transverse aortic arch in an arch view

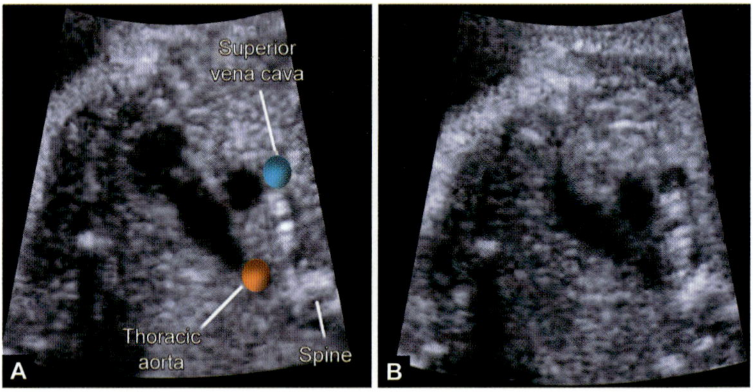

Figures 12.66A and B Images showing superior vena cava and thoracic aorta

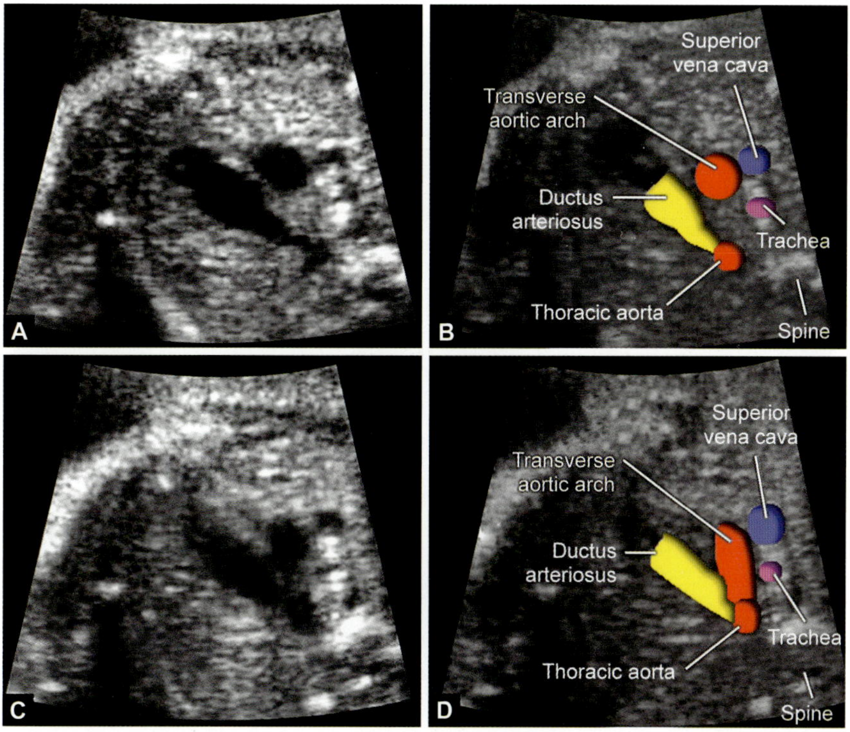

Figures 12.67A to D Two-dimensional and labeled images showing various structures in a tracheal view

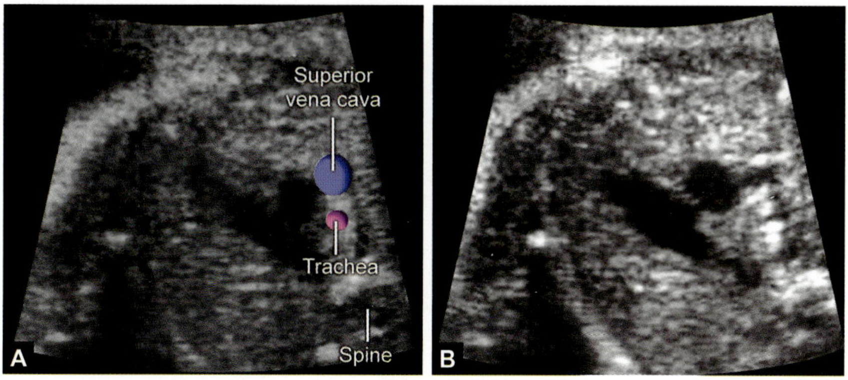

Figures 12.68A and B Superior vena cava and trachea in a tracheal view

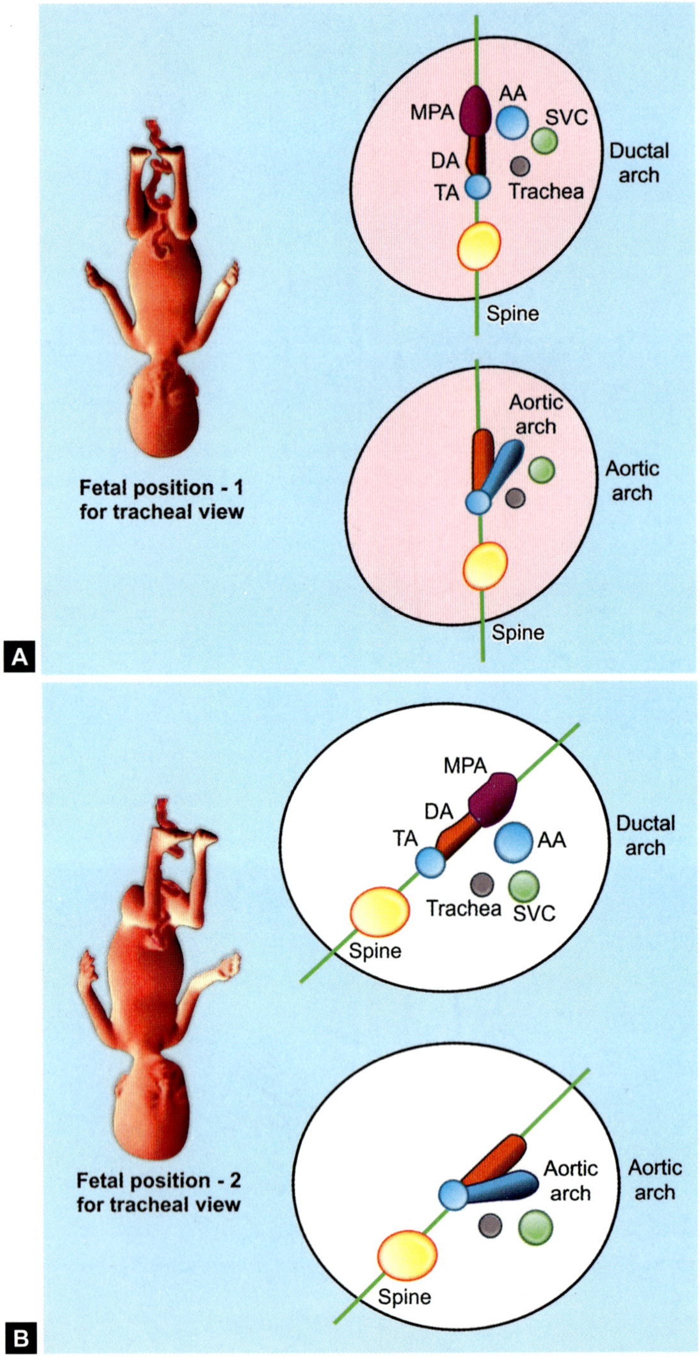

Figures 12.69A and B

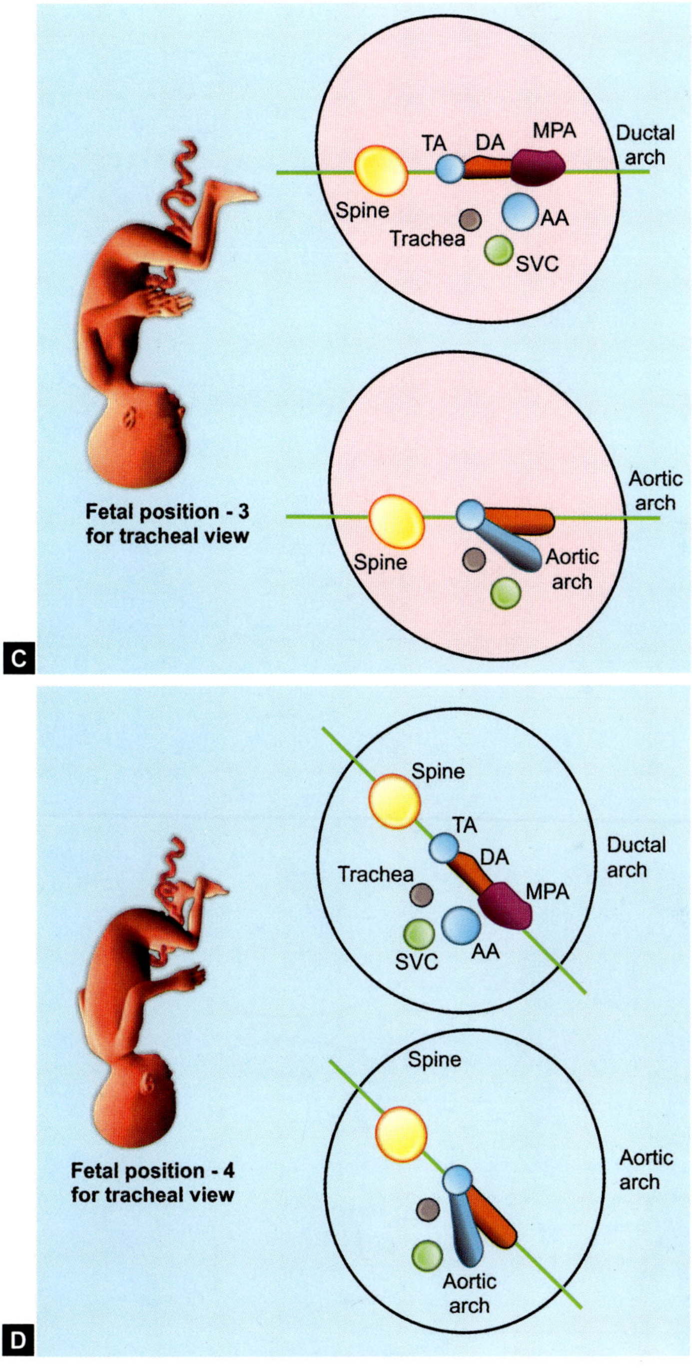

Figures 12.69C and D

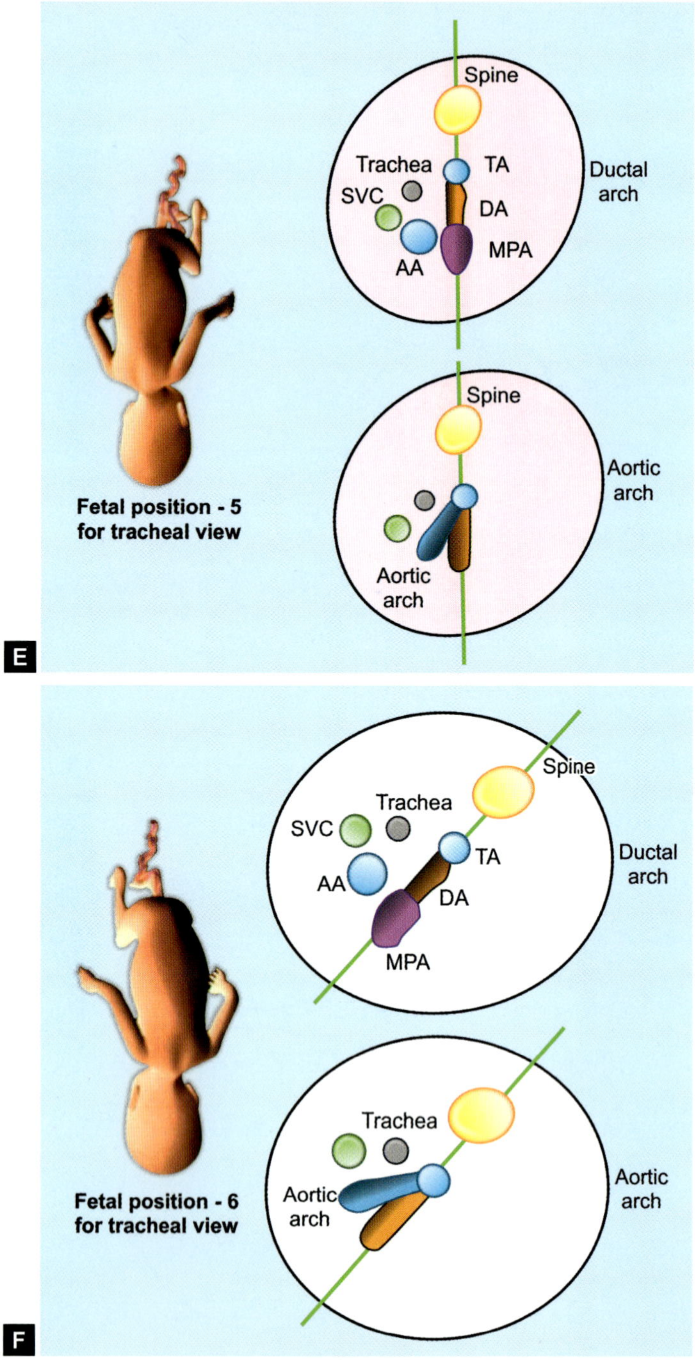

Figures 12.69E and F

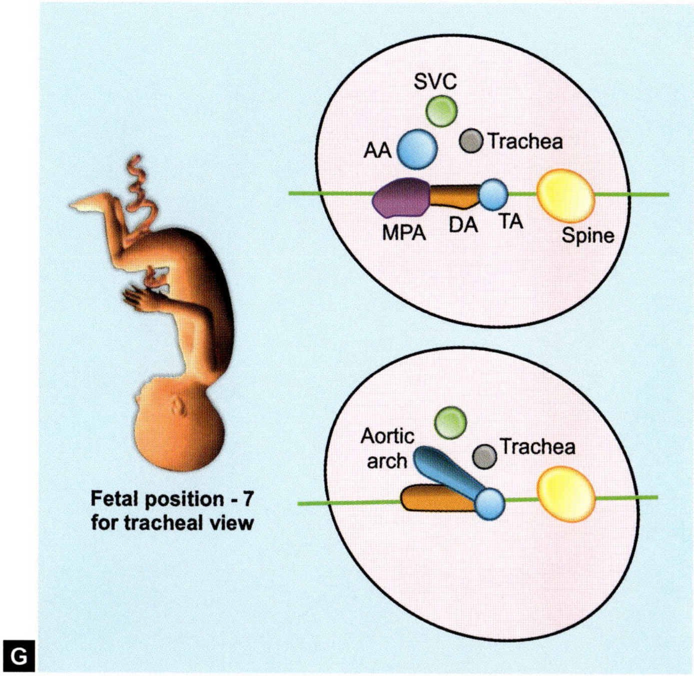

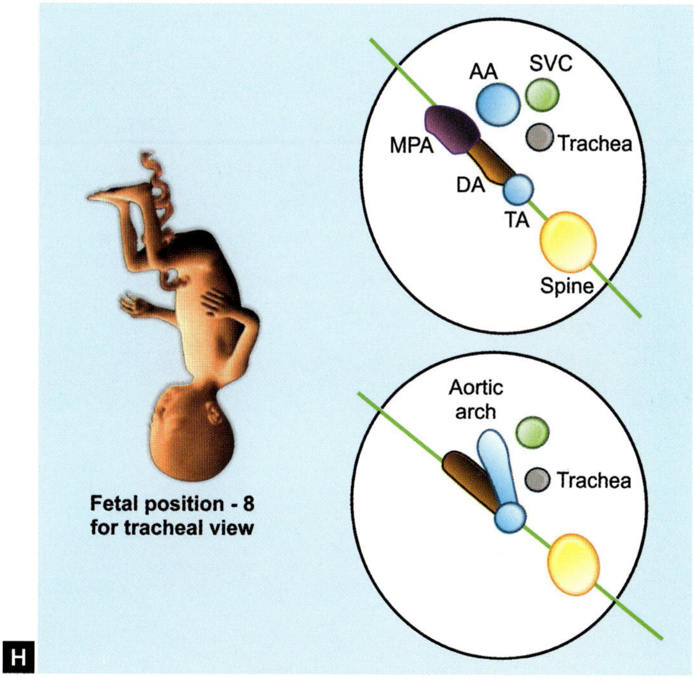

Figures 12.69G and H

Figures 12.69A to H Tracheal view in various fetal positions

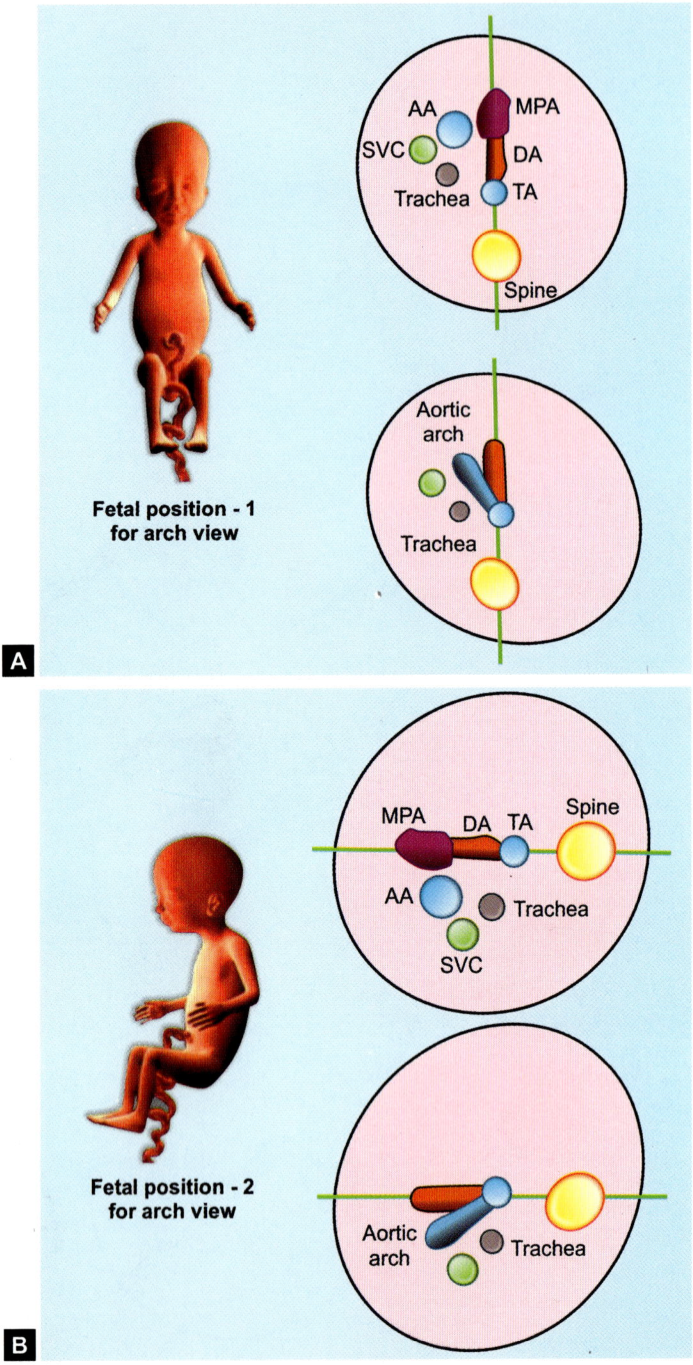

Figures 12.70A and B

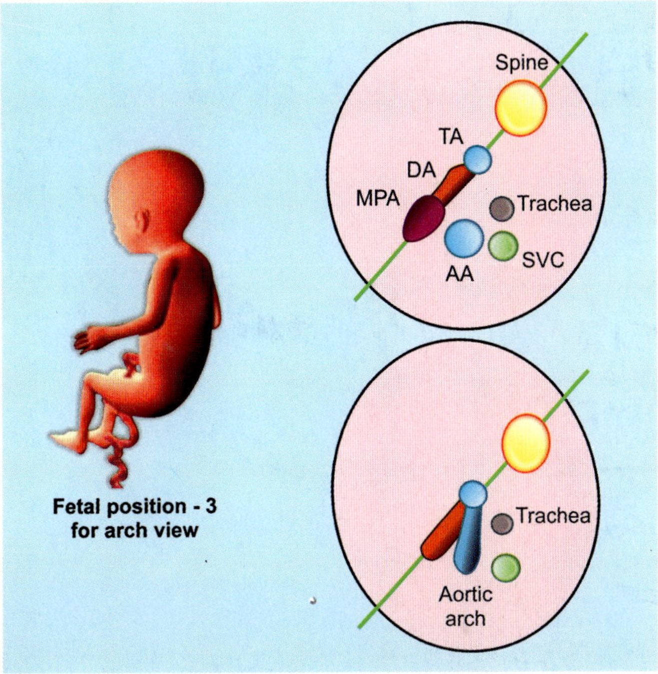

C

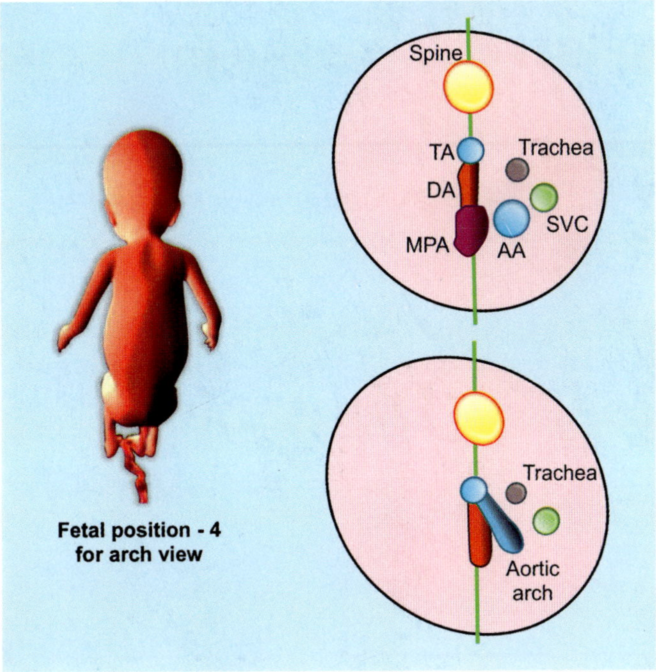

D

Figures 12.70C and D

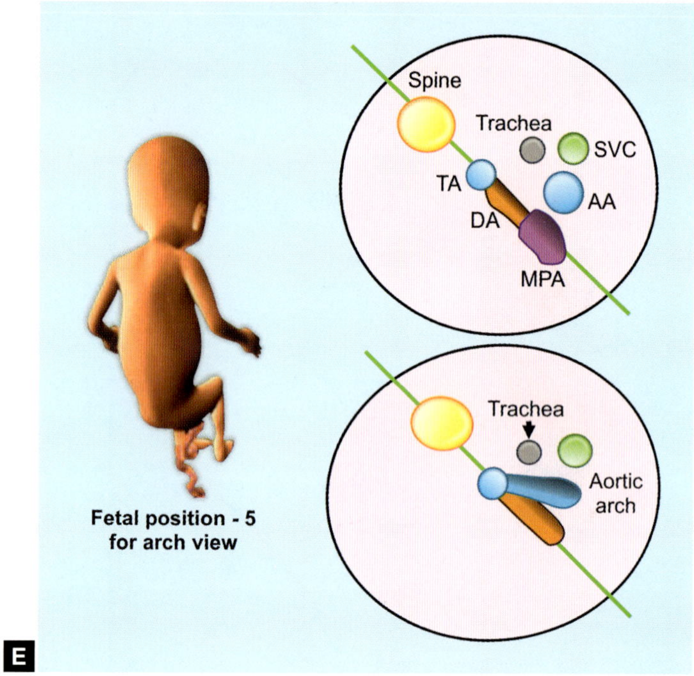

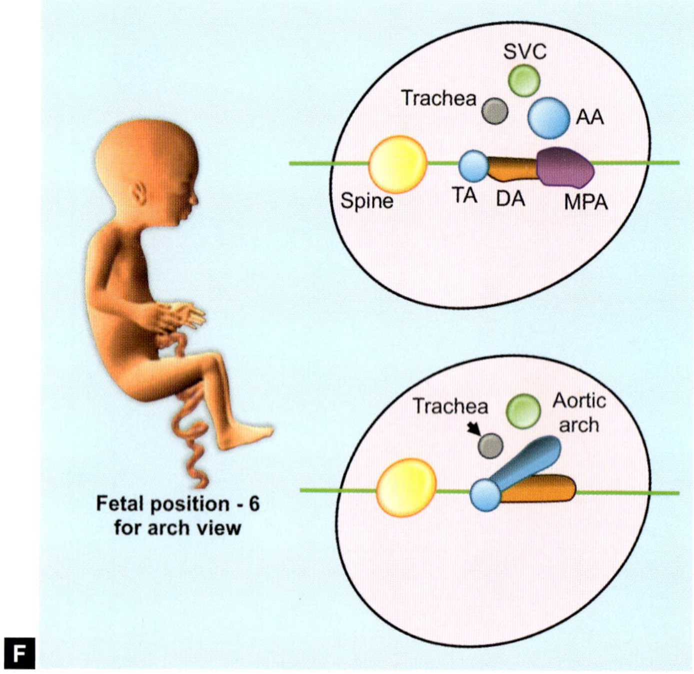

Figures 12.70E and F

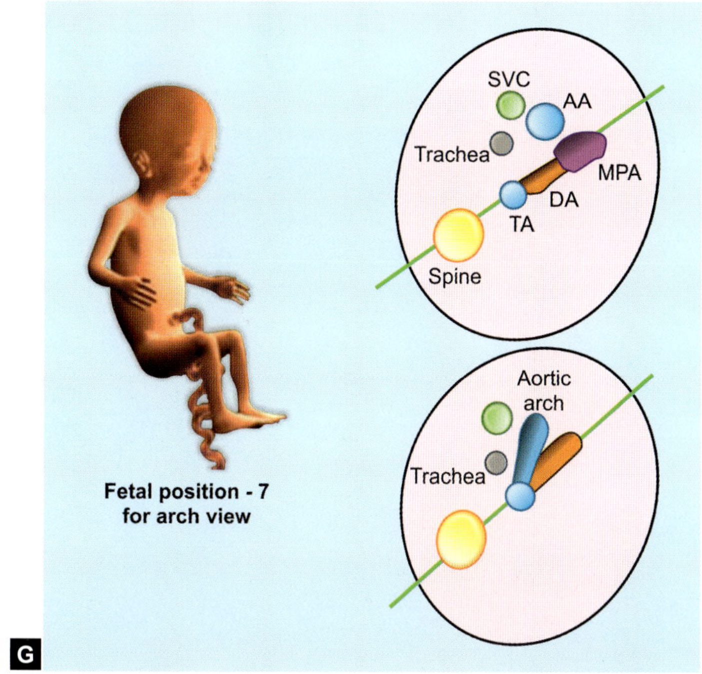

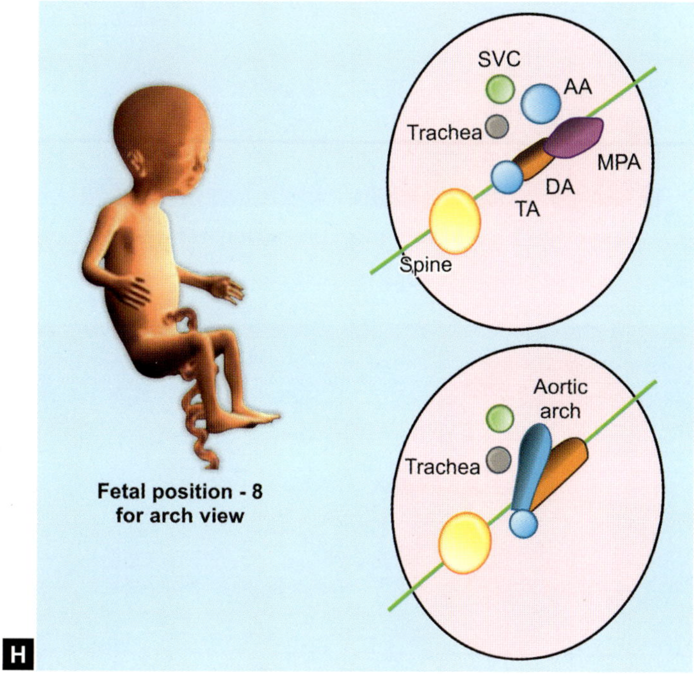

Figures 12.70G and H

Figures 12.70A to H Arch view in various fetal positions

ADDITIONAL VIEWS OF THE HEART (FIGURES 12.71 TO 12.81)

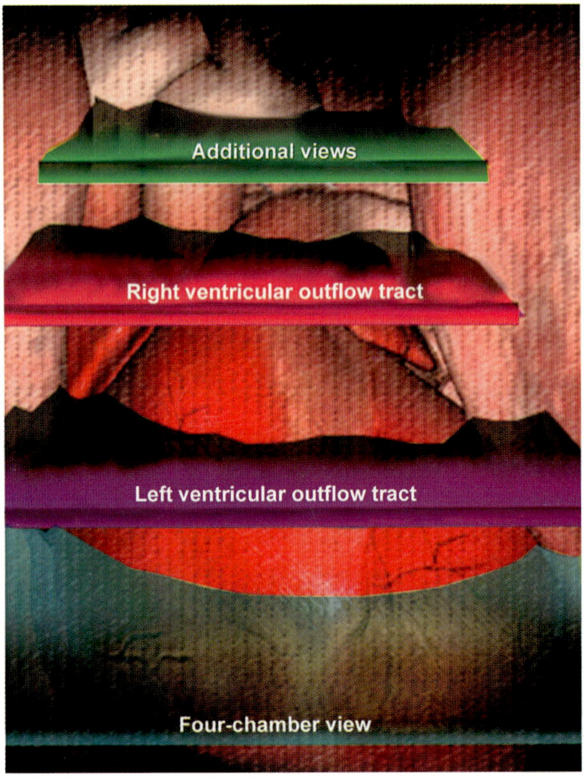

Figure 12.71 Levels for various ultrasound heart views

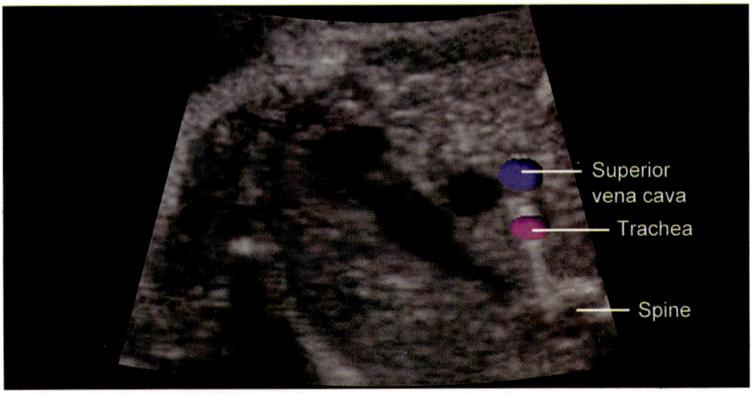

Figure 12.72 Three-vessel tracheal view

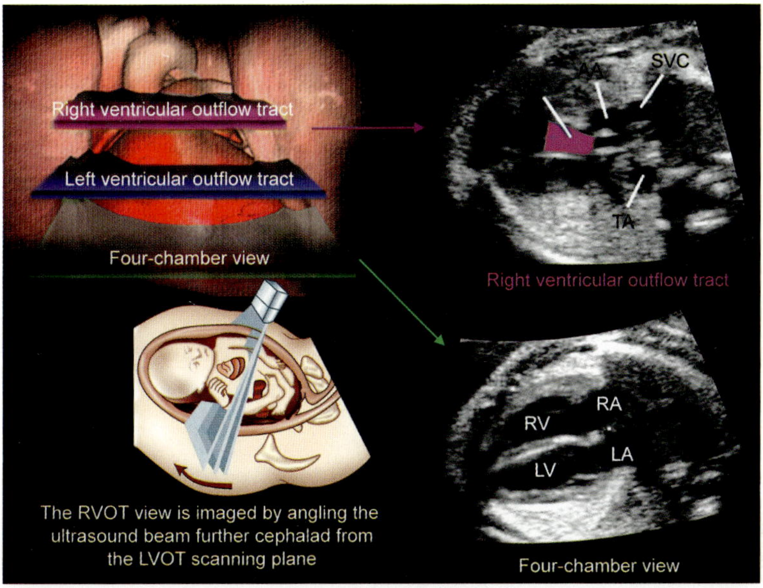

Figure 12.73 Right ventricular outflow tract

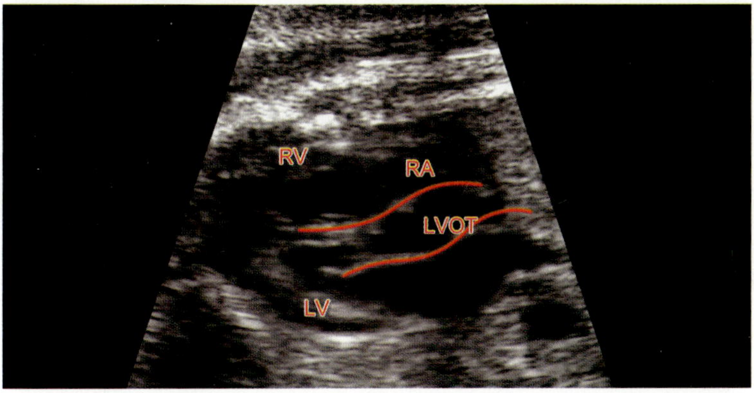

Figure 12.74 Left ventricular outflow tract

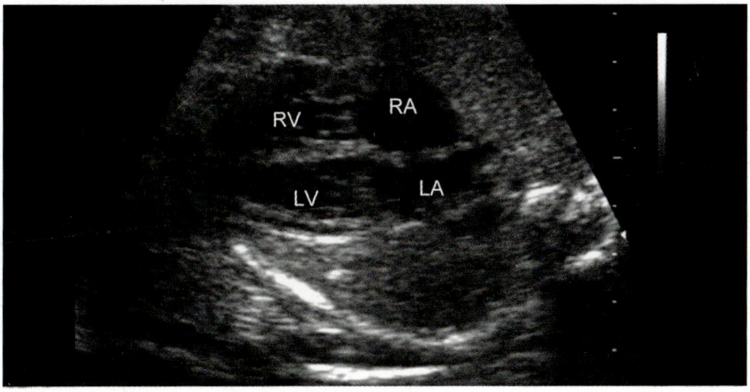

Figure 12.75 Four-chamber view

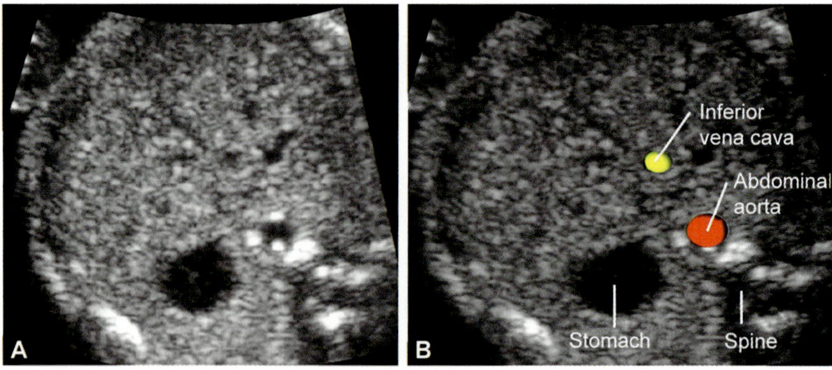

Figures 12.76A and B (A) Two-dimensional image showing inferior vena cava and abdominal aorta; (B) Labeled image

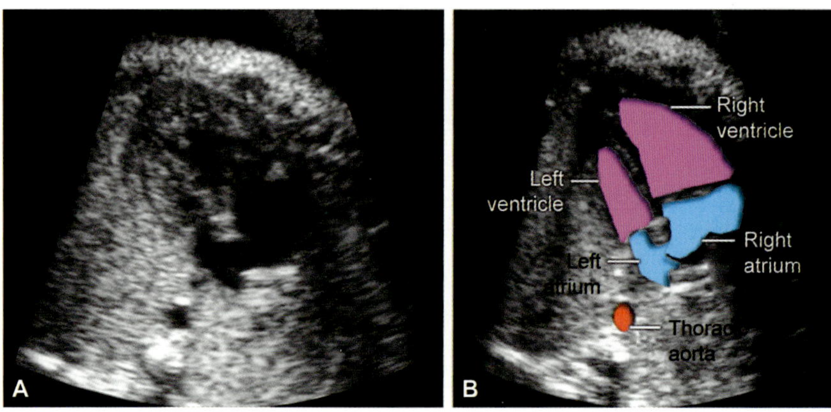

Figures 12.77A and B (A) Two-dimensional image showing four-chamber heart with thoracic aorta; (B) Labeled image

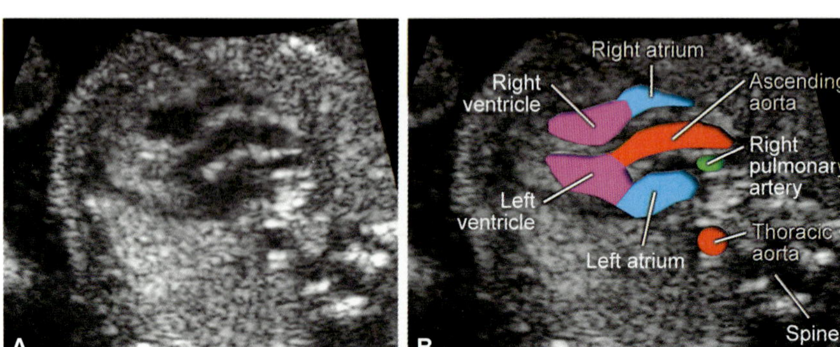

Figures 12.78A and B (A) Two-dimensional image showing five-chamber view; (B) Labeled image

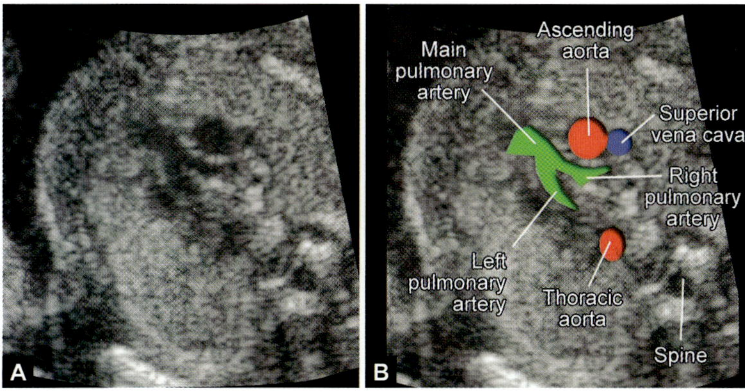

Figures 12.79A and B (A) Two-dimensional image showing right ventricular outflow tract; (B) Labeled image

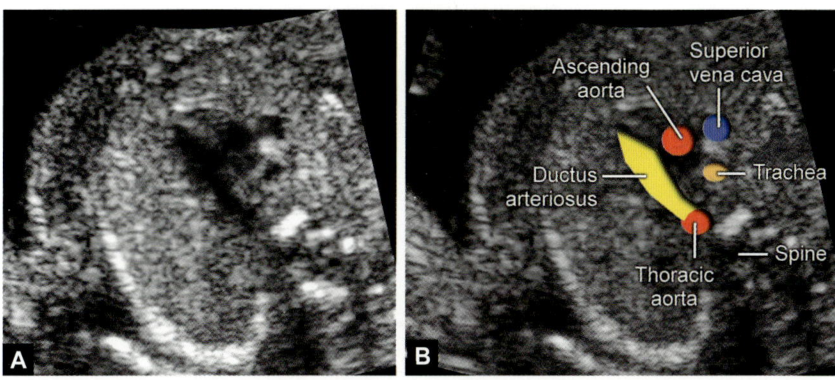

Figures 12.80A and B (A) Ductus arteriosus in a tracheal view; (B) Labeled image

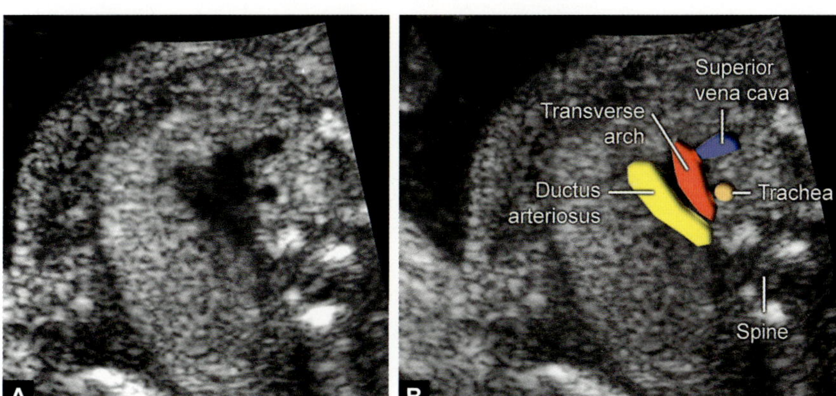

Figures 12.81A and B (A) Two-dimensional image showing ductus arteriosus and transverse arch in an arch view; (B) Labeled image

FETAL HEART DISSECTION (FIGURES 12.82 TO 12.102)

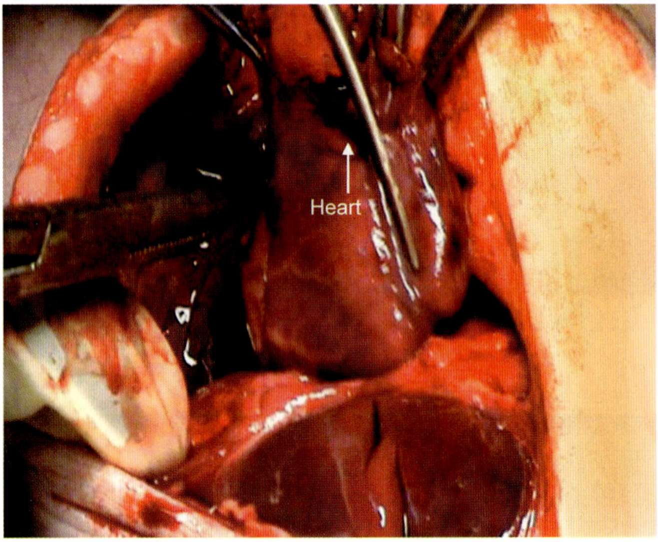

Figure 12.82 A fetal heart dissection

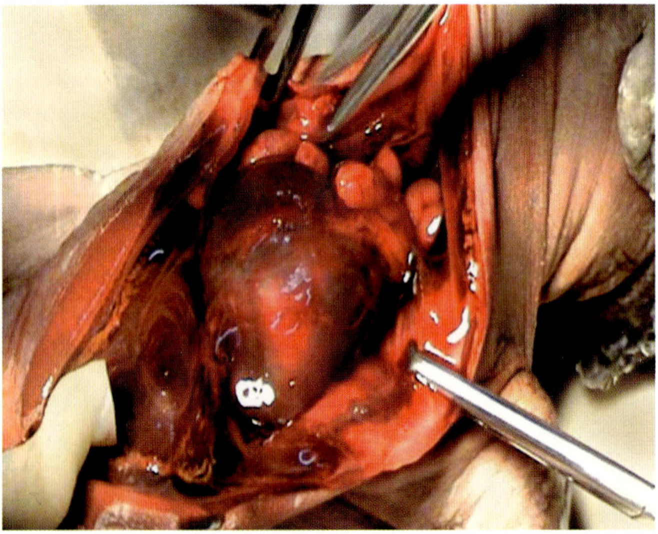

Figure 12.83 The anterior surface of the heart with dissected neck

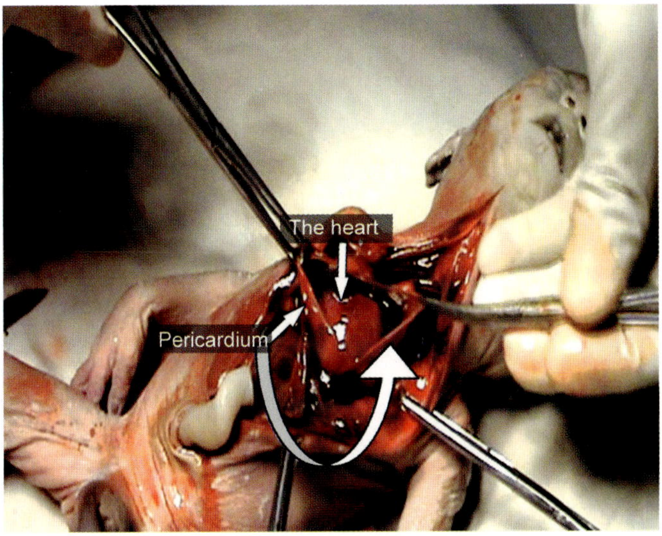

Figure 12.84 The opened pericardium with anterior surface of the heart

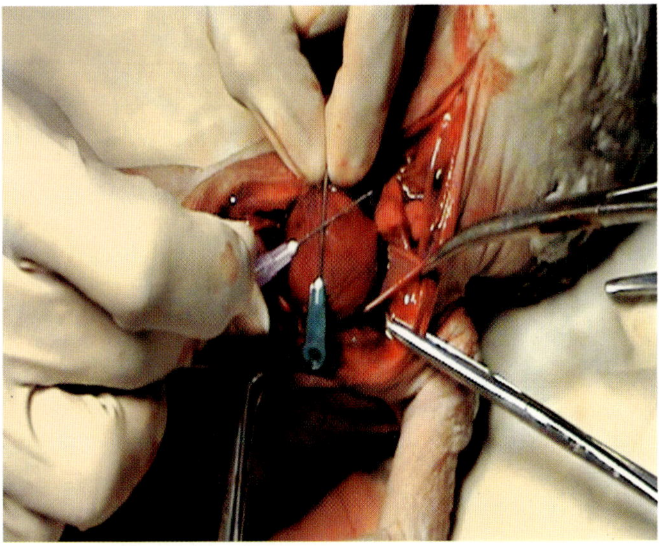

Figure 12.85 The assessment of the cardiac axis

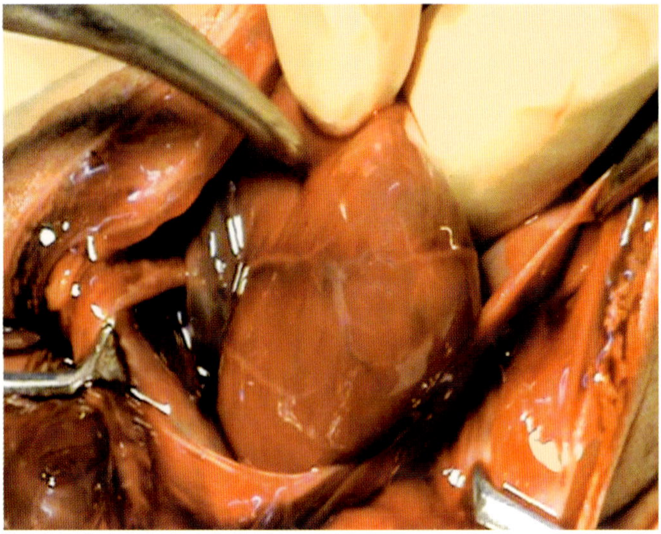

Figure 12.86 Anterolateral surface of the heart with right auricle

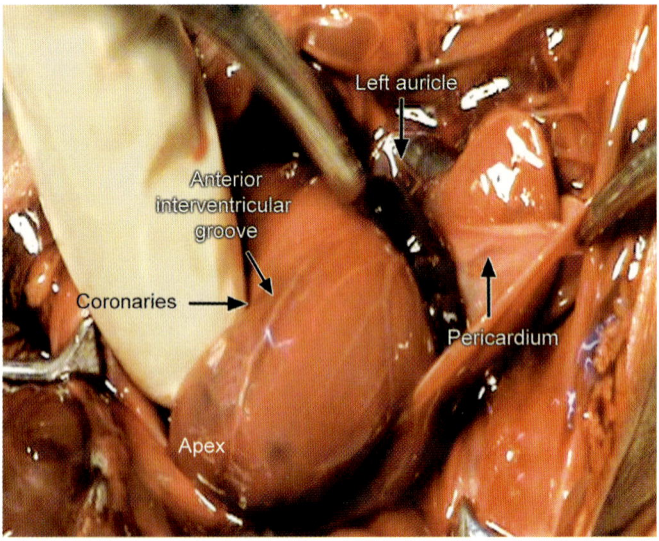

Figures 12.87 Left auricle, anterior interventricular groove and pericardium

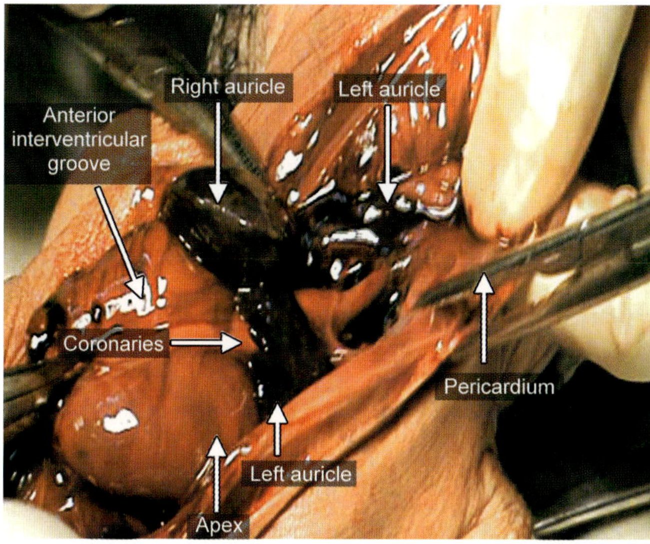

Figure 12.88 The auricles and anterior interventricular groove

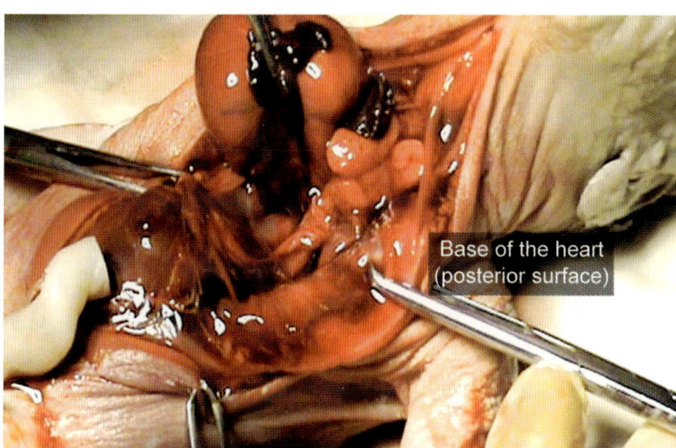

Figure 12.89 The posterior surface of the heart

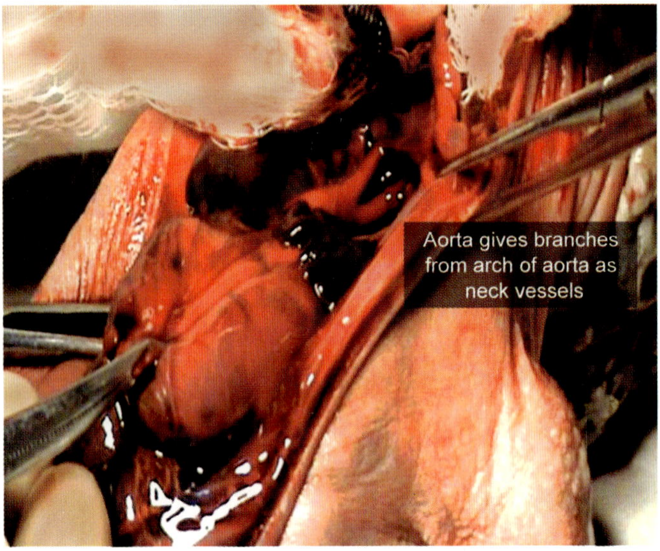

Figure 12.90 Aortic arch with two main branches

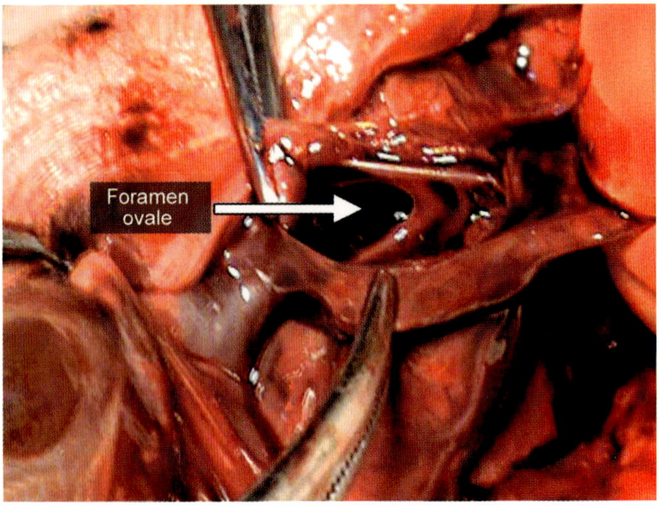

Figure 12.91 Foramen ovale opening from RA to LA

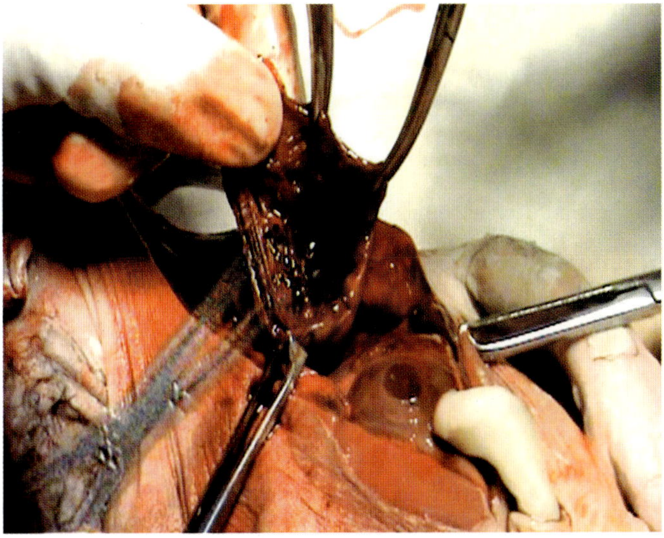

Figure 12.92 Opened right auricle

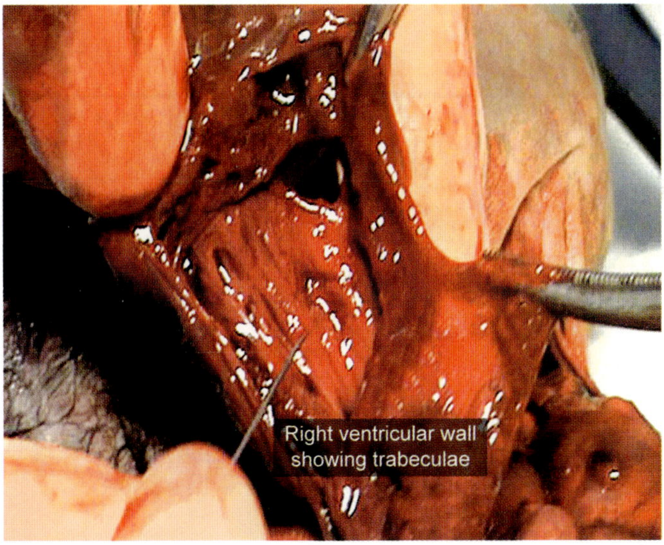

Figure 12.93 Opened right ventricle (dirty chamber)

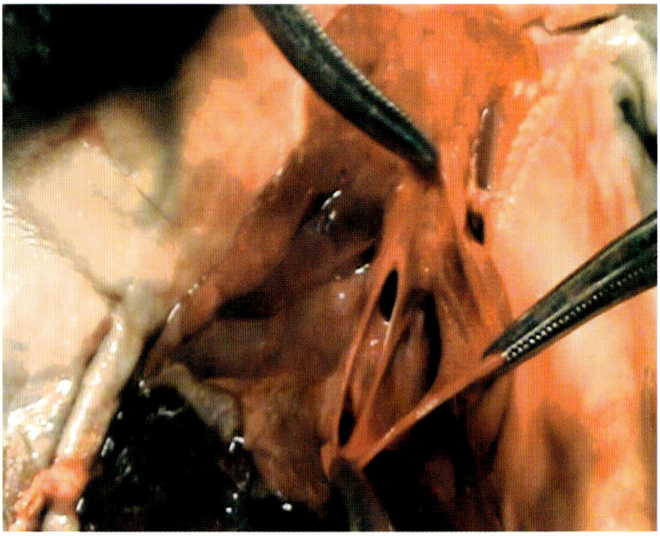

Figure 12.94 Opened aortic and pulmonary valves

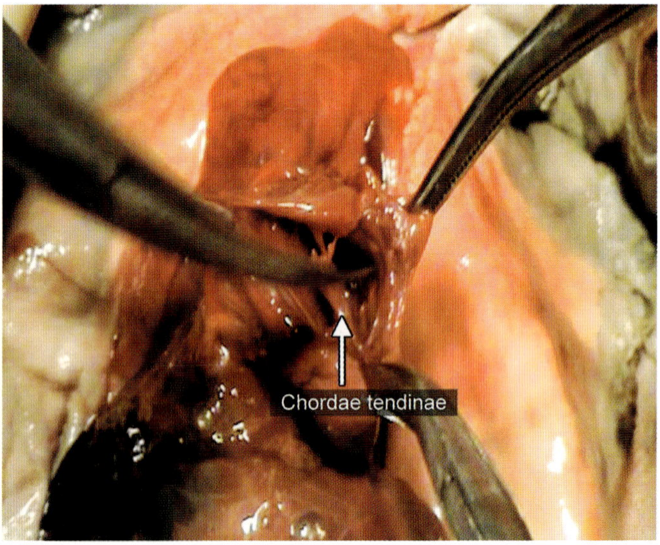

Figure 12.95 Opened ventricle and chordae tendinae

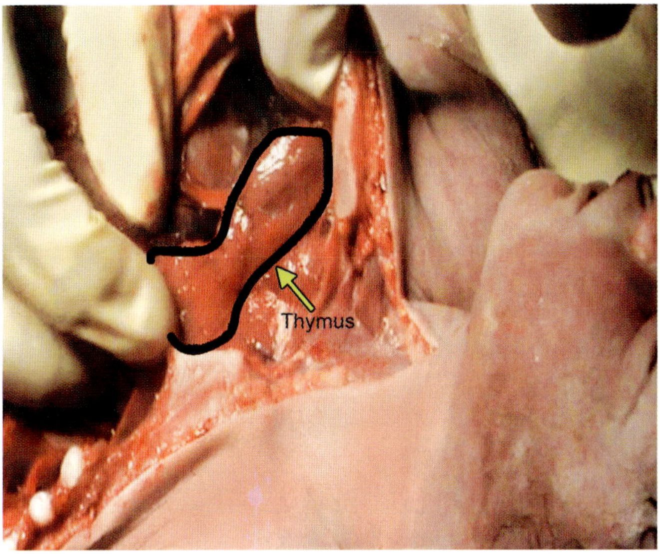

Figure 12.96 Thymus

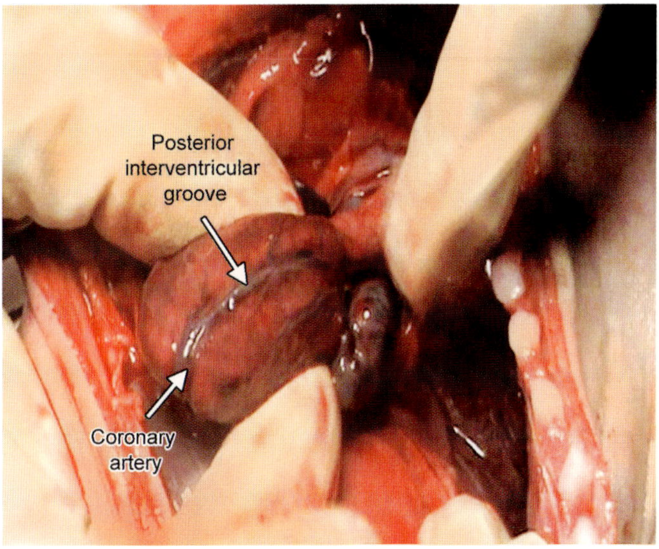

Figure 12.97 Posterior interventricular groove with coronary artery

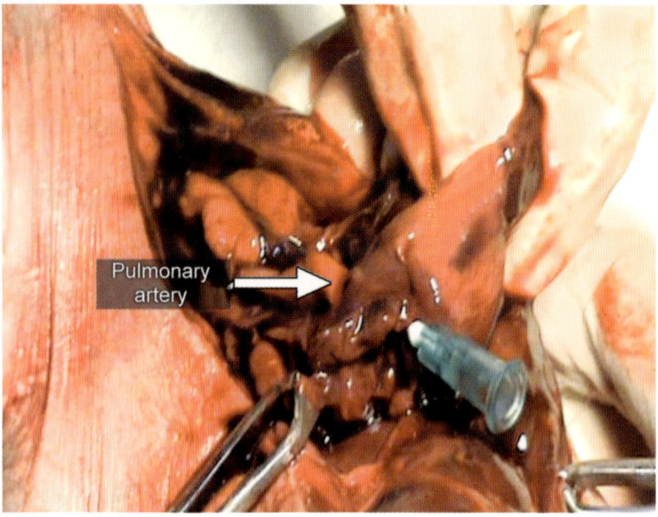

Figure 12.98 Origin of the pulmonary artery from the right ventricle

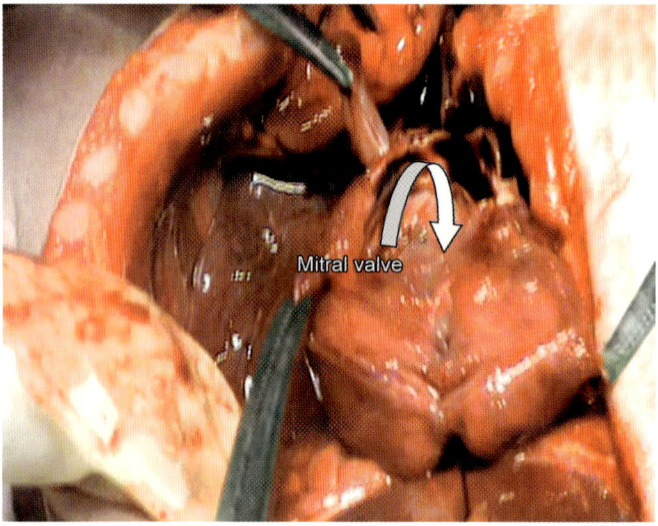

Figure 12.99 Mitral valve in the opened left ventricular chamber

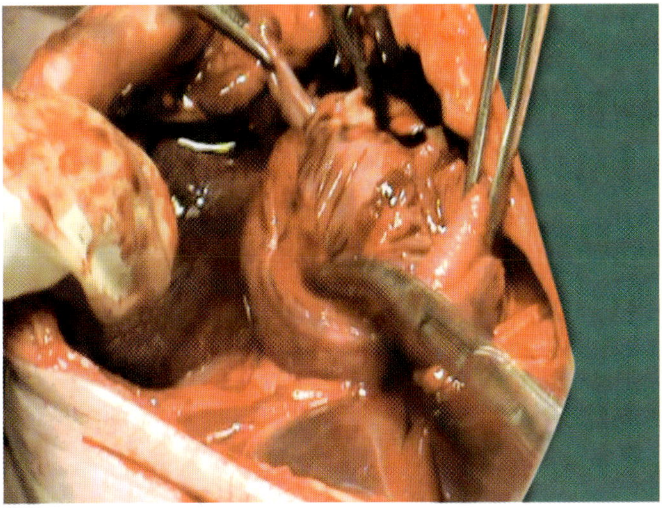

Figure 12.100 The opened right ventricle

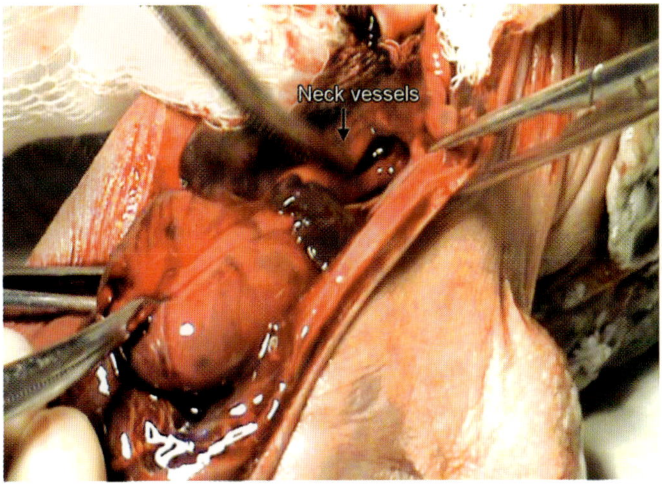

Figure 12.101 Dissected neck vessels

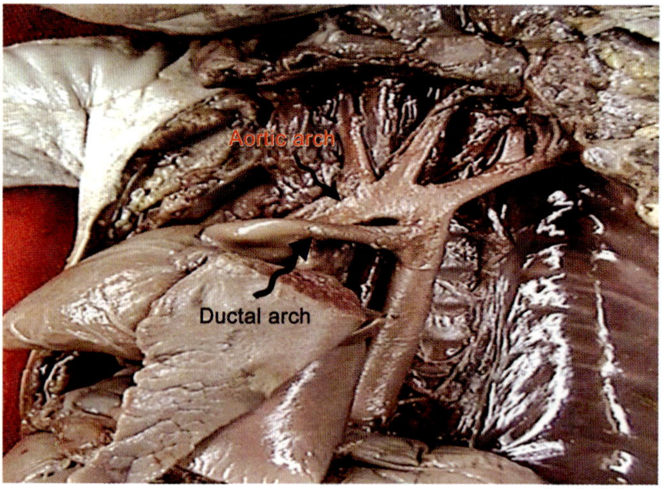

Figure 12.102 Ductal arch

NUTSHELL

1. This chapter gives us an idea regarding normal heart images.
2. Images of fetal echo gives and idea regarding how to use contrast, focal zone, difference between high frequency and low frequency, use of harmonics and cut section of heart at level of four-chamber view.
3. How to get normal axis of heart and normal and assessment of fetal situs and four chamber in color for easy understanding of every structure.
4. Outflow tract in color and different fetus position of tract.
5. Additional view such as tracheal and arch view for PAS..., pulmonary, aorta and superior vena cava.
6. Fetal heart dissection for correlation with sonography images, and how gets proper images.

13

Normal Heart Images

This chapter gives an idea regarding different normal heart images (Figs 13.1 to 13.90

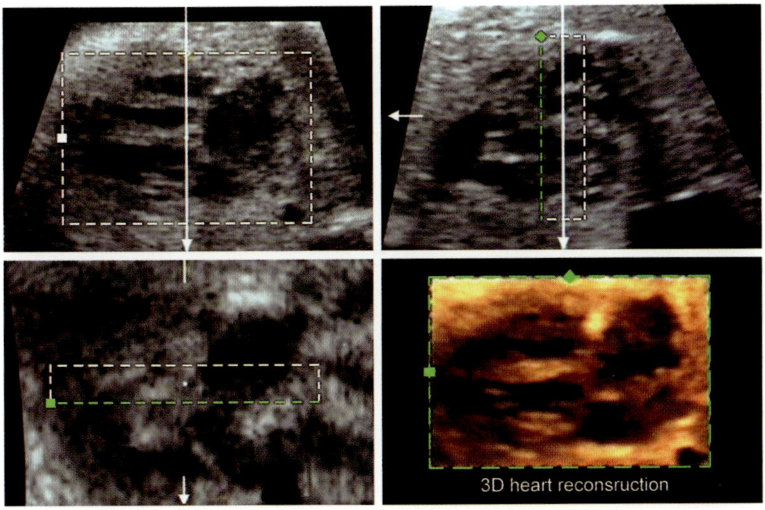

Figure 13.1 Three-dimensional cusp

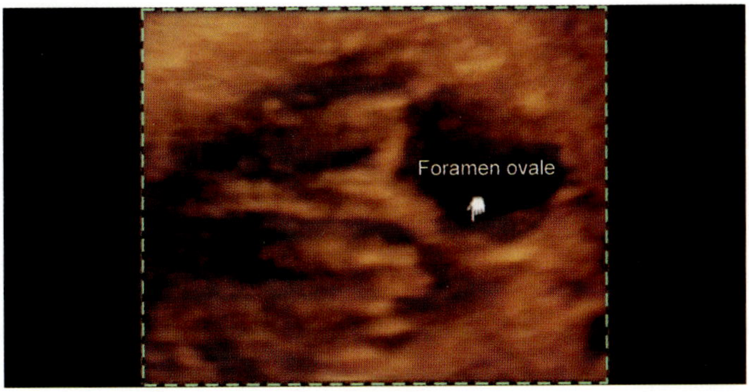

Figure 13.2 Three-dimensional foramen ovale

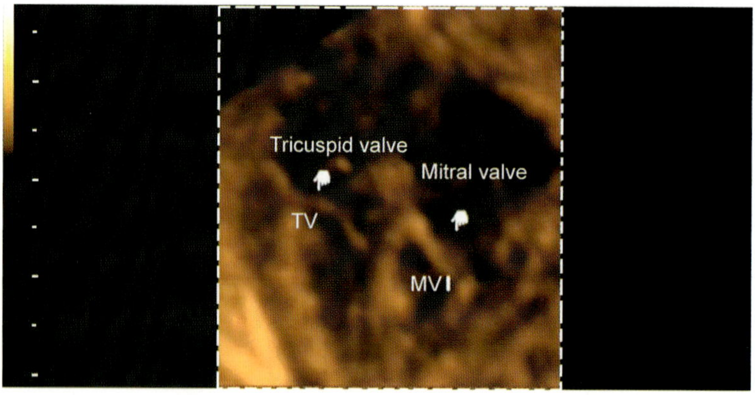

Figure 13.3 Three-dimensional heart surface

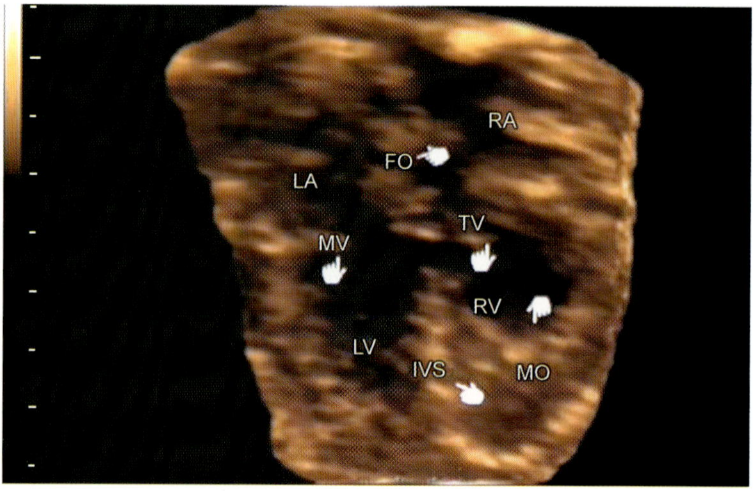

Figure 13.4 Three-dimensional heart with labeling

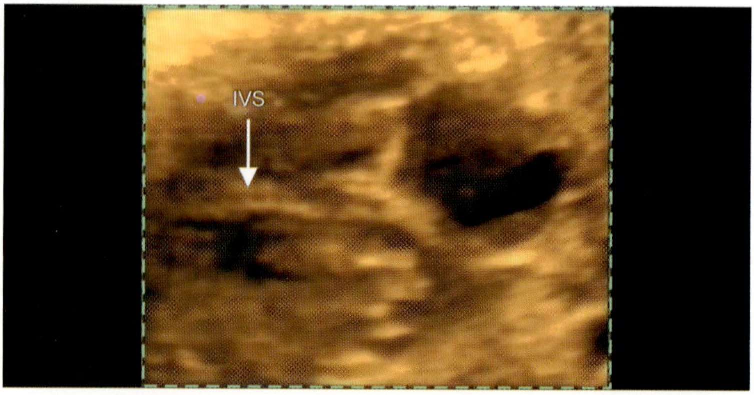

Figure 13.5 Three-dimensional heart showing IVS

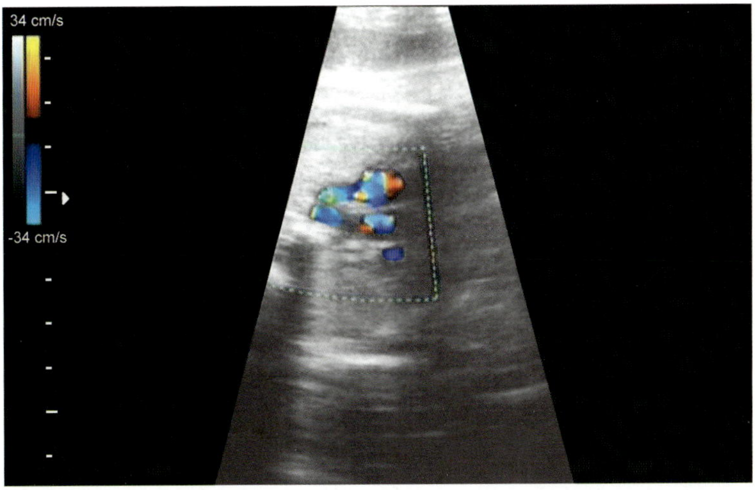

Figure 13.6 Three vessels view with color

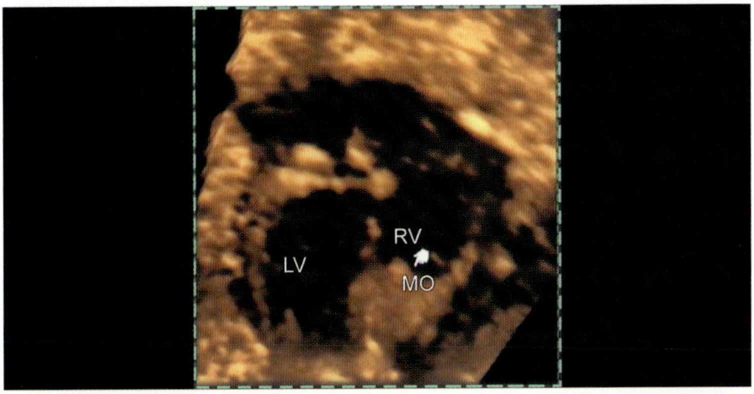

Figure 13.7 Three-dimensional heart showing moderator band

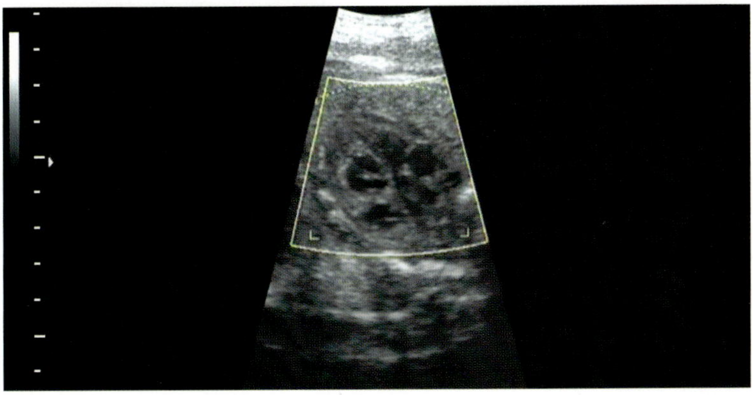

Figure 13.8 Three-dimensional sectional image: Step 1

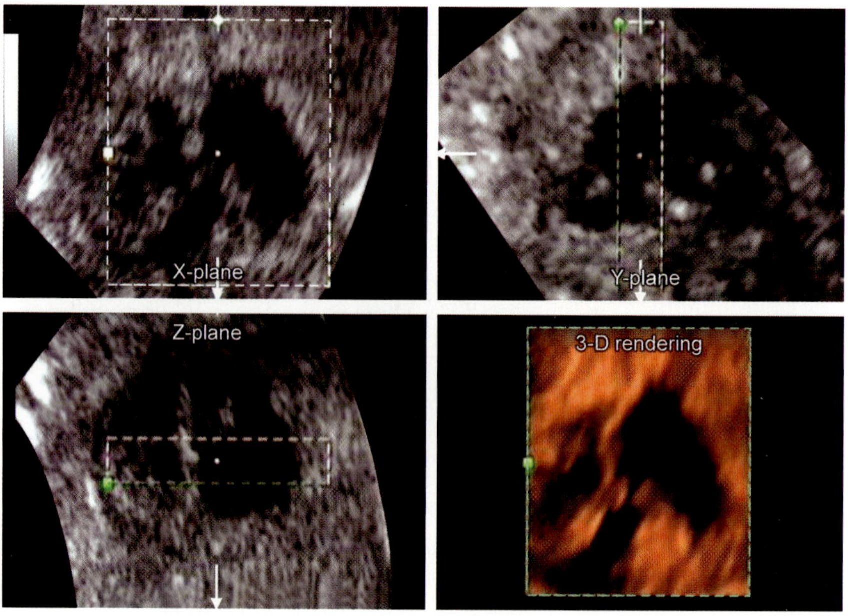

Figure 13.9 Three-dimensional sectional image: Step 2

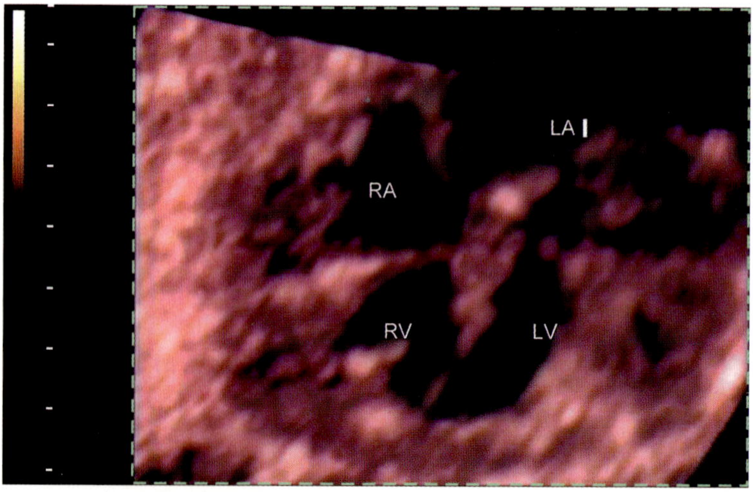

Figure 13.10 Three-dimensional sectional image: Step 3

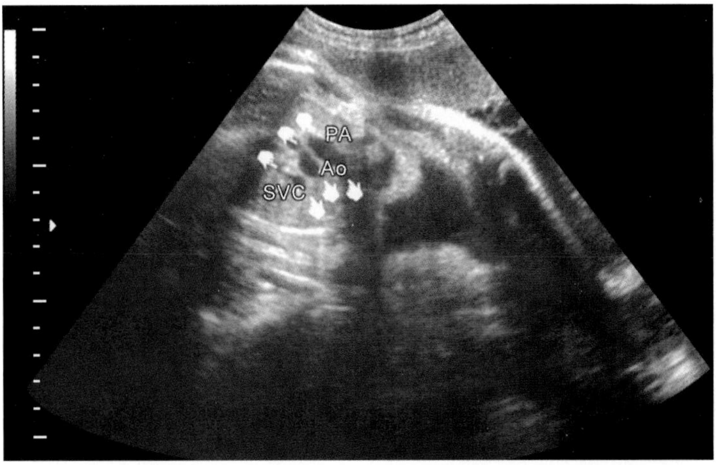

Figure 13.11 Labeled image showing triple vessels

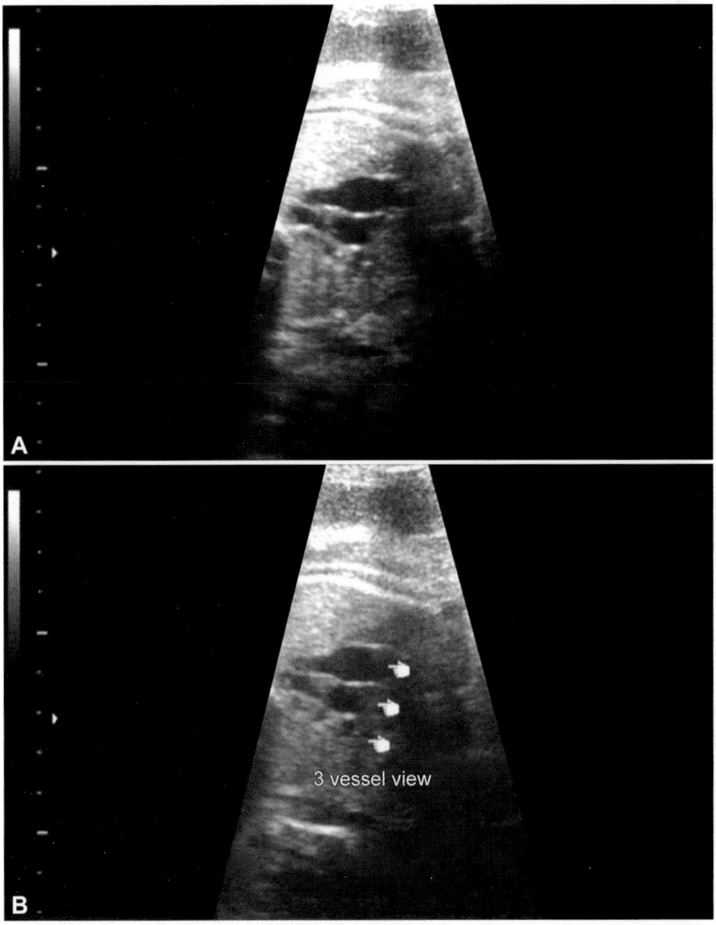

Figures 13.12A and B Three-vessel view

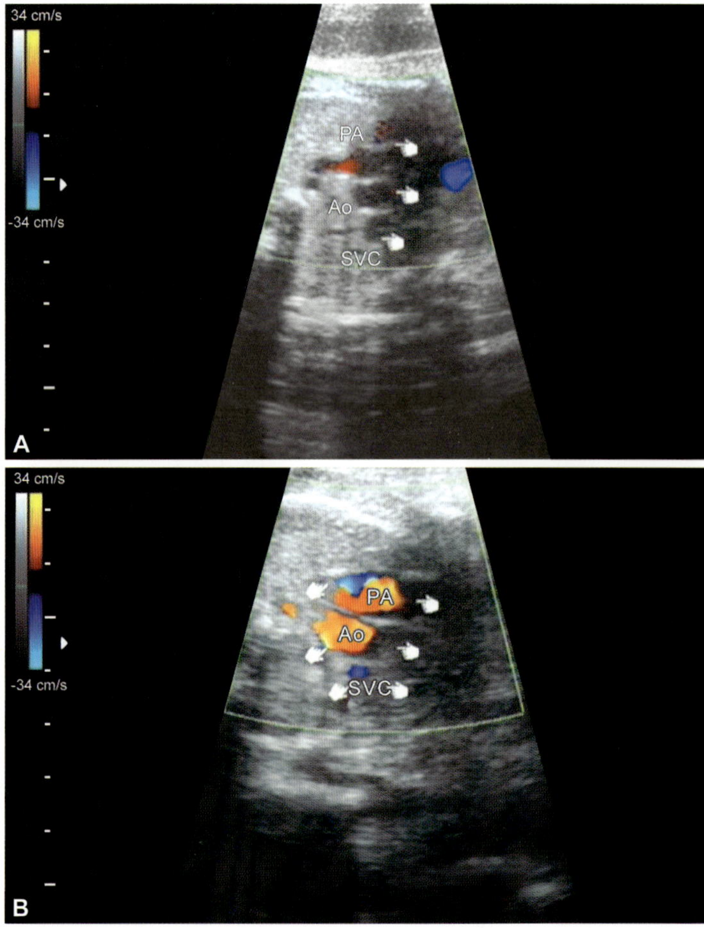

Figures 13.13A and B Three-vessel view with color Doppler

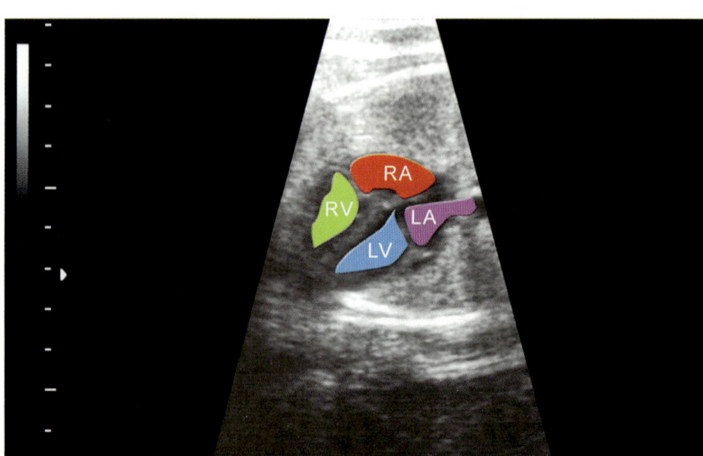

Figure 13.14 Four-chamber view of the heart

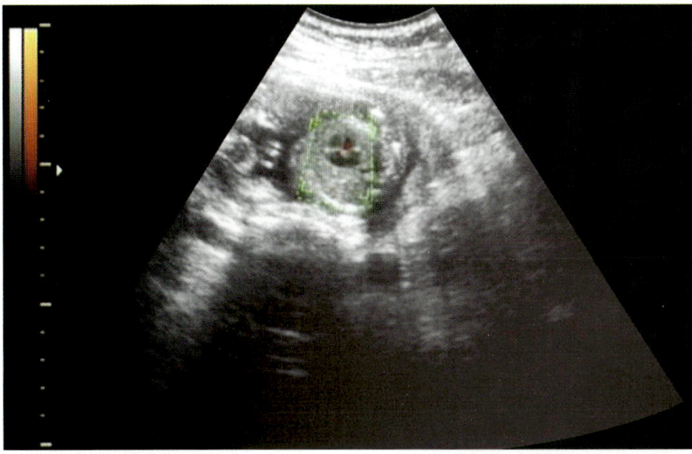

Figure 13.15 Four-chamber heart in two dimensions

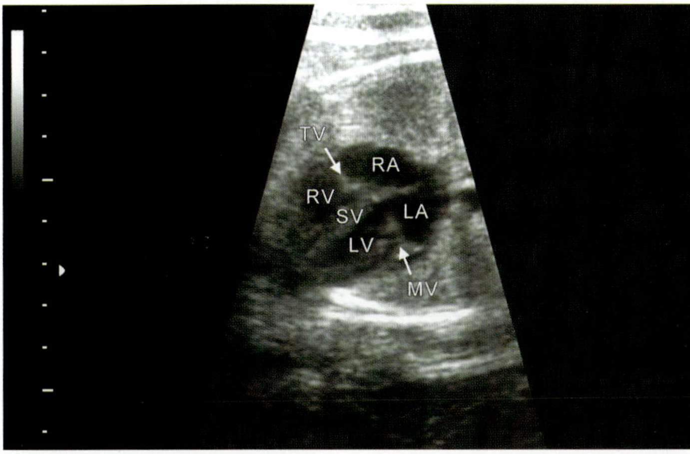

Figure 13.16 Four-chamber view

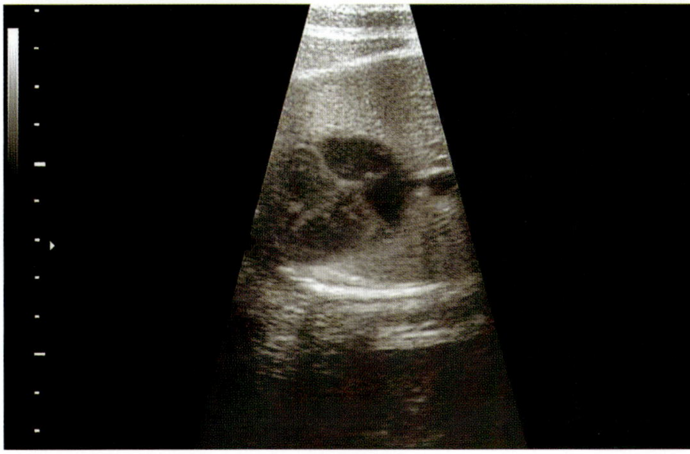

Figure 13.17 Four-chamber sepia

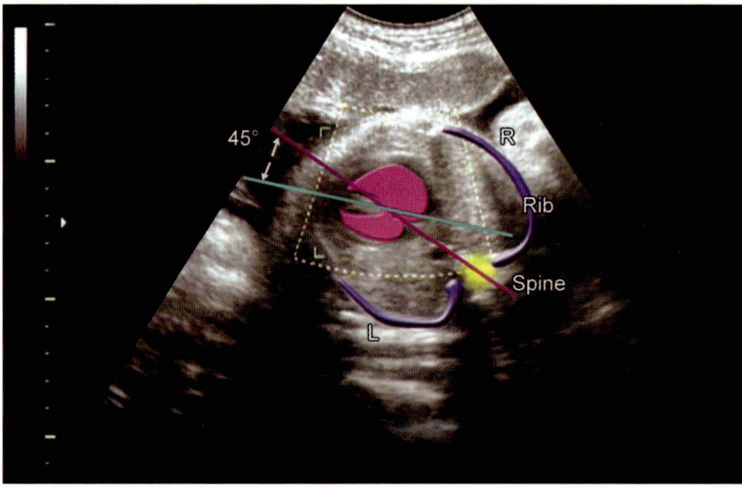

Figure 13.18 Cardiac axis

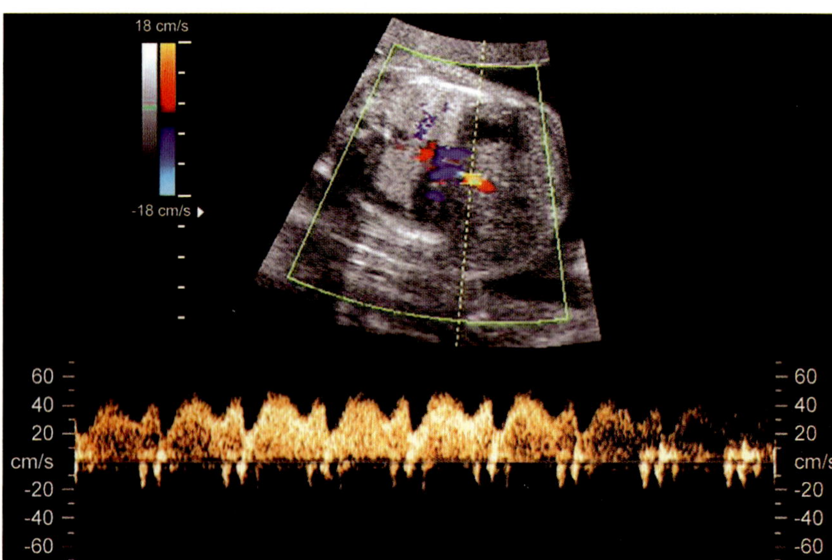

Figure 13.19 Ductus venosus waveform

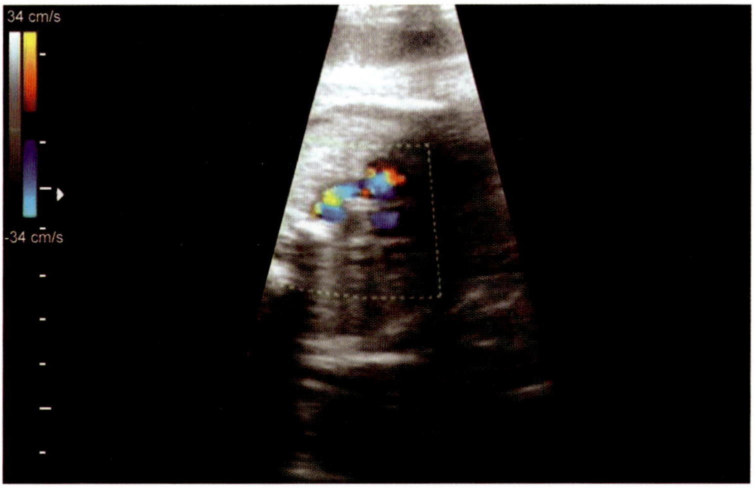

Figure 13.20 Color aliasing

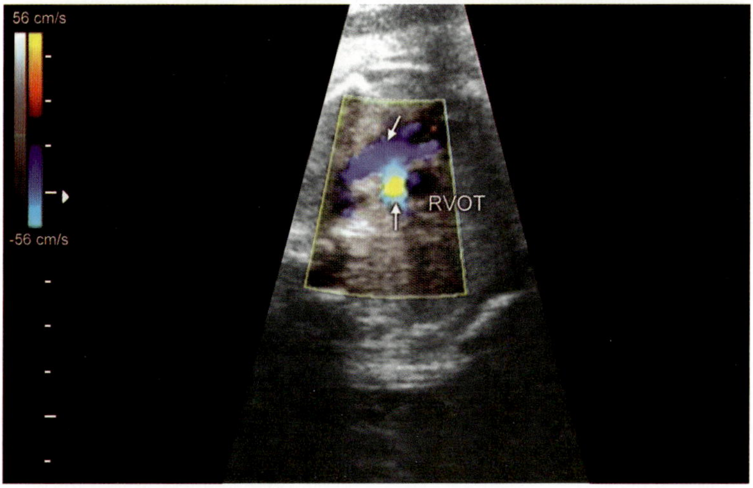

Figure 13.21 Color aliasing in right ventricular outflow tract

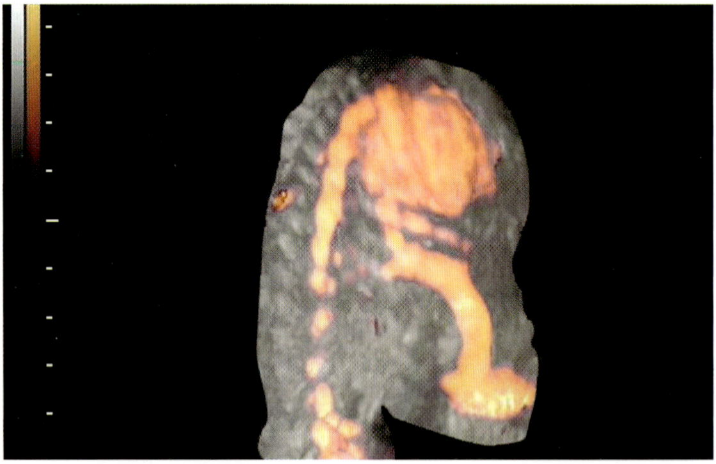

Figure 13.22 Aortic arch: Ground glass appearance

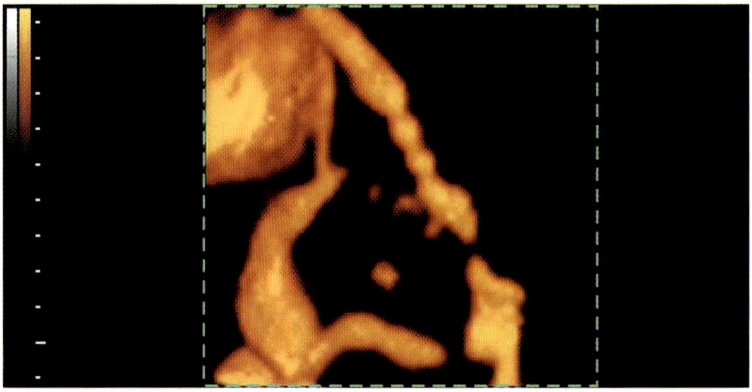

Figure 13.23 Arch of aorta with power Doppler

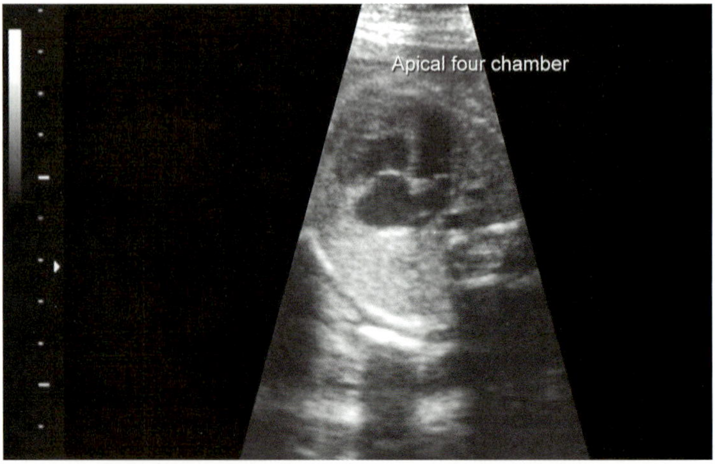

Figure 13.24 Apical four-chamber view in two dimensions

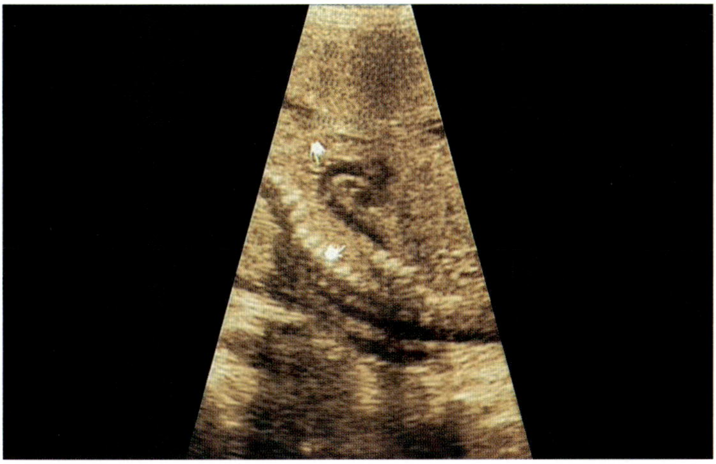

Figure 13.25 Arch sepia

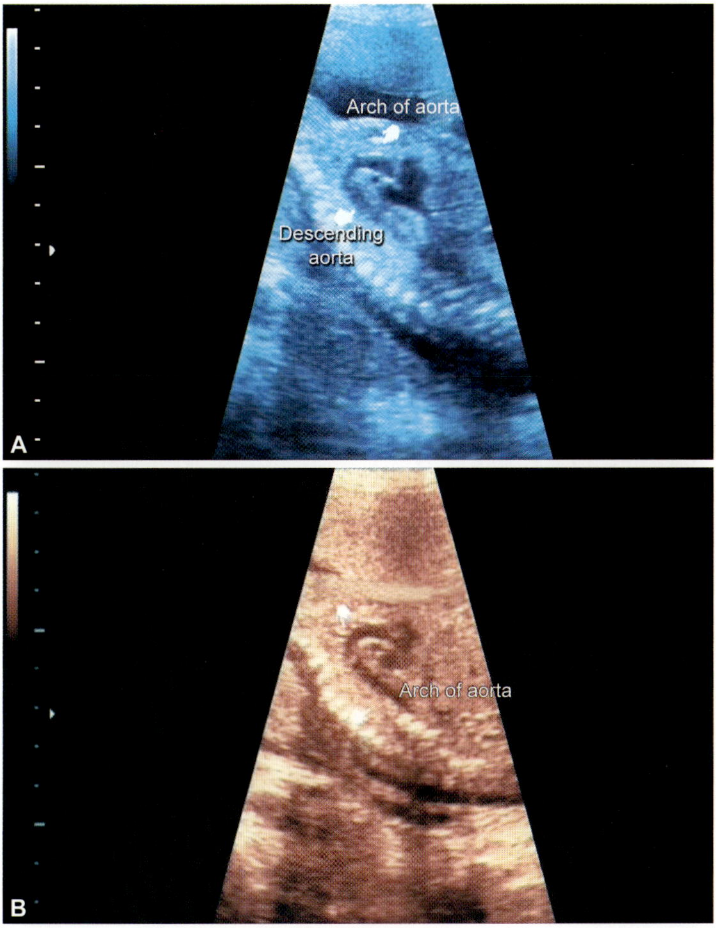

Figures 13.26A and B

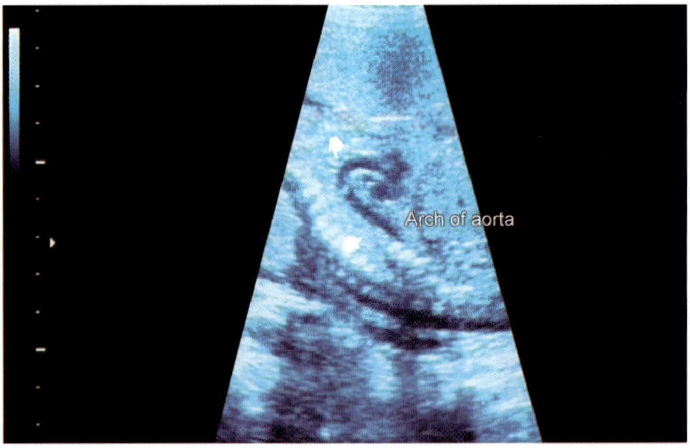

Figure 13.26C
Figures 13.26A to C Arch of aorta

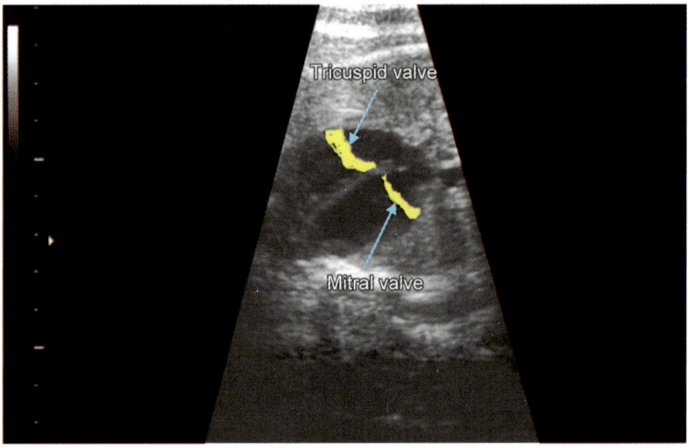

Figure 13.27 Atrioventricular valves

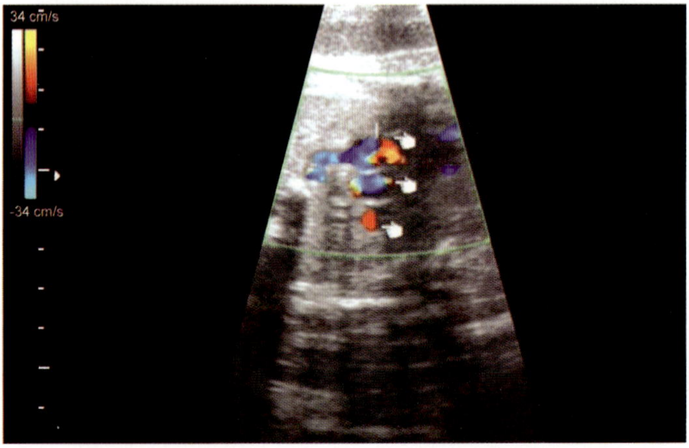

Figure 13.28 Three-vessel view with color Doppler

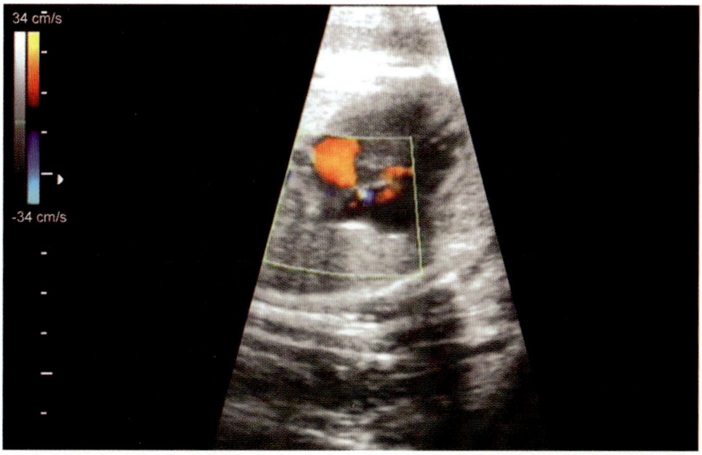

Figure 13.29 Color aliasing

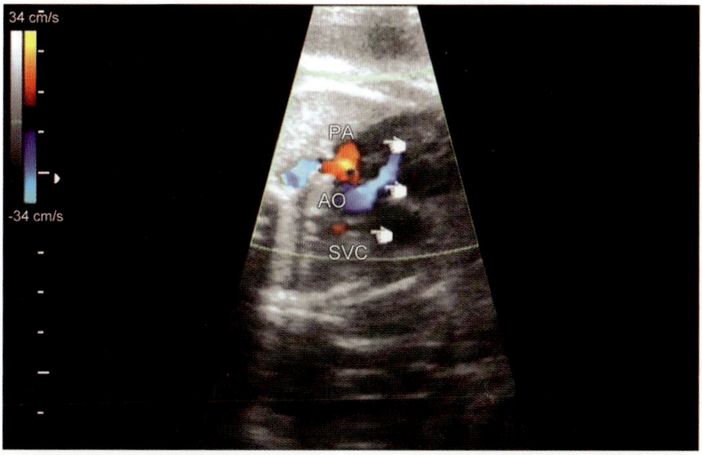

Figure 13.30 Crossing vessels in color

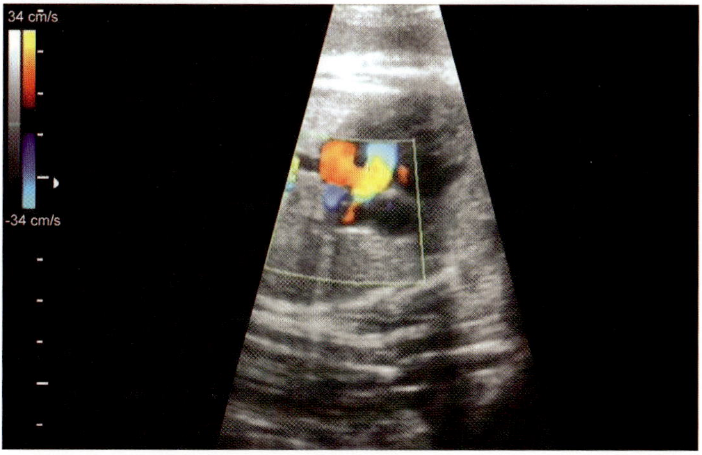

Figure 13.31 Aliasing in crossing vessels

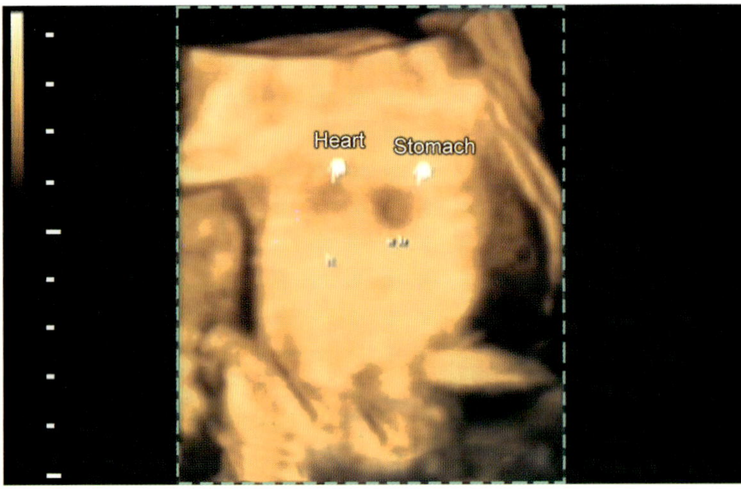

Figure 13.32 Diaphragmatic hernia

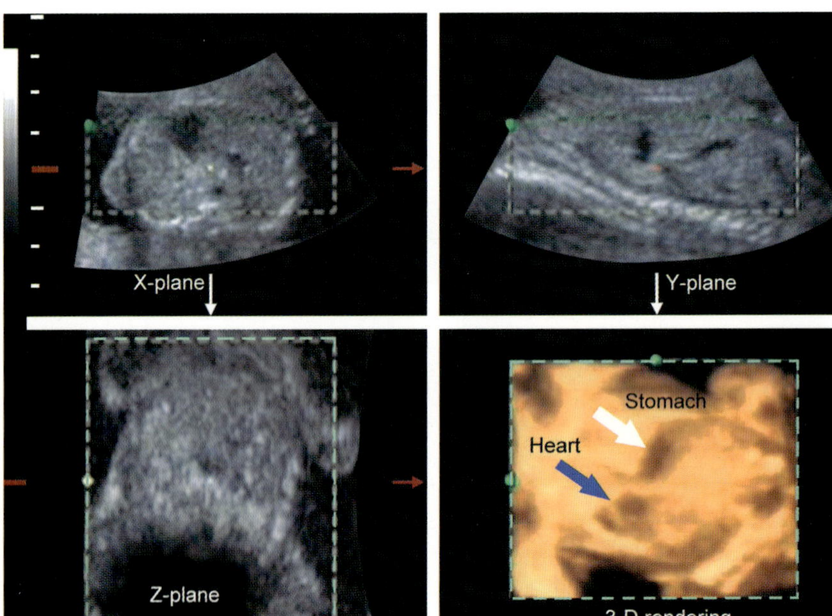

Figure 13.33 Diaphragmatic hernia in three dimensions

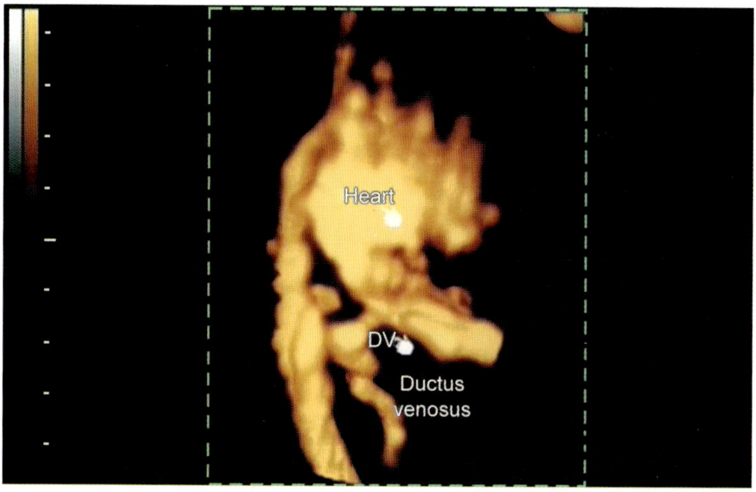

Figure 13.34 Ductus venosus power Doppler

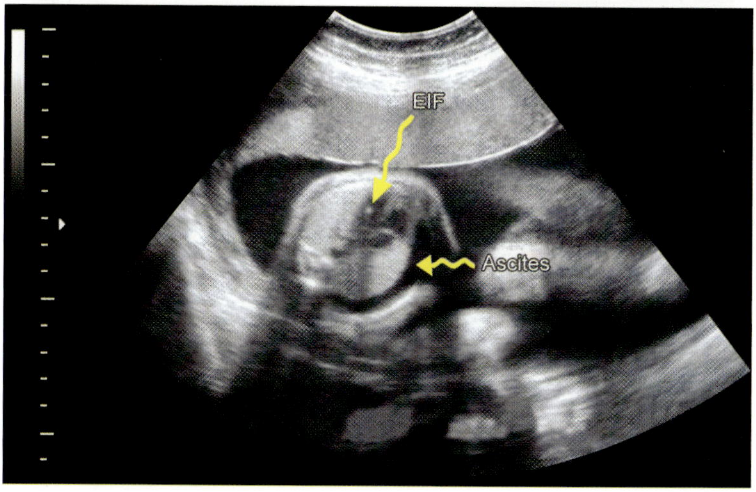

Figure 13.35 Echogenic intracardiac focus (EIF) with ascites

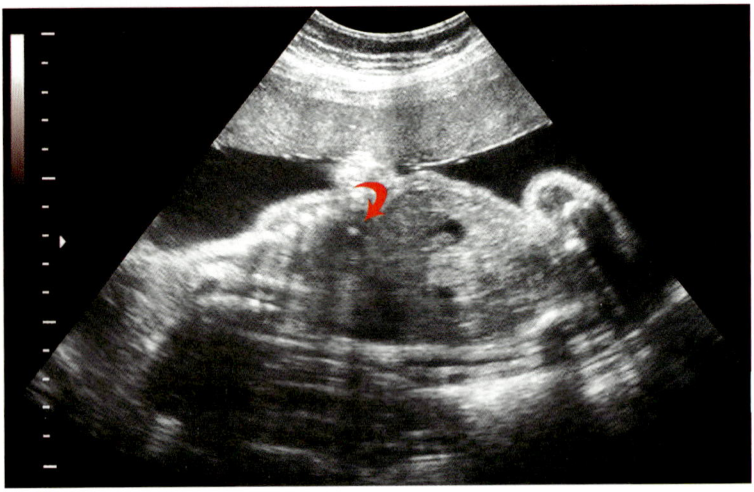

Figure 13.36 Echogenic focus (lateral view)

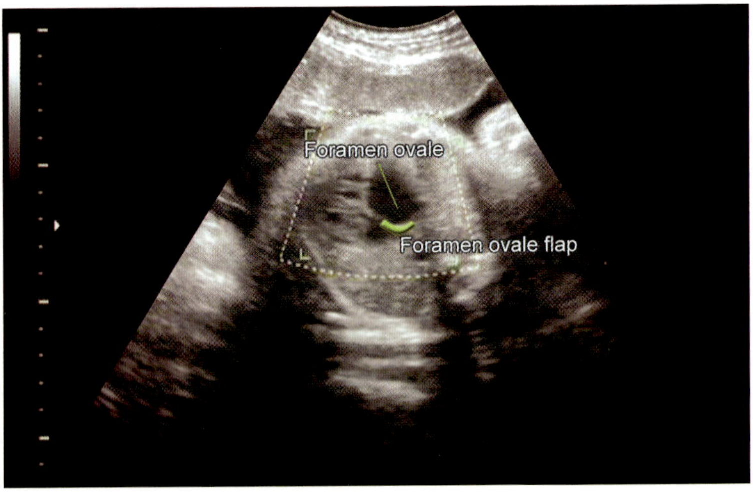

Figure 13.37 Foramen ovale

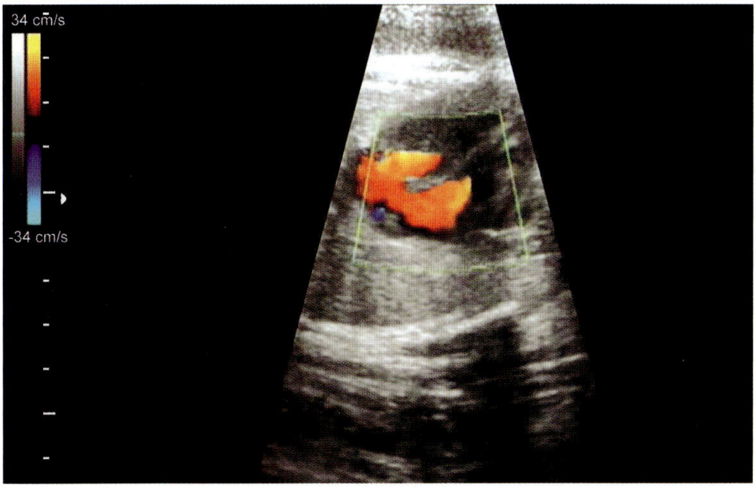

Figure 13.38 Flow through the AV valves

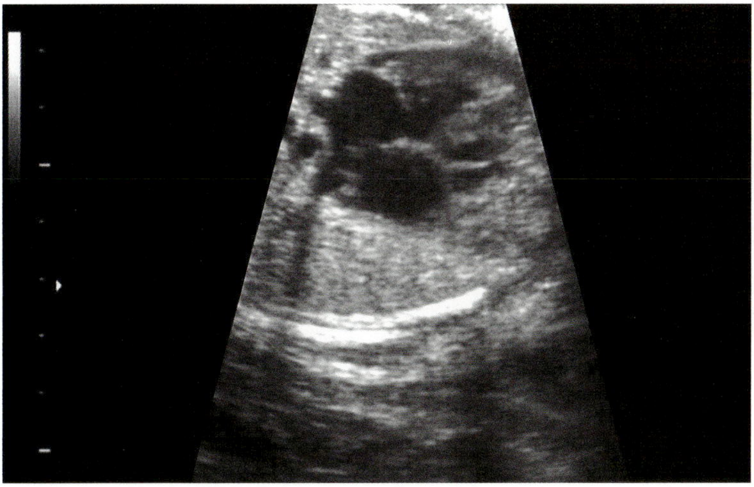

Figure 13.39 Foramen ovale—open

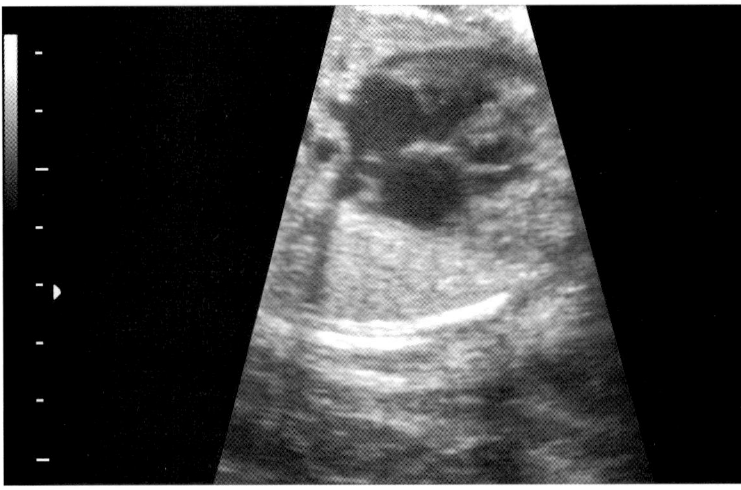

Figure 13.40 Foramen ovale—closing

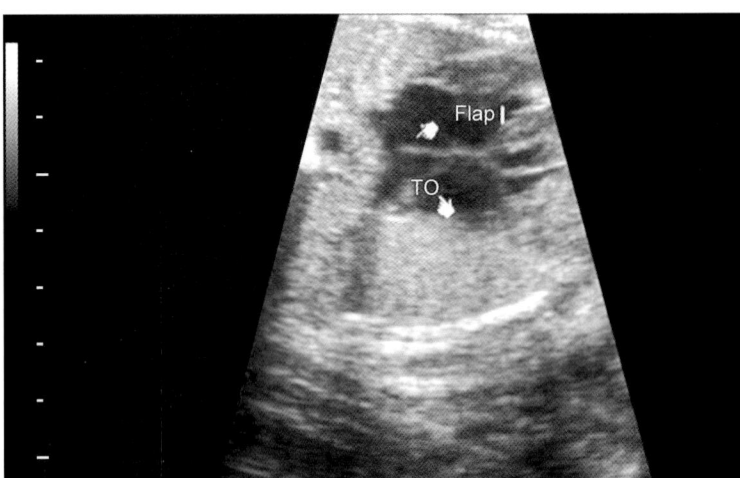

Figure 13.41 Foramen ovale with flap

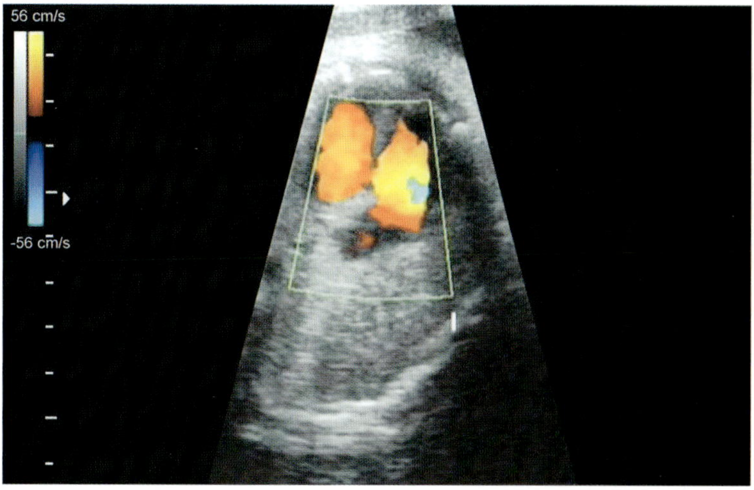

Figure 13.42 Both ventricles with color aliasing

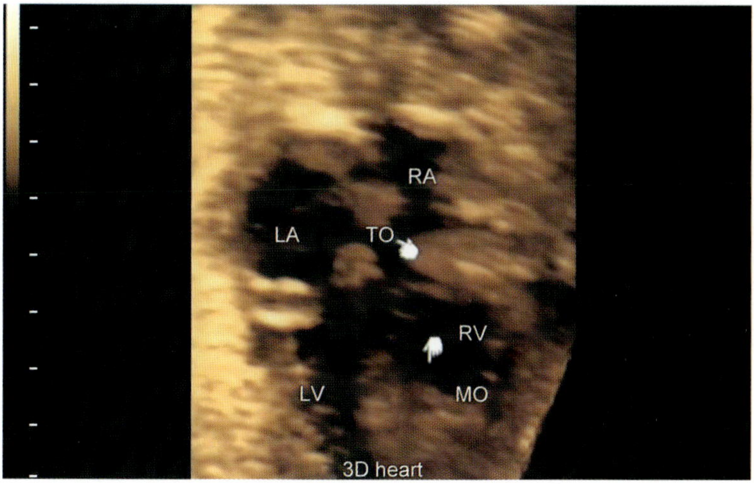

Figure 13.43 Three-dimensional heart

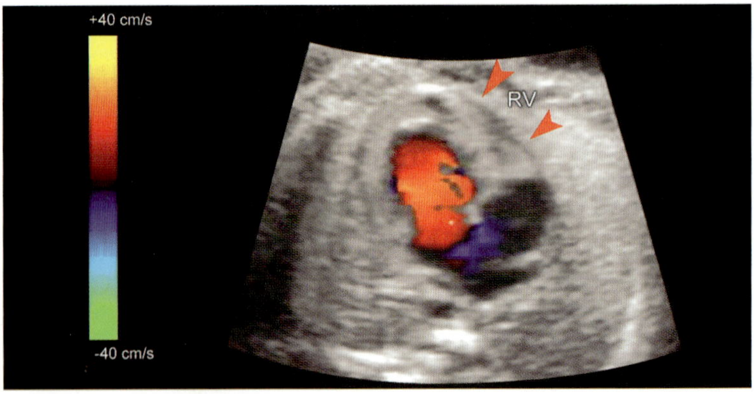

Figure 13.44 Hypoplastic right ventricle

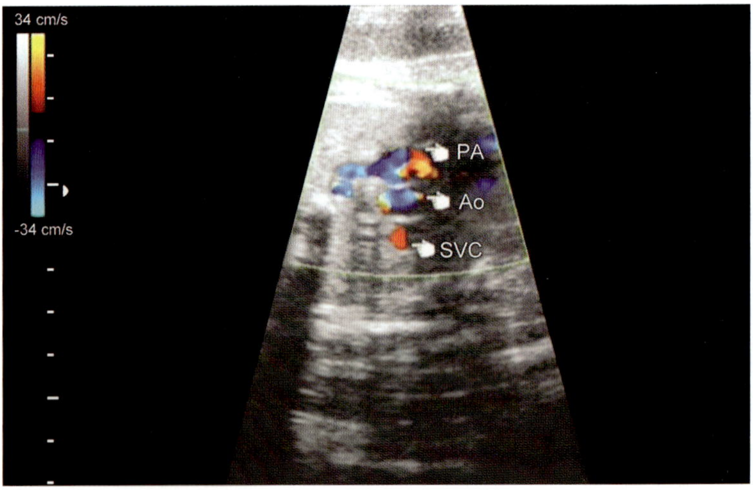

Figure 13.45 Labeled image showing three vessels in color

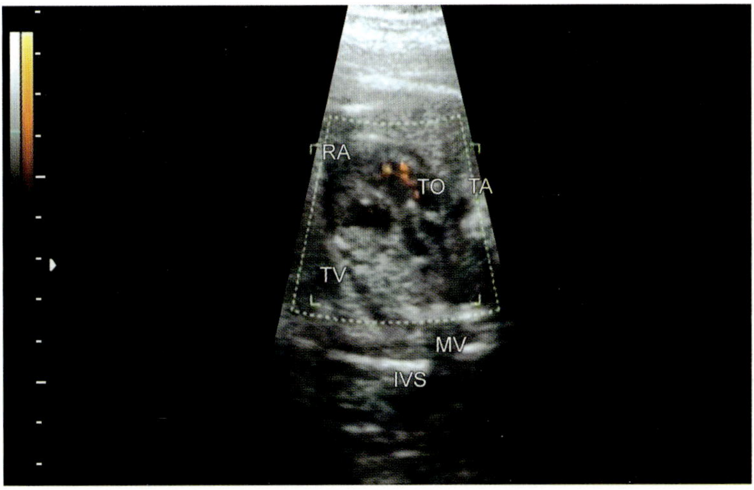

Figure 13.46 Left ventricular outflow tract (LVOT) in power angio

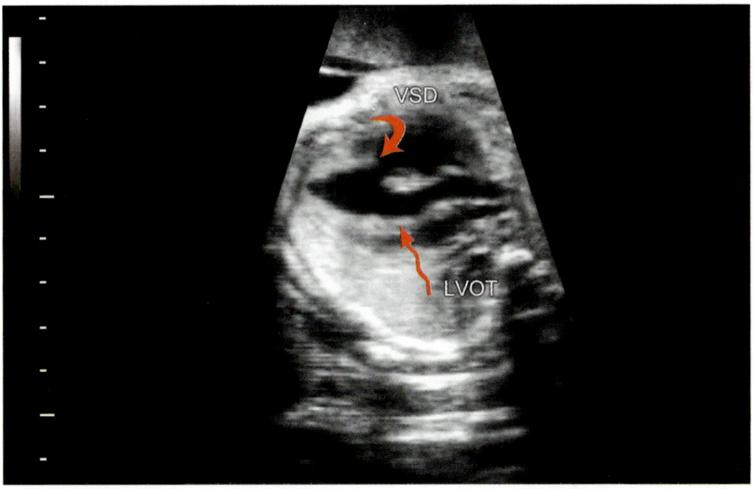

Figure 13.47 Ventricular septal defect with left ventricular outflow tract (LVOT)

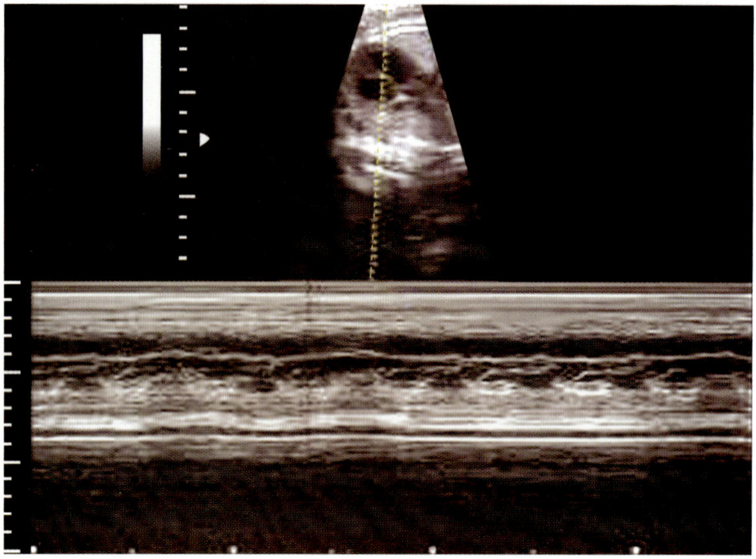

Figure 13.48 M-mode Echo

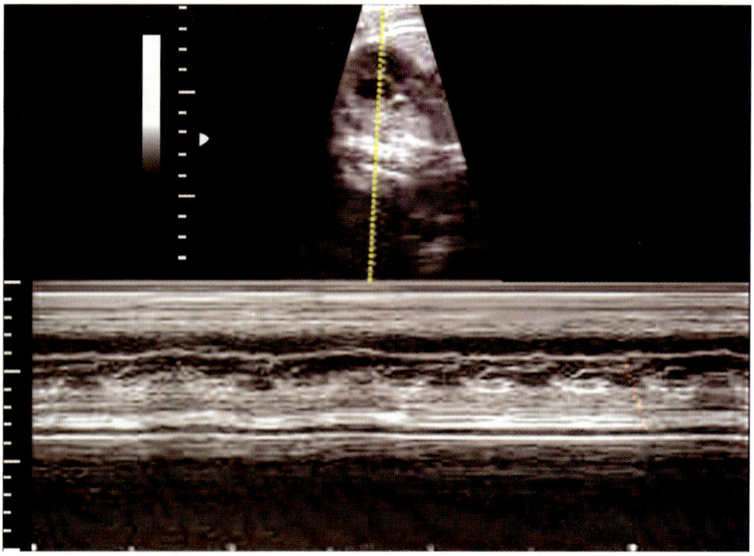

Figure 13.49 M-mode Doppler

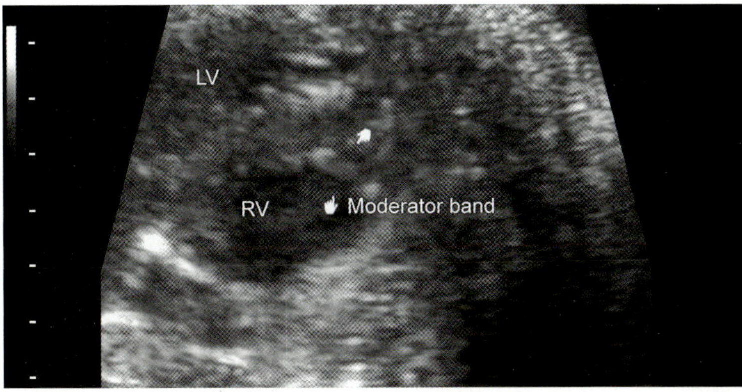

Figure 13.50 Moderator band

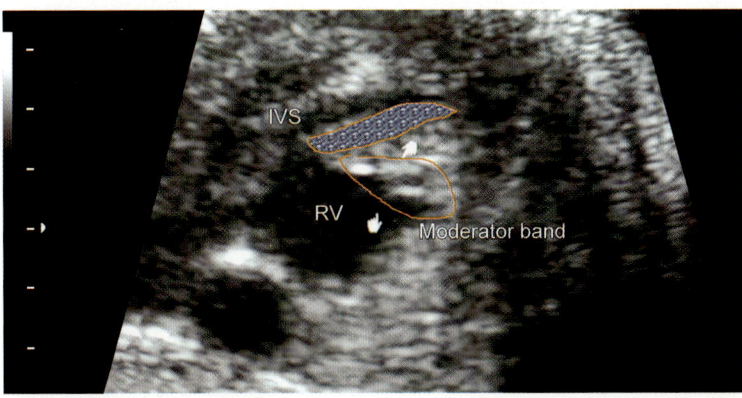

Figure 13.51 Labeled image showing the moderator band

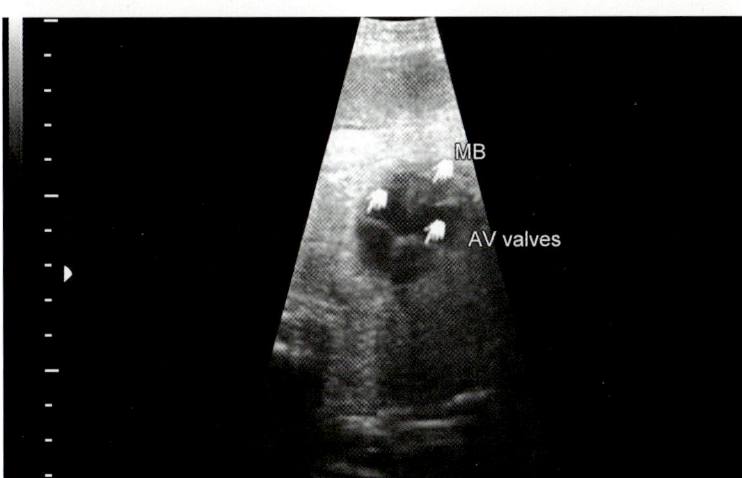

Figure 13.52A

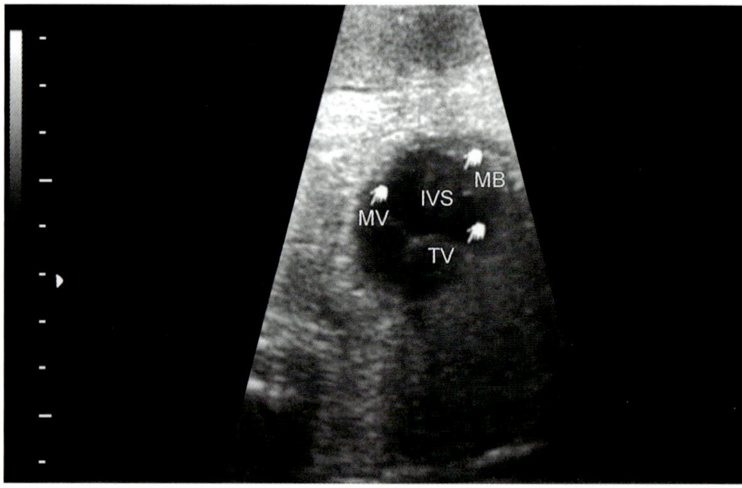

Figure 13.52B

Figures 13.52A and B Moderator band in four-chamber view

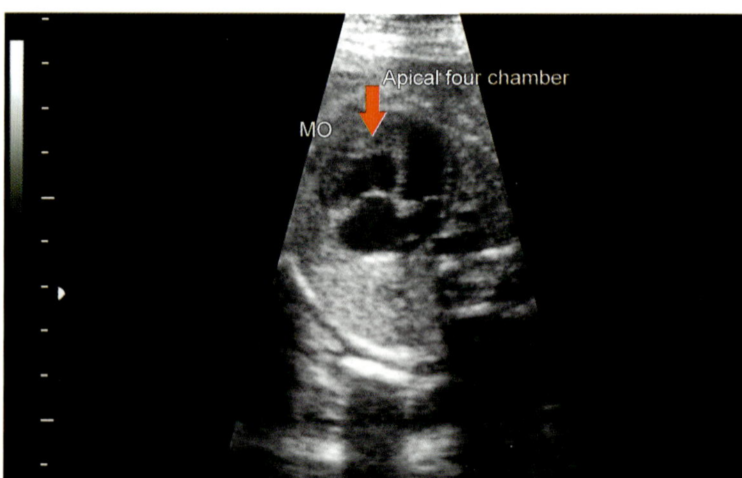

Figure 13.53 Moderator band in apical four-chamber

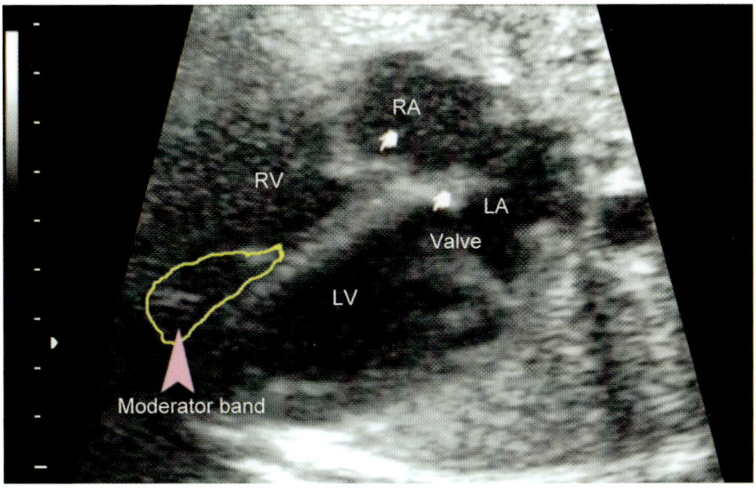

Figure 13.54 Labeled image of moderator band

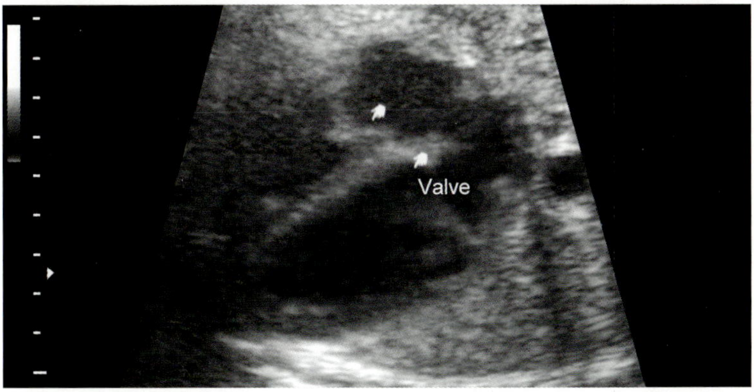

Figure 13.55 Two-dimensional four-chamber view with valve

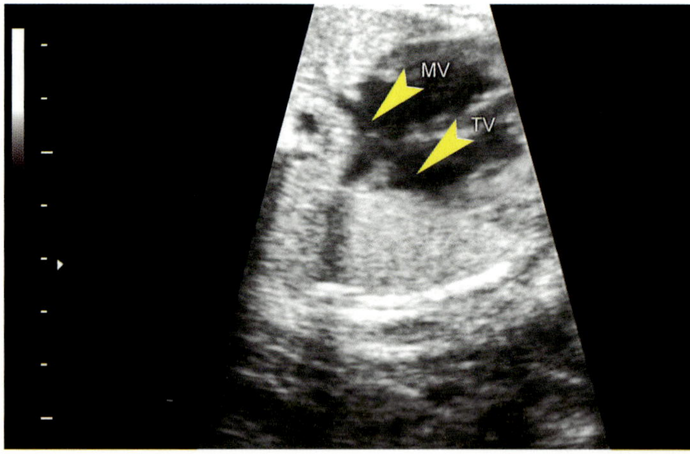

Figure 13.56 Open atrioventricular valves

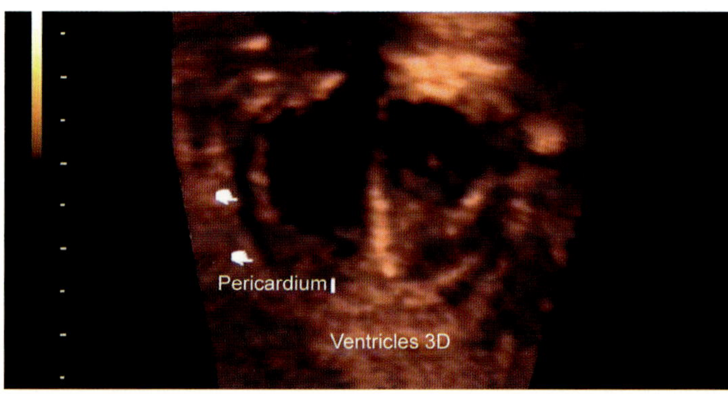

Figure 13.57 Pericardium in 3D heart

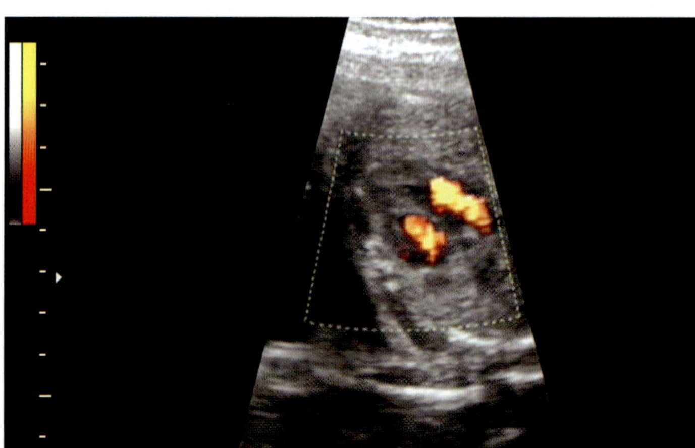

Figure 13.58 Power angio in heart

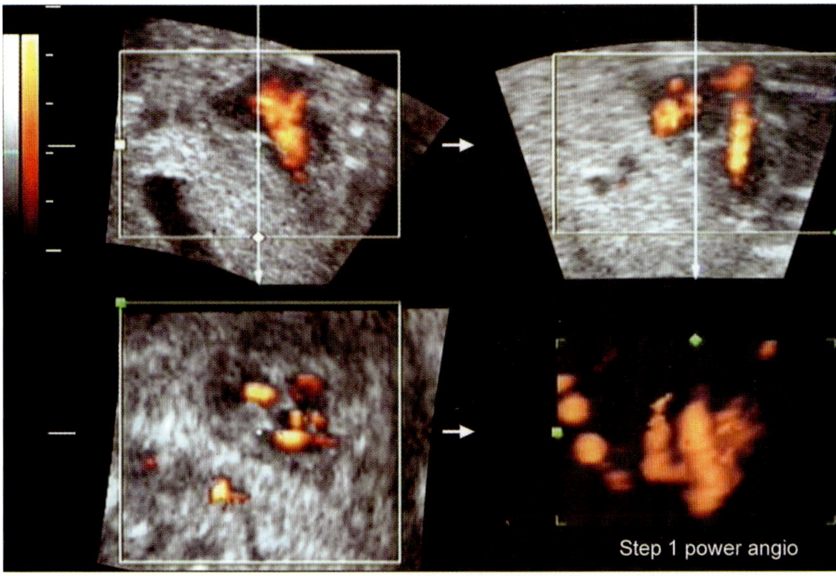

Figure 13.59 Power angio: Step 1

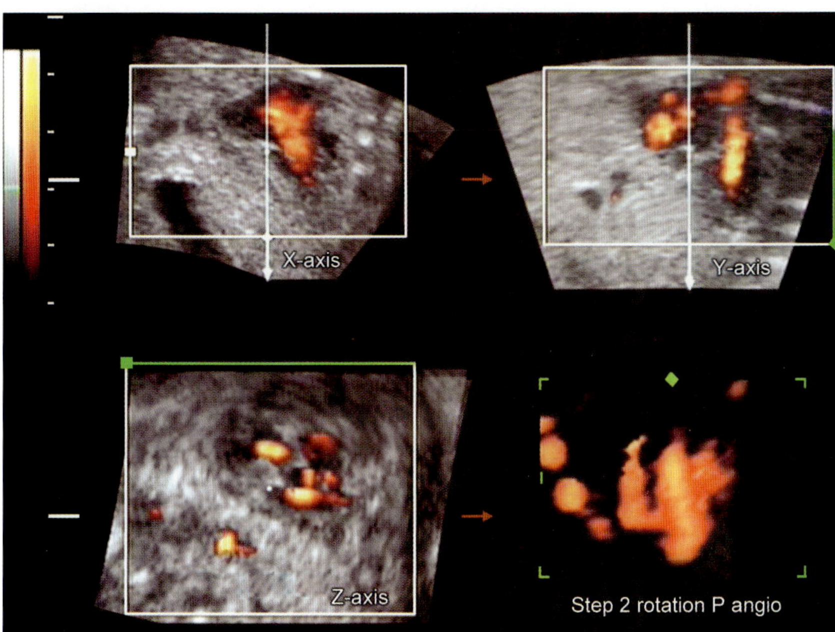

Figure 13.60 Power angio: Step 2, rotation

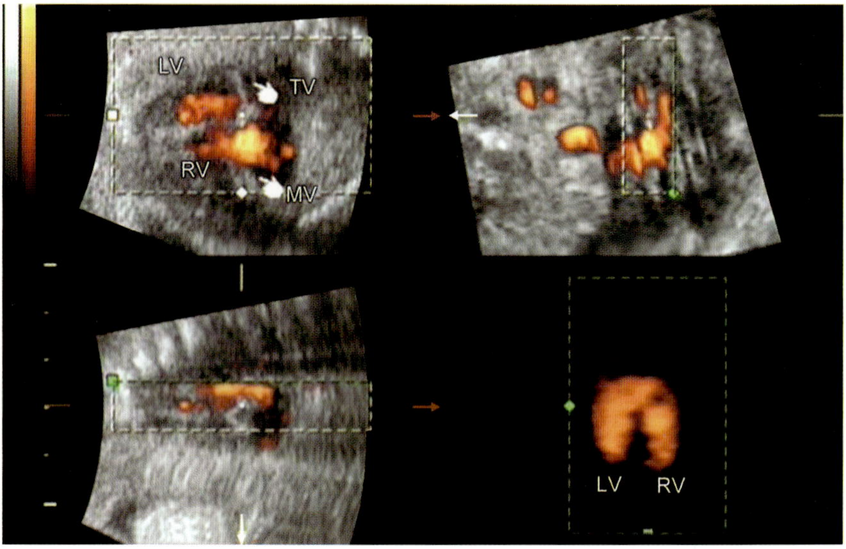

Figure 13.61 Final rotation of both the ventricles in power angio: Step 3

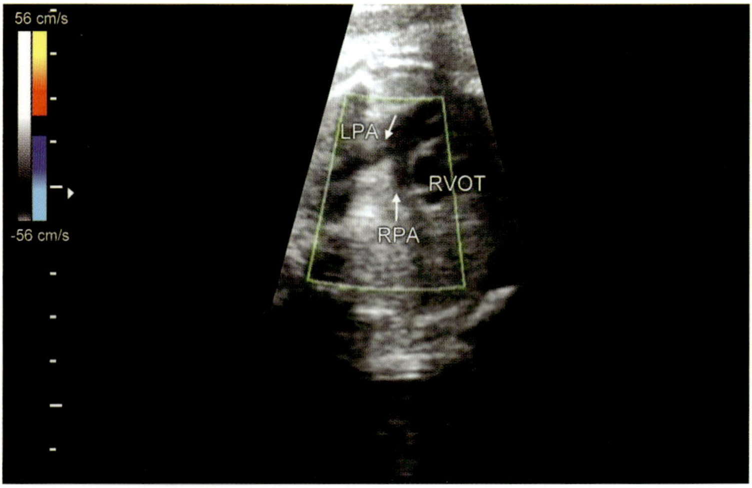

Figure 13.62A

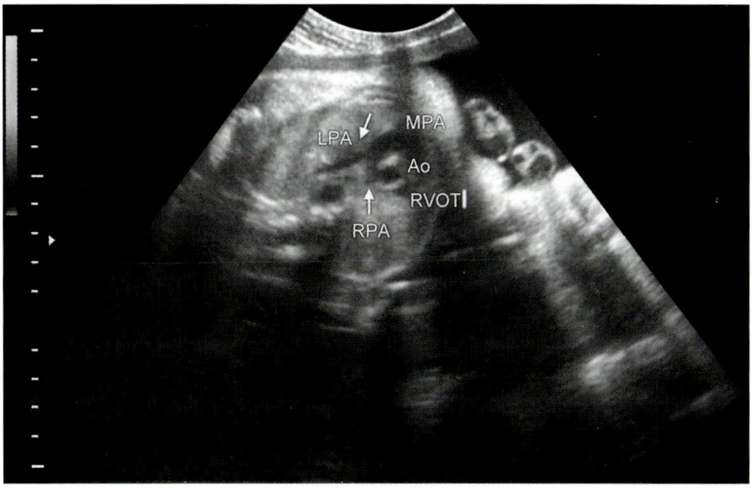

Figure 13.62B

Figures 13.62A and B Right ventricular outflow tract (RVOT)

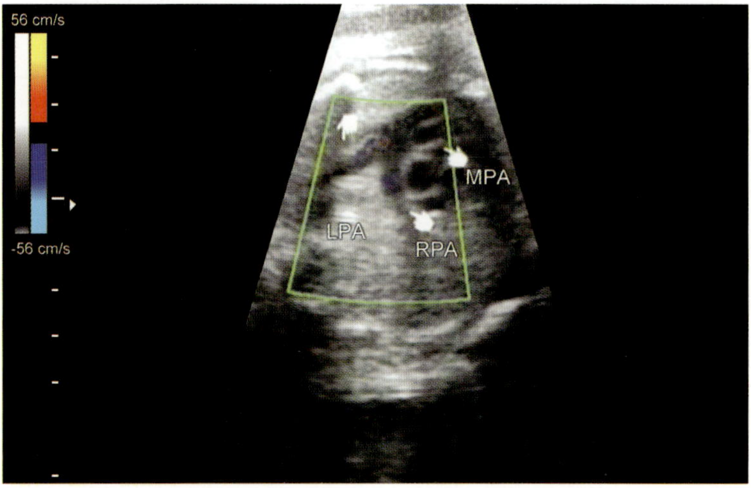

Figure 13.63 Right ventricular outflow tract (MPA, LPA, RPA)

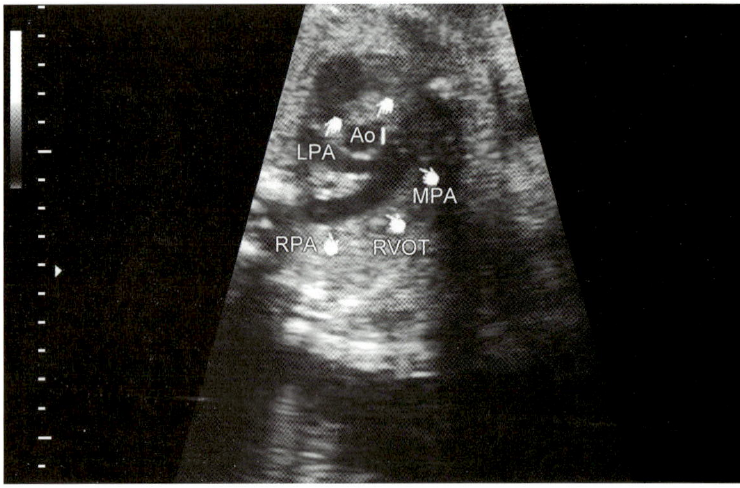

Figure 13.64 Right ventricular outflow tract—two-dimensional

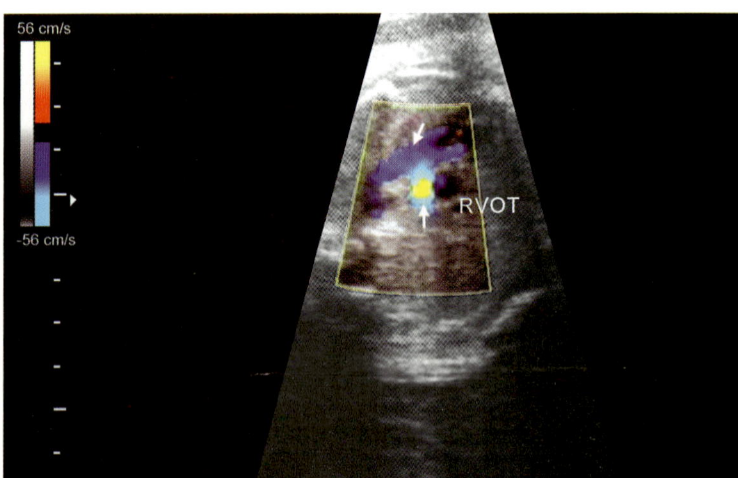

Figure 13.65 Right ventricular outflow tract in color Doppler

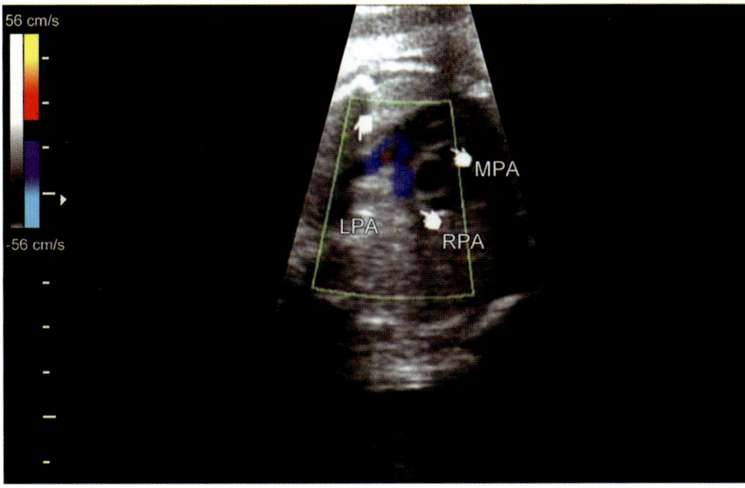

Figure 13.66 Labeled image in color, RVOT

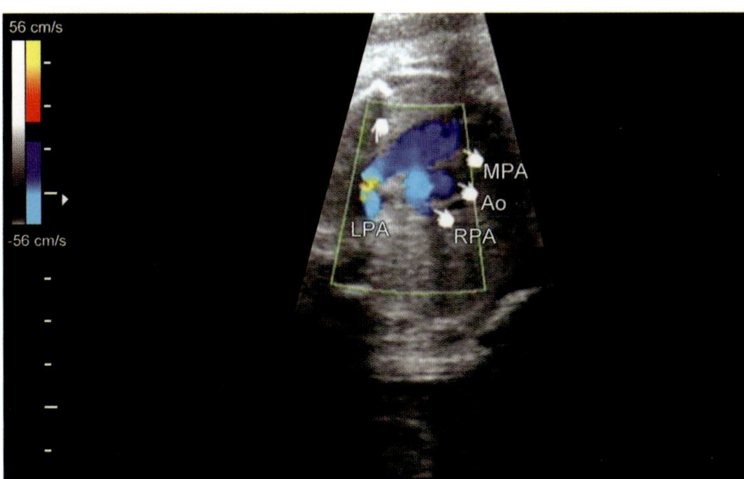

Figure 13.67 Labeled image of RVOT with color Doppler

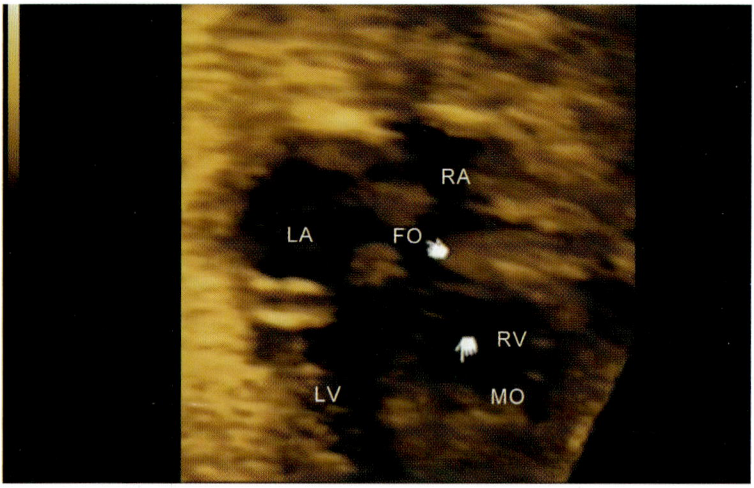

Figure 13.68 Schematic heart 3D

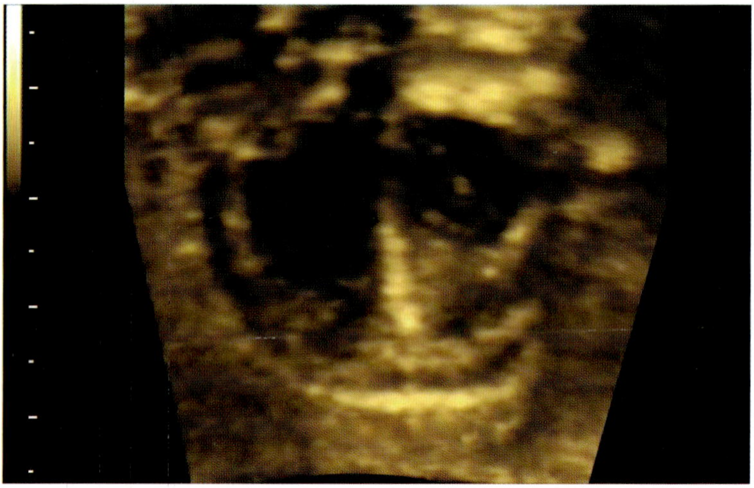

Figure 13.69 Ventricles 3D

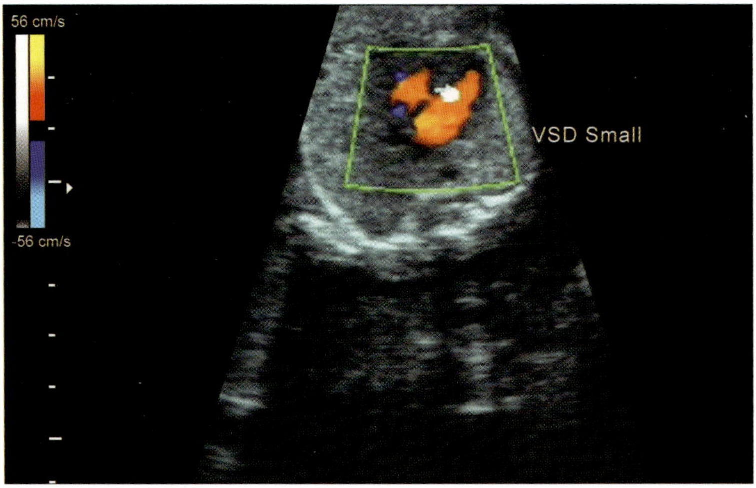

Figure 13.70 Small VSD

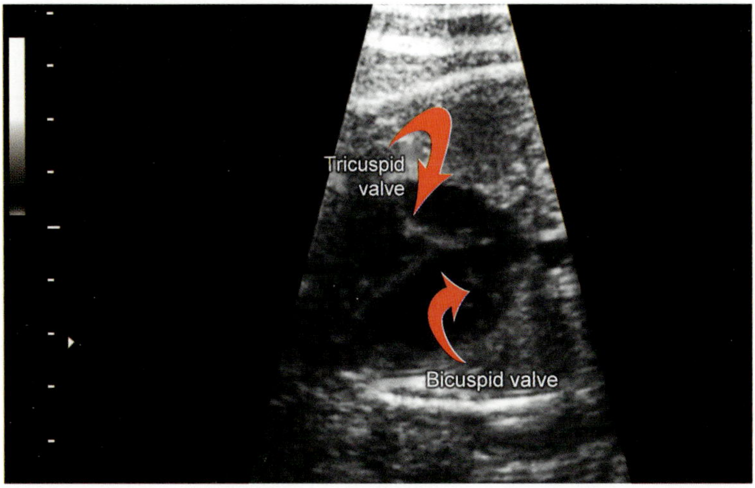

Figure 13.71 Valves labeled

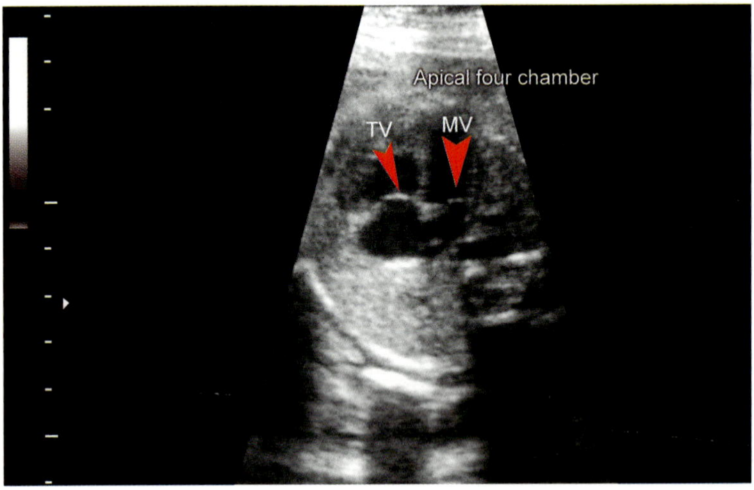

Figure 13.72 Valvular offset

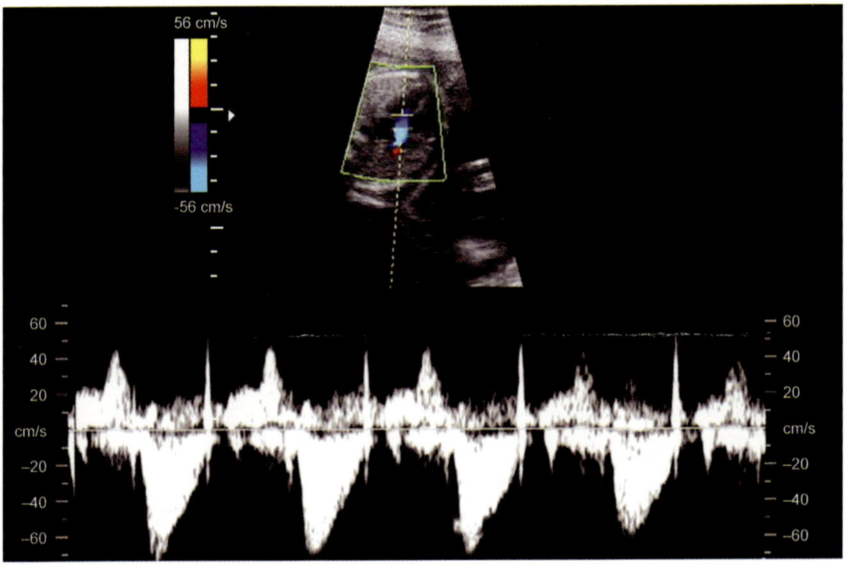

Figure 13.73 Valvular spectral Doppler

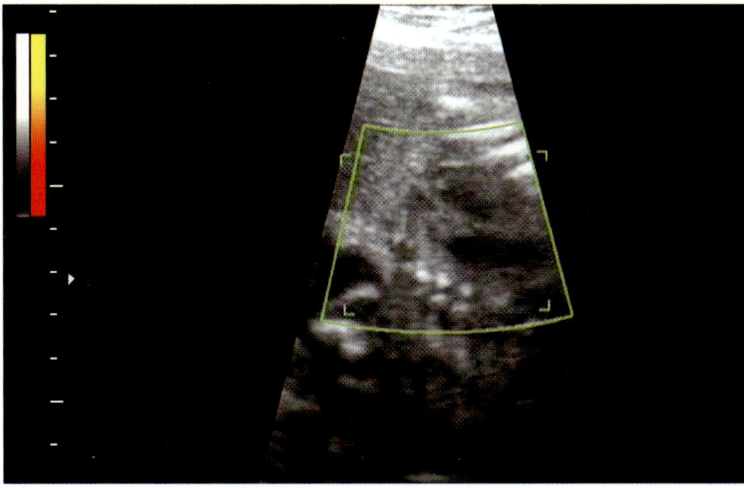

Figure 13.74 *Step 1:* Vascular tree power angio

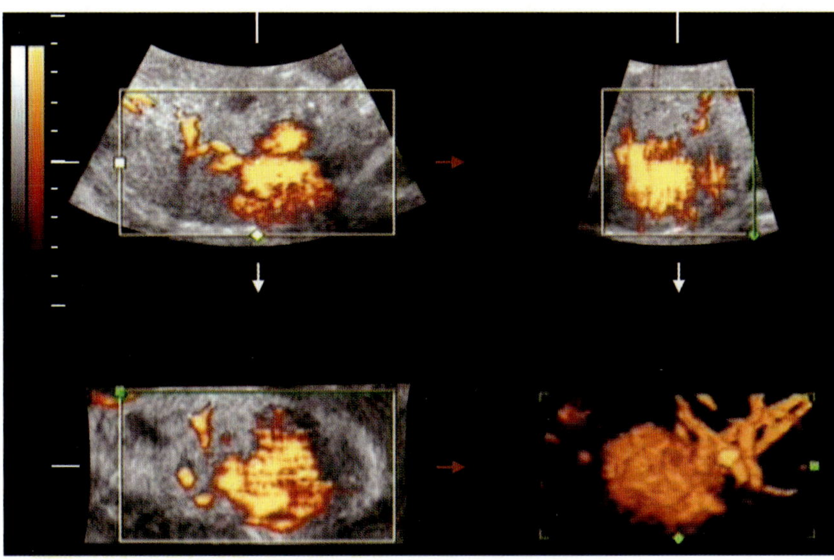

Figure 13.75 *Step 2:* Vascular tree 3D rendering

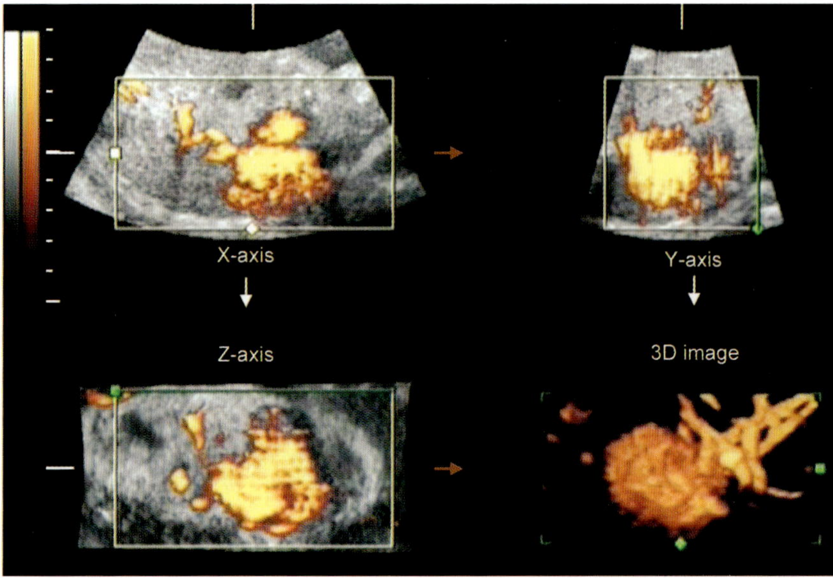

Figure 13.76 *Step 3:* Vascular tree final 3D image

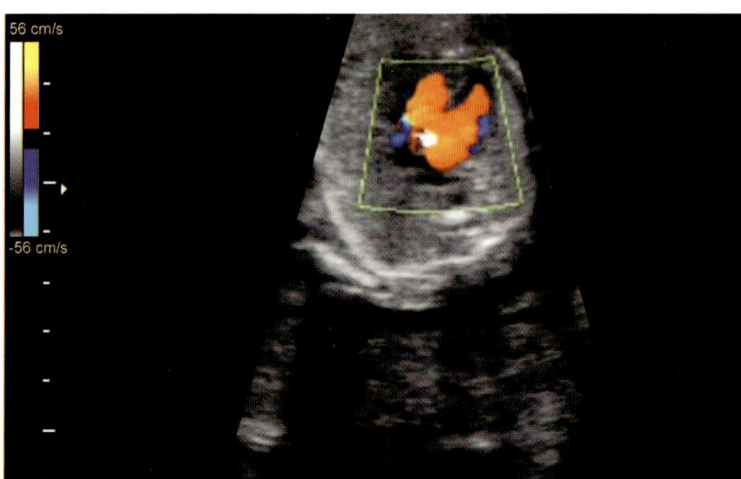

Figure 13.77 Ventricular septal defect with Doppler

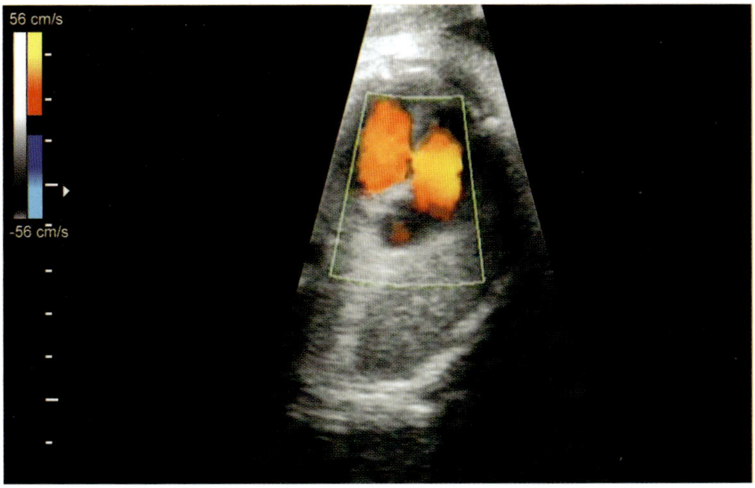

Figure 13.78 Ventricles in color Doppler

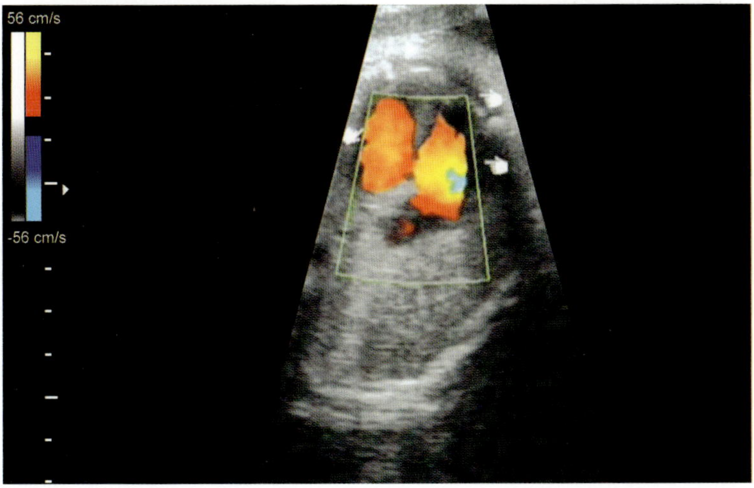

Figure 13.79 Ventricles in color Doppler and aliasing

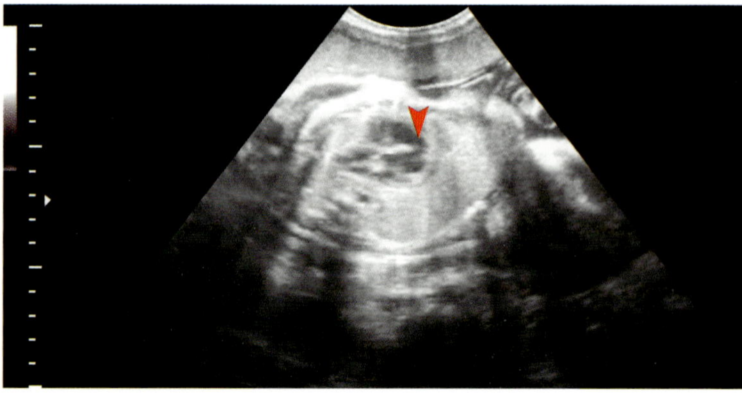

Figure 13.80 Large VSD

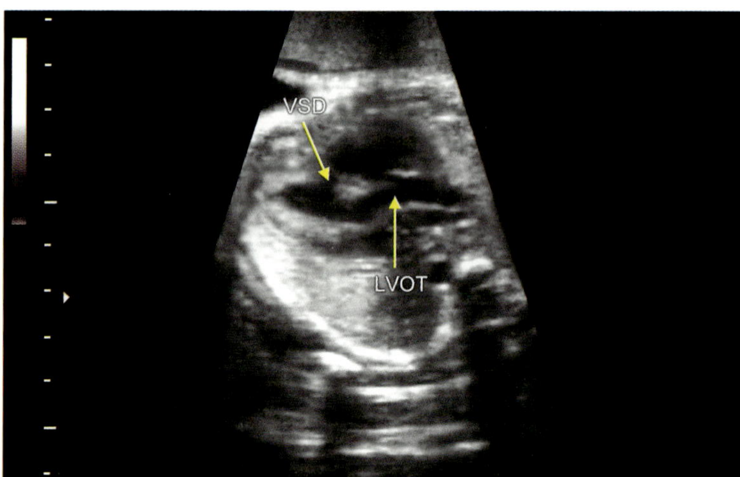

Figure 13.81 Large VSD with left ventricular outflow tract

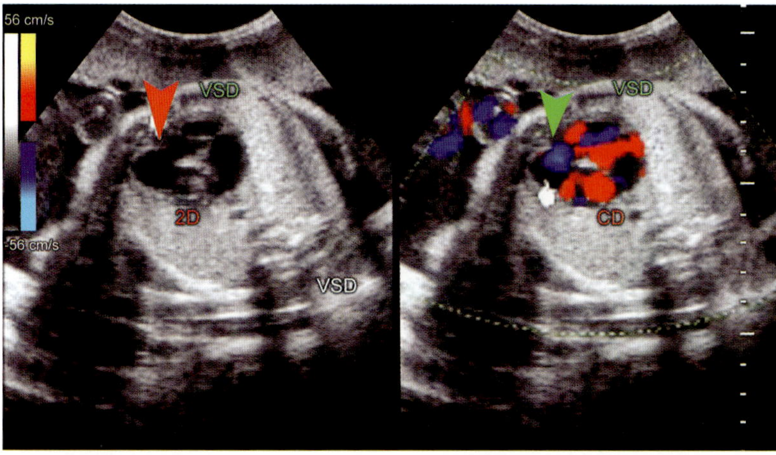

Figure 13.82 Ventricular septal defect with 2D and color Doppler

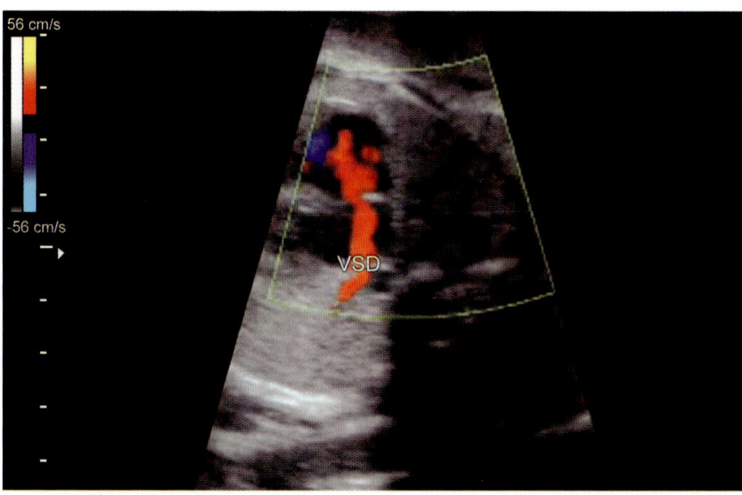

Figure 13.83 Ventricular septal defects

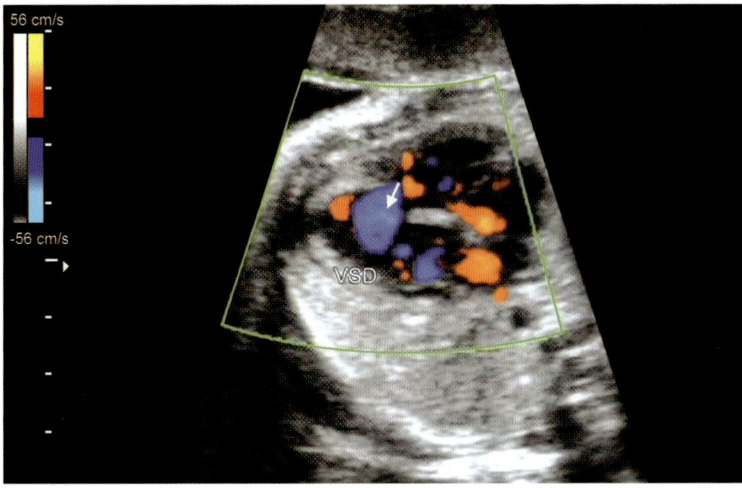

Figure 13.84 Ventricular septal defects with color Doppler

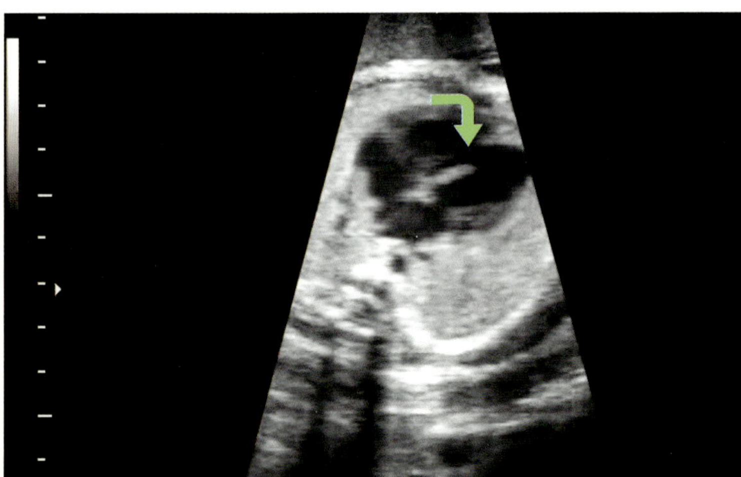

Figure 13.85 Ventricular septal defect: Large

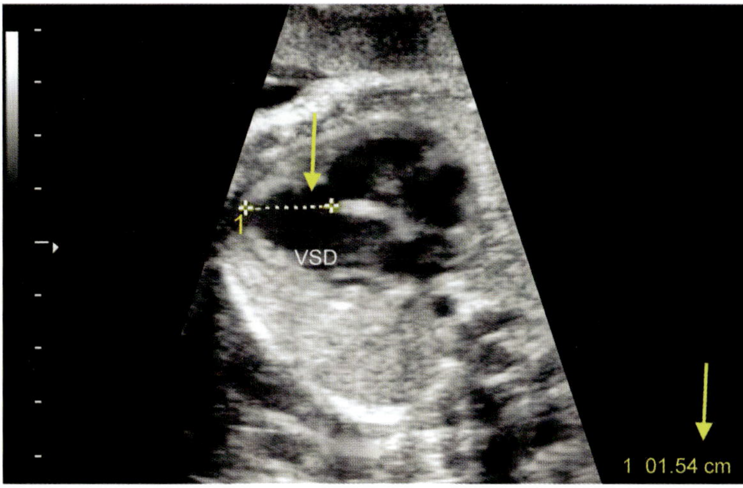

Figure 13.86 Measurement of septal defect

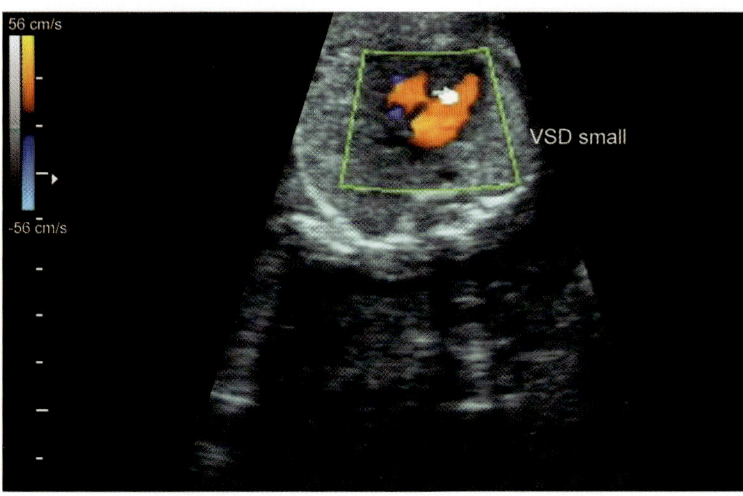

Figure 13.87 Ventricular septal defect: Small

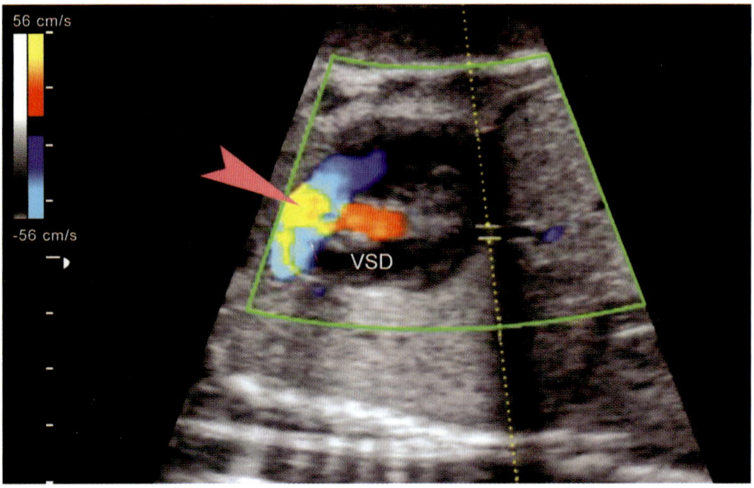

Figure 13.88 Aliasing in VSD

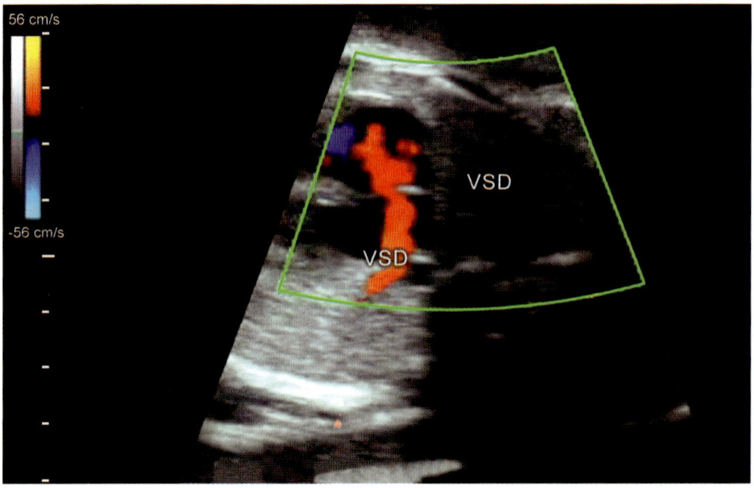

Figure 13.89 Large VSD with color Doppler

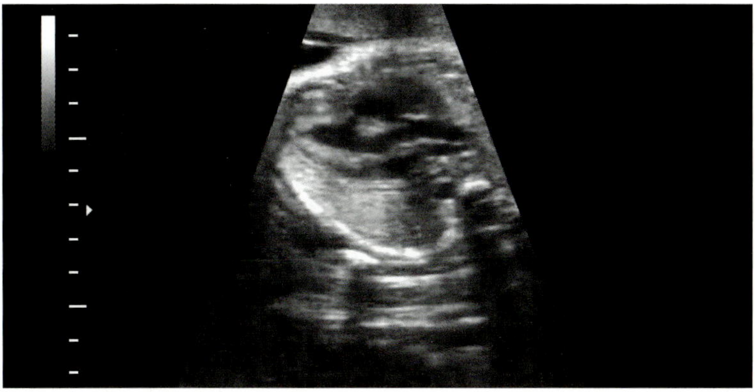

Figure 13.90 Ventricular septal defect with zoom

NUTSHELL

1. We have all images in 3D heart software for easy understanding like 3D valve cusp, foramen ovale, 3D heart reconstructive, IAS, moderator band.
2. Take 3-step action for 3D heart reconstruction step 1, take good section of heart in 2D mode, put 3D box in it step 2 take good sweep with steady hand ... we will get x, y, z plane images, take rotation of axis to get good 3D rendering image and label it.
3. Three-vessel view is PAS, i.e. pulmonary artery, aorta and superior vena cava we have to see for alignment, size and position.
4. Four-chamber view is basic view taken with different color and we can have cardiac axis measurement also.
5. Ductus venosus is vessel of millennium and there are easy way to get at level of color aliasing, 3D rendering images of ductus are well explained earlier.
6. Arch of aorta is well demonstrated in different color for easy understanding.
7. Color Doppler shows all view in color with crossing vessel.
8. Diaphragmatic hernia shown in 3D and rendering images in Figures 13.32 and 13.33.
9. Echogenic focus in heart has got chromosomal problem, if associated with some more soft marker, isolated echogenic focus in heart is better to be not mention, it will increase worry of parents.
10. Foramen ovale is shunt in heart which allows flow of blood from RA $\geq$ to LA and Figures 13.39 to 13.41 show all motion of it—open, close and flap.
11. Color gives us an idea regarding ventricular filling normally both ventricle should fill normally equal but in hypoplastic right heart we cannot see color in right ventricle in Figure 13.44.
12. LVOT in power angio and color mode gives clear idea.
13. VSD will be clearly seen in Figure 13.47.
14. M-mode is for easy understanding of wall motion and size of atria and ventricle.

15. Moderator band see at base of right ventricle and it is a diagnostic sign for it.
16. Both valve move freely and seen four-chamber view.
17. Ventricle can be reconstructed in rendering image by three step (Figures 13.59 to 13.61).
18. RVOT is beautifully seen in Figures 13.62A and B and also seen in 2D and color up to Figure 13.67.
19. Both ventricle seen clearly in Figure 13.69 with moderator band.
20. Vascular tree seen in power angio mode in Figure 13.74.
21. VSD is seen clearly when color used and zoom.

14

Fetal Heart Images (Abnormal)

This chapter gives an idea regarding different abnormal fetal heart images and how it look in 2D and 3D with color and in transurethral incision (TUI) images.

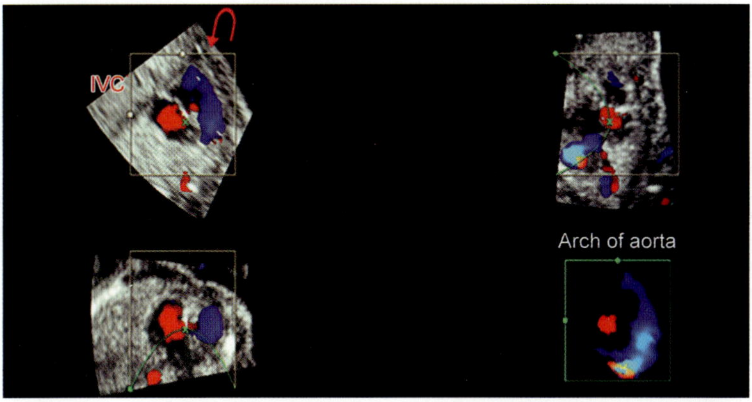

Figure 14.1 Hypoplastic left heart syndrome (HLHS) in multiplaner image with color rendering mode shows no color in left heart and shows arch of aorta with color aliasing

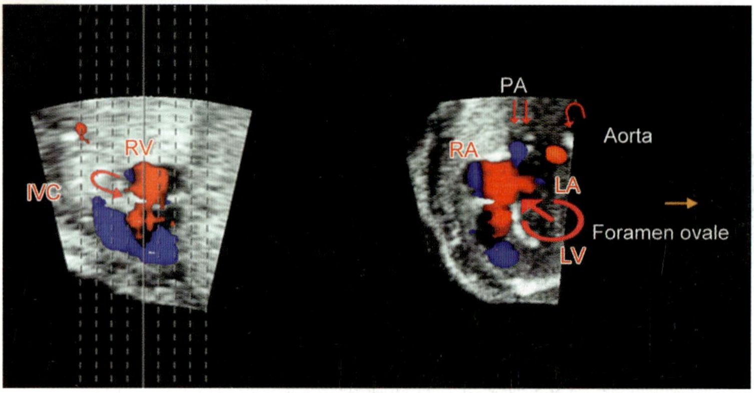

Figuer 14.2 HLHS with color image shows no color in left heart with land mark of foramen ovale

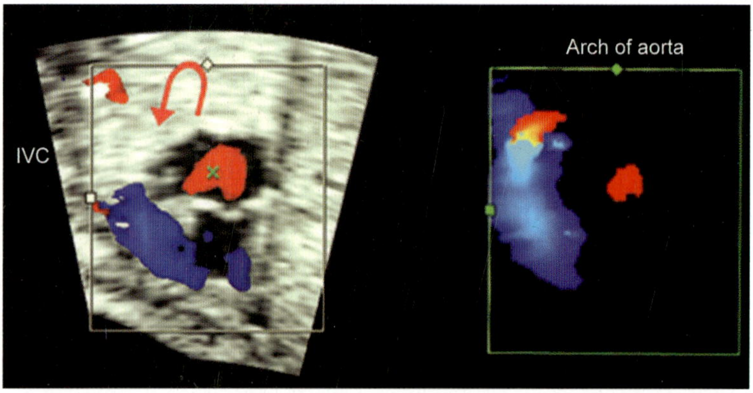

Figure 14.3 HLHS with color rendering shows arch of aorta and interventricular septum

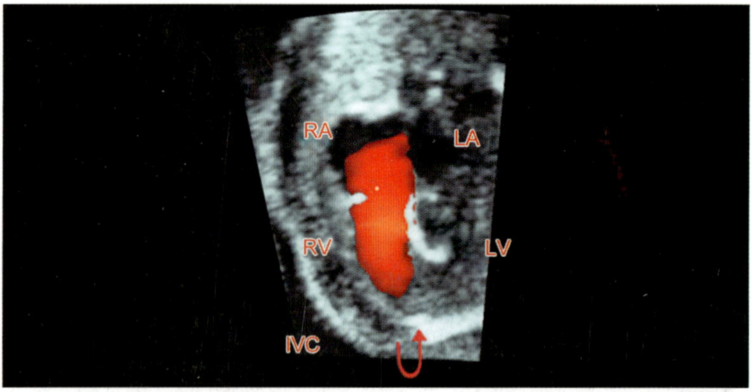

Figure 14.4 This is classical image of HLHS and shows right atrium, left atrium and right ventricle full of color while left ventricle has no color

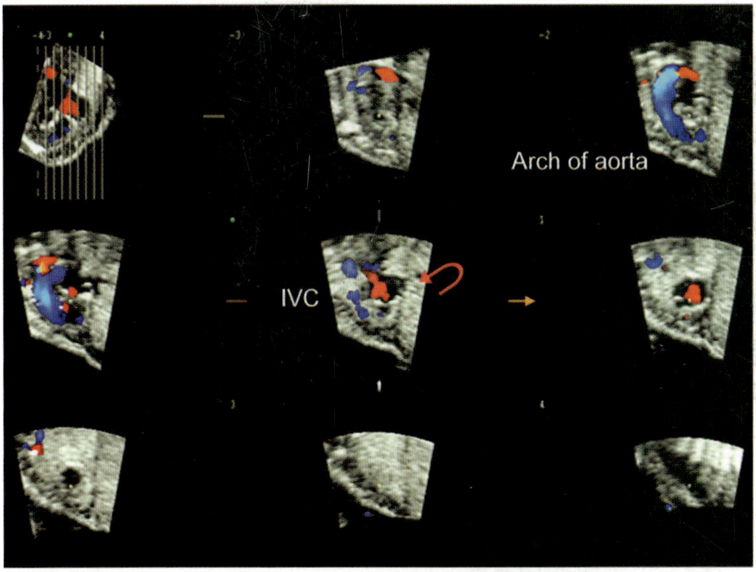

Figure 14.5 TUI of HLHS showing different 9 images at different cutting levels like stomach bubble in image 7 and IVC in image 5

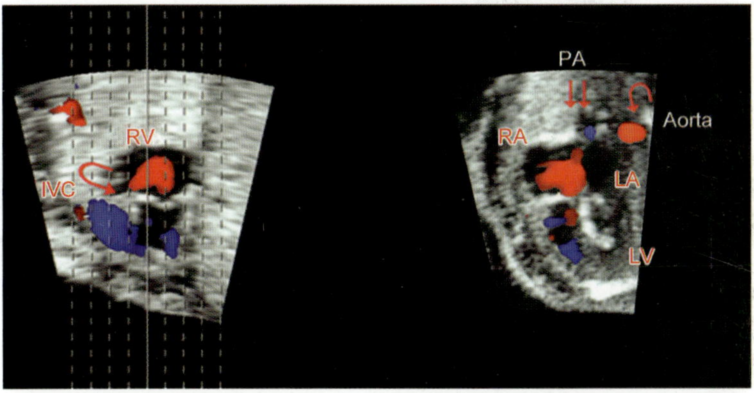

Figure 14.6 HLHS in relation with right ventricle in different angles

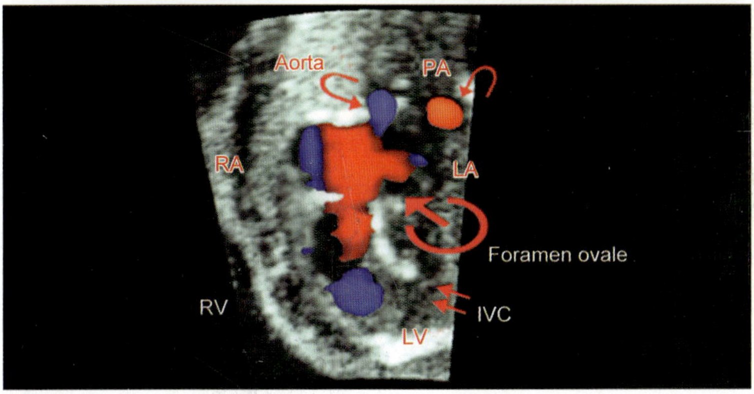

Figure 14.7 HLHS with label

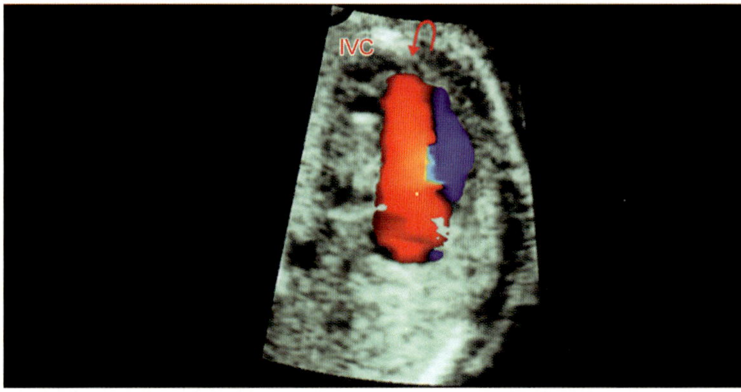

Figure 14.8 Landmark image of HLHS with clear no color flow in left heart with color aliasing flow in right heart

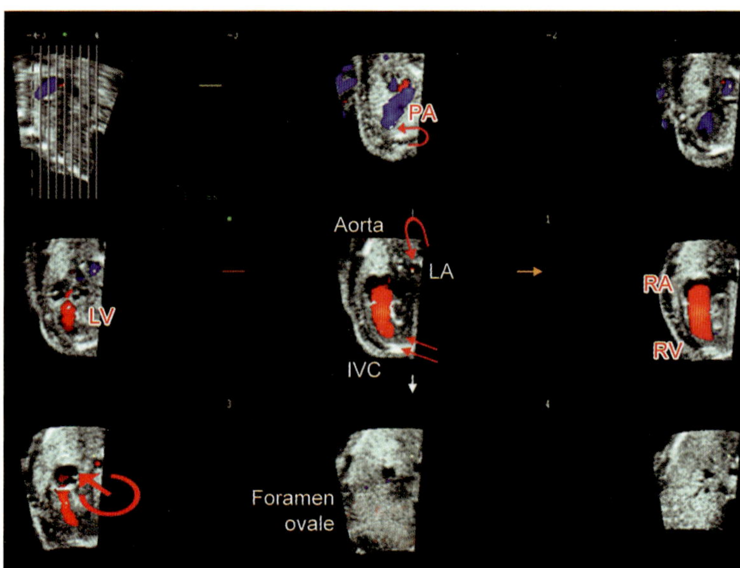

Figure 14.9 Tomographic ultrasound imaging (TUI) of HLHS with no color pickup in left heart in every image with labeling

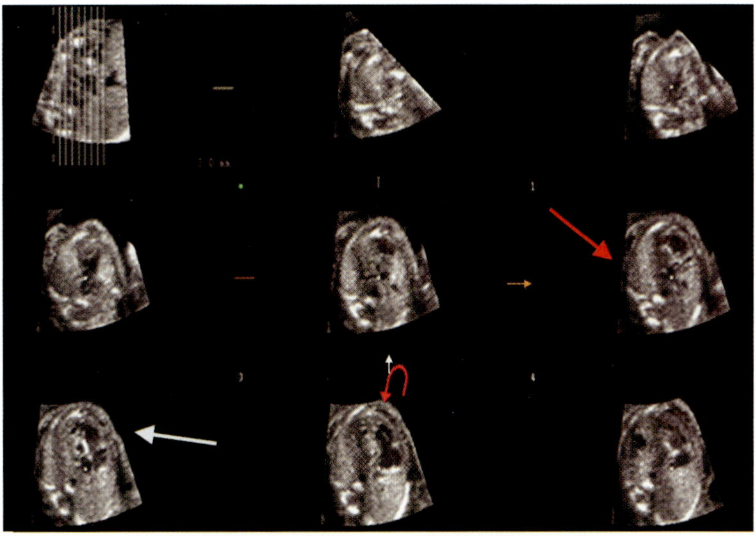

Figure 14.10 HLHS without color and can be seen as hypoechoic left ventricle compare to hyperechoic right ventricle

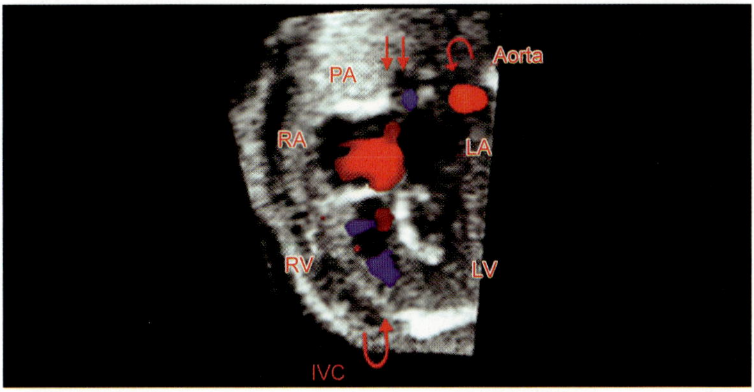

Figure 14.11 Hypoplastic left leart syndrome (HLHS) with surrounding label

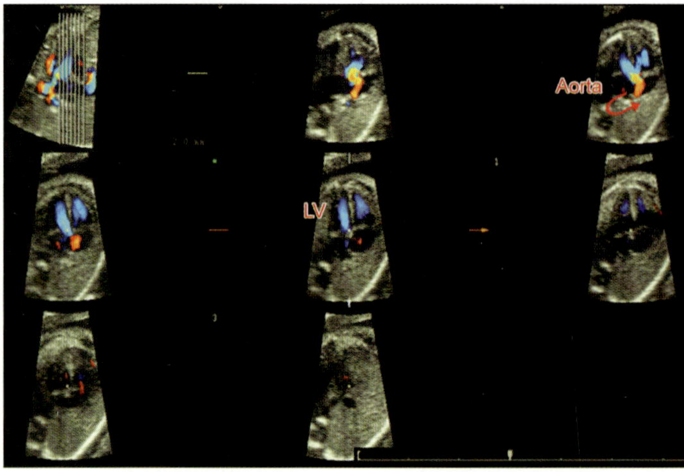

Figure 14.12 Tetralogy of Fallot in TUI shows over-riding of aorta

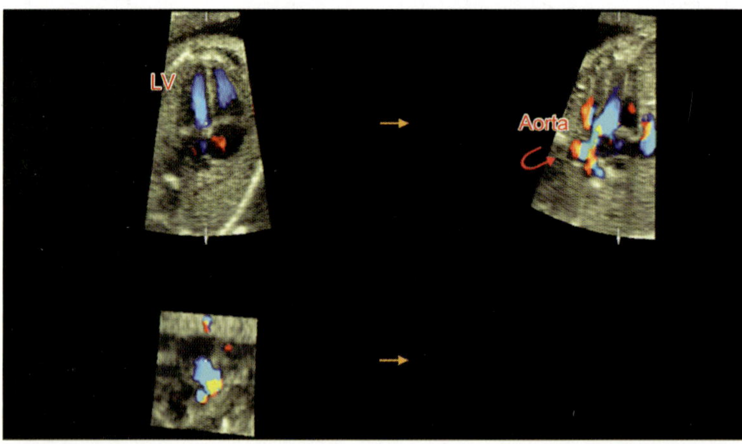

Figure 14.13 Tetralogy of Fallot (TOF) In color shows over-riding of aorta

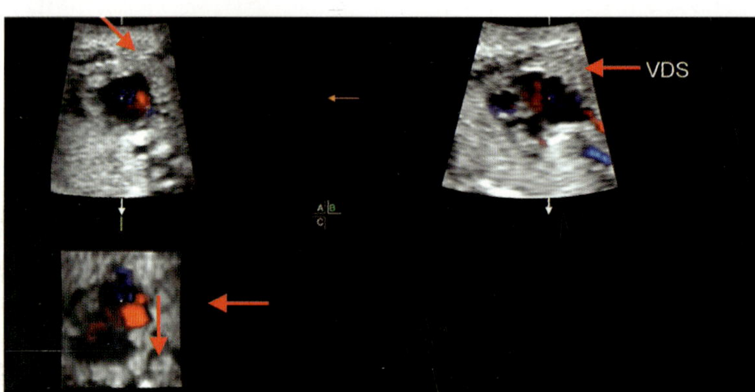

Figure 14.14 Ventricular septal defect in TOF with right ventricular hypertrophy

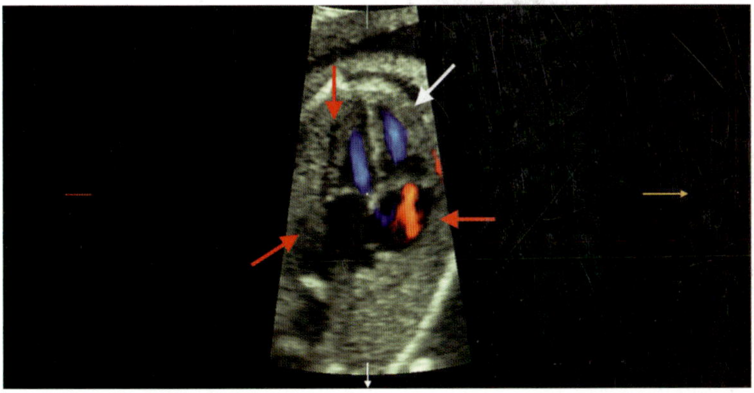

Figure 14.15 Normal four-chamber view in TOF

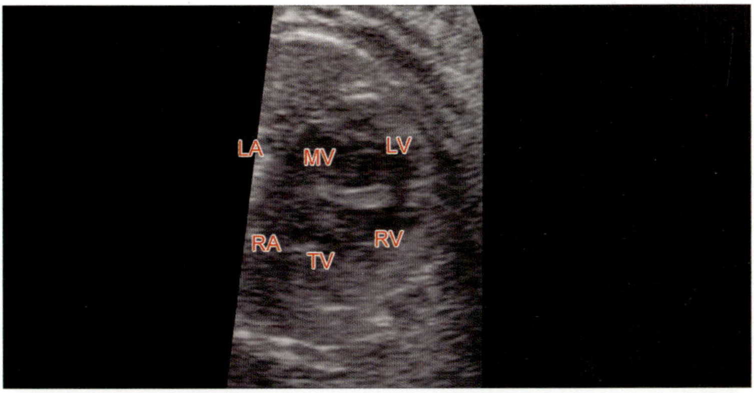

Figure 14.16 Ventricular septal defect

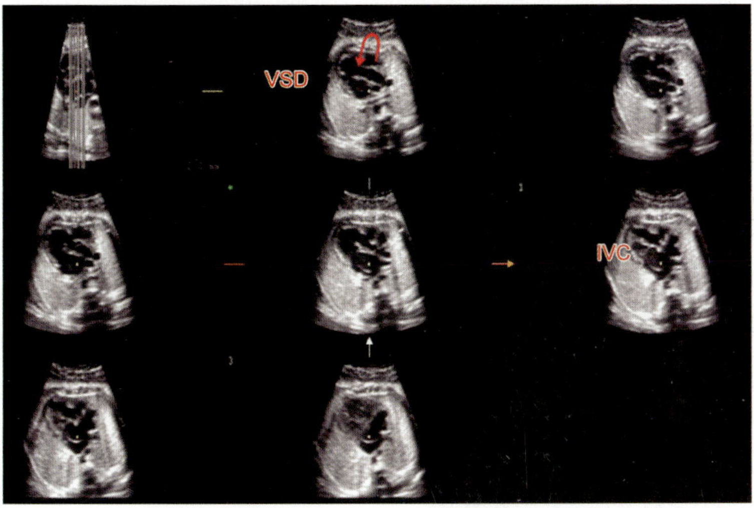

Figure 14.17 VSD in TUI shows VSD in IVS

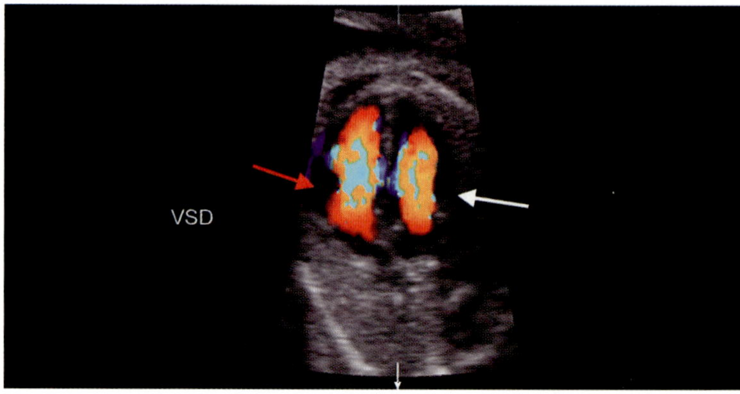

Figure 14.18 VSD seen tetralogy of Fallot with color aliasing

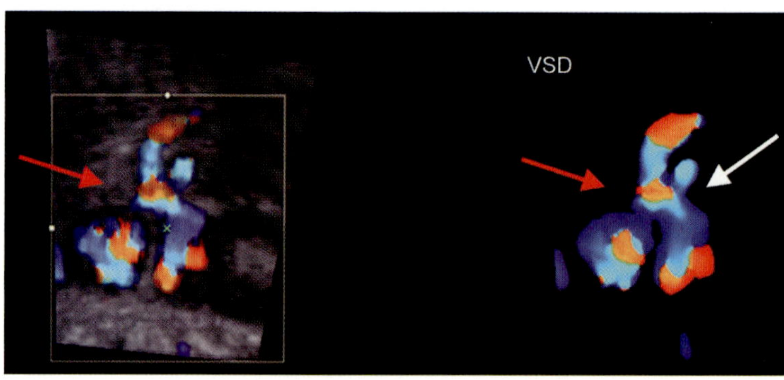

Figure 14.19 VSD in TOF with color aliasing in color angio

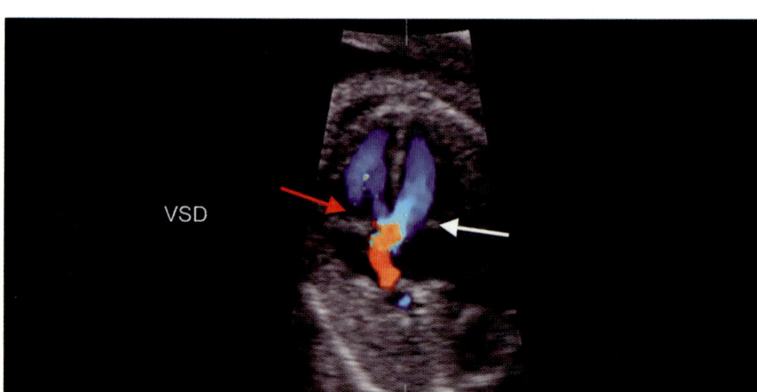

Figure 14.20 VSD with regurgitation flowing right ventricle in TOF

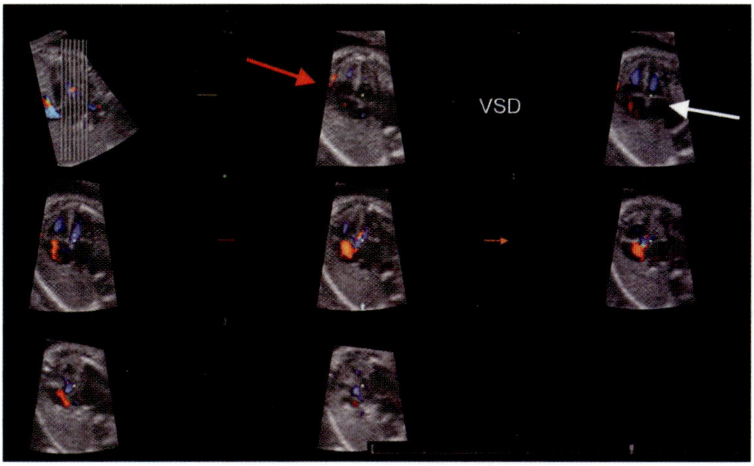

Figure 14.21 VSD with TUI in TOF

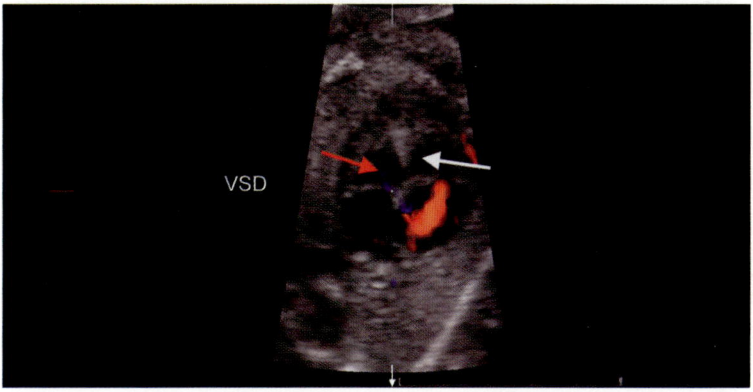

Figure 14.22 VSD seen in TOF

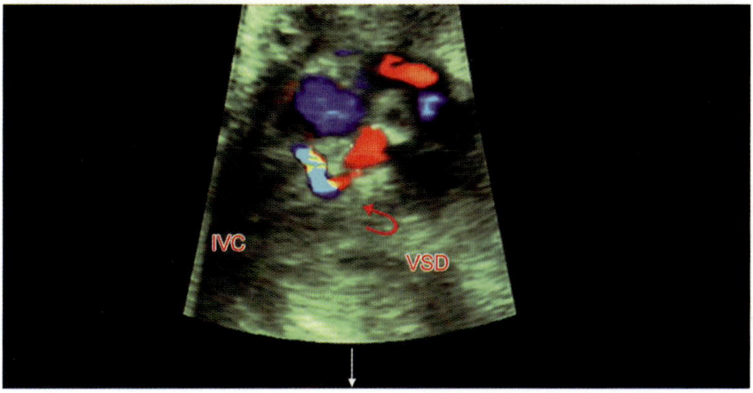

Figure 14.23 VSD in color true diagnostic

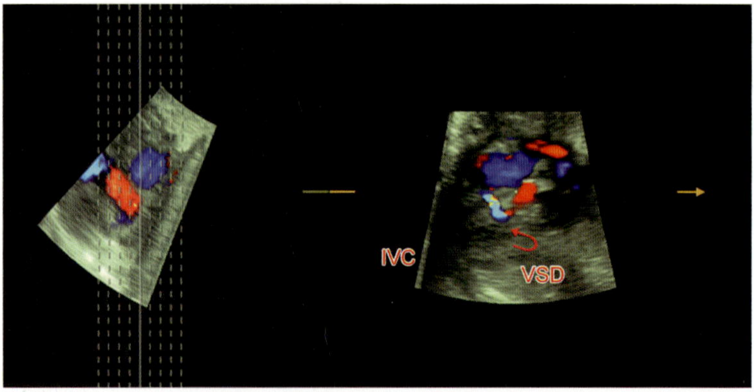

Figure 14.24 VSD in color with TUI

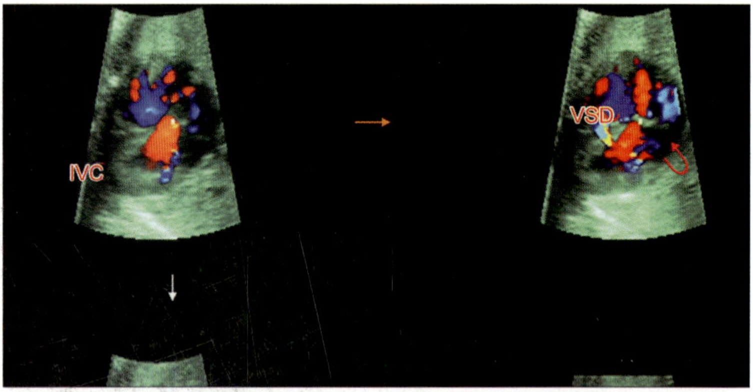

Figure 14.25 VSD in color with different angle

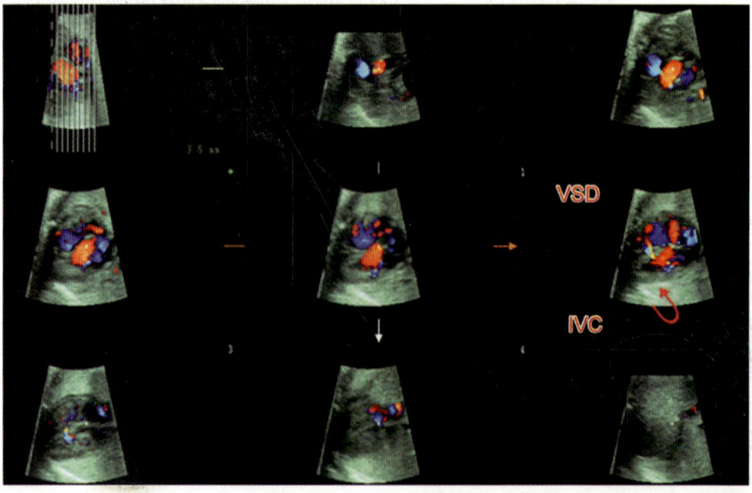

Figure 14.26 VSD in TUI

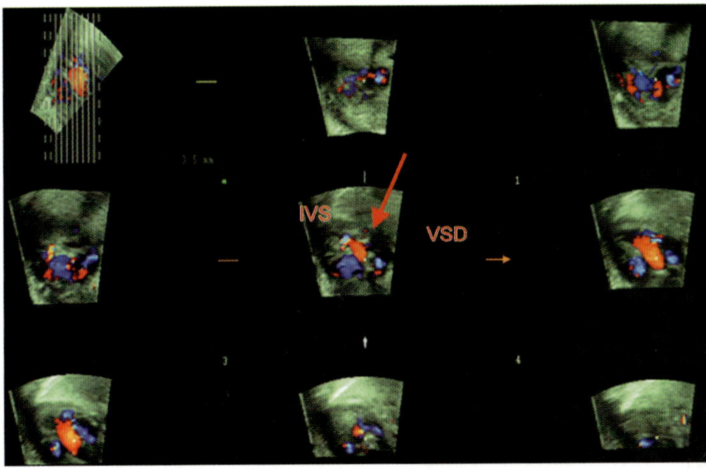

Figure 14.27 VSD in TUI with different cut

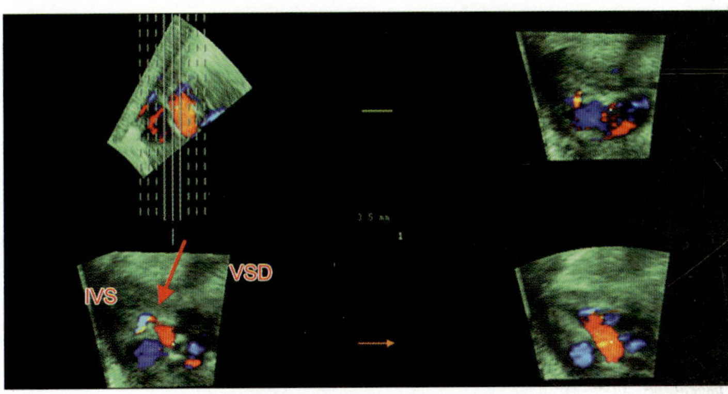

Figure 14.28 VSD with lateral angulation

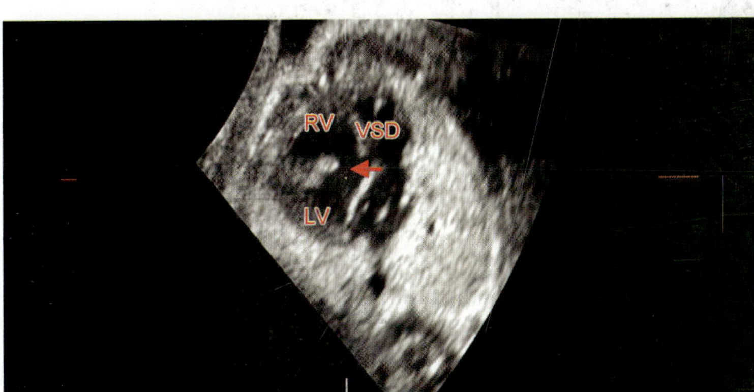

Figure 14.29 Large VSD in 2D

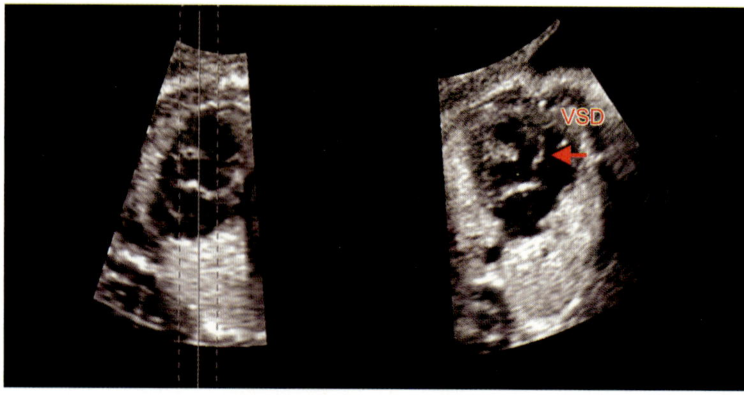

Figure 14. 30 Large VSD in 2D

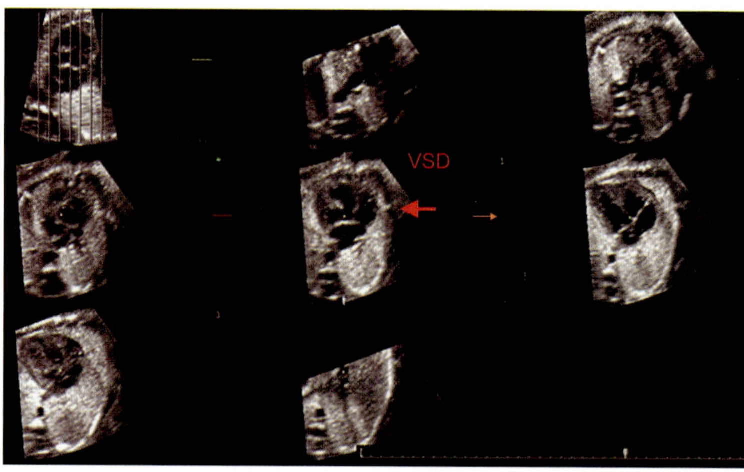

Figure 14.31 Large VSD in TUI

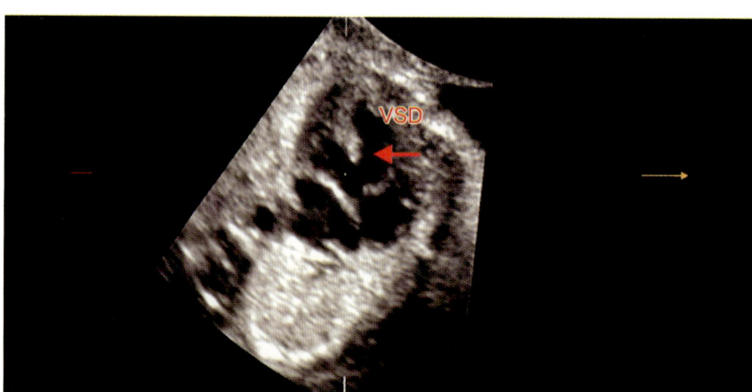

Figure 14.32 Large VSD gap in 2D

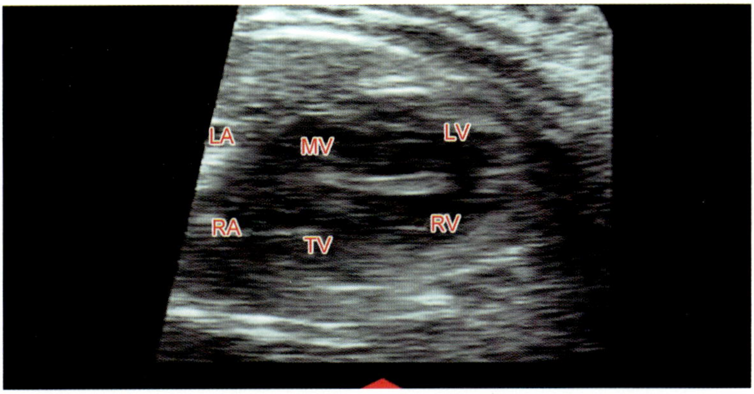

Figure 14.33 Large VSD in 2D

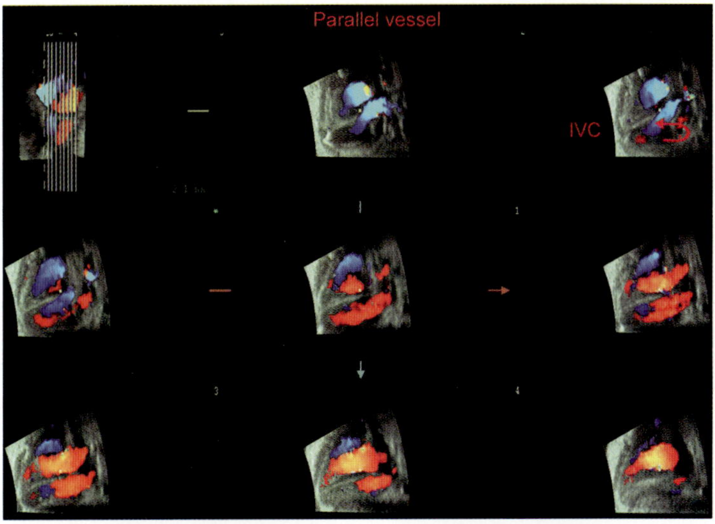

Figure 14.34 Transposition of the great vessel see both tract running parellel to each other, normallly they cross at 90°

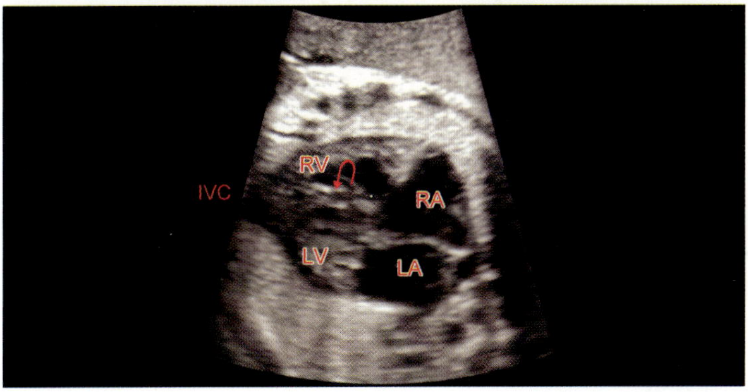

Figure 14.35 Normal four-chamber view in transposition of the great vessel (TGA)

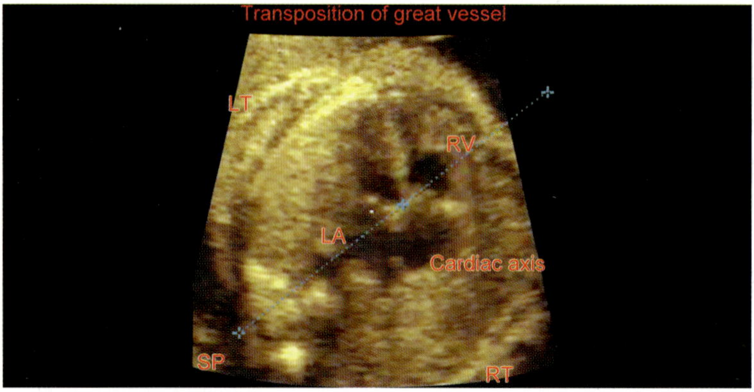

Figure 14.36 TGA with normal cardiac axis

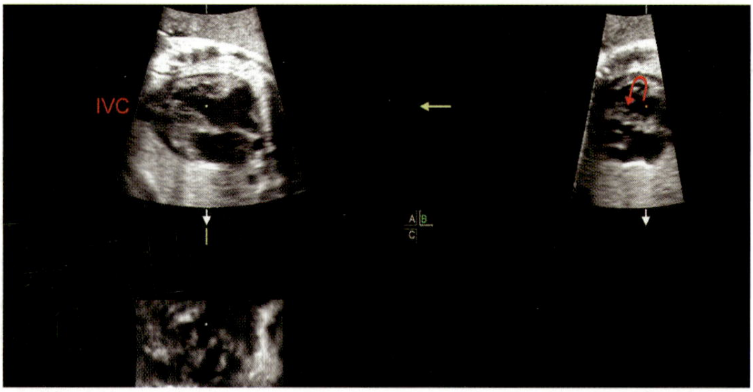

Figure 14.37 Normal four-chamber view in TGA

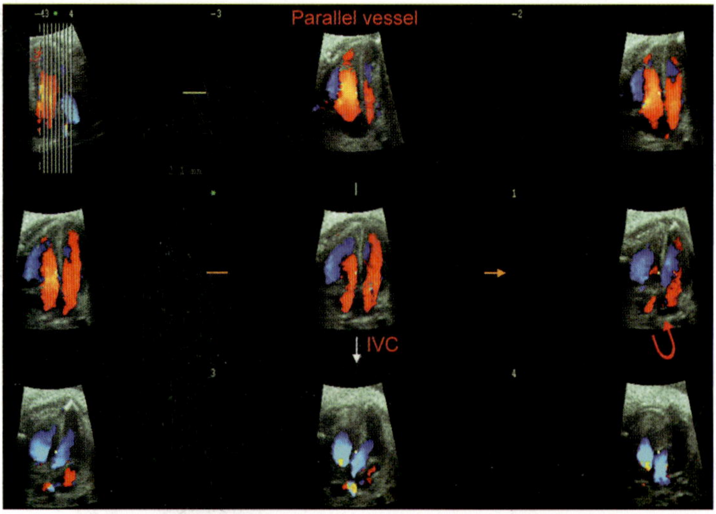

Figure 14.38 See both tract RVOT and LVOT in parrerel line in TGA

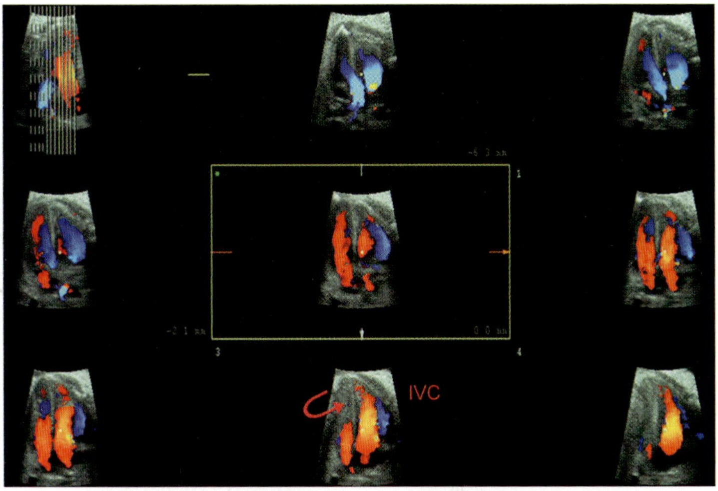

Figure 14.39 Both great vessel aorta and pulmonary are arising form right ventricle and left ventricle

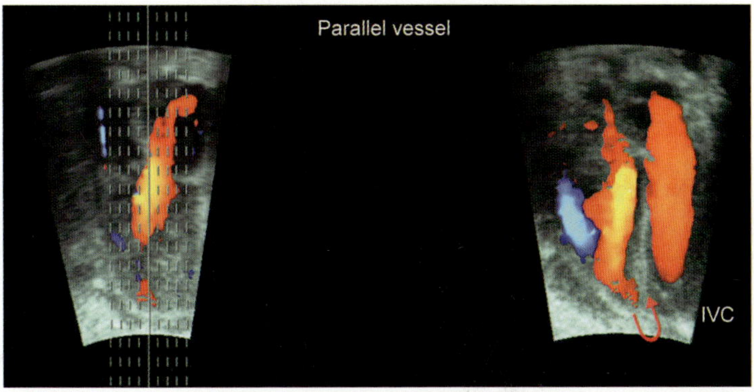

Figure 14.40 Aorta from right ventricle and pulmonary from left ventricle both are paralled

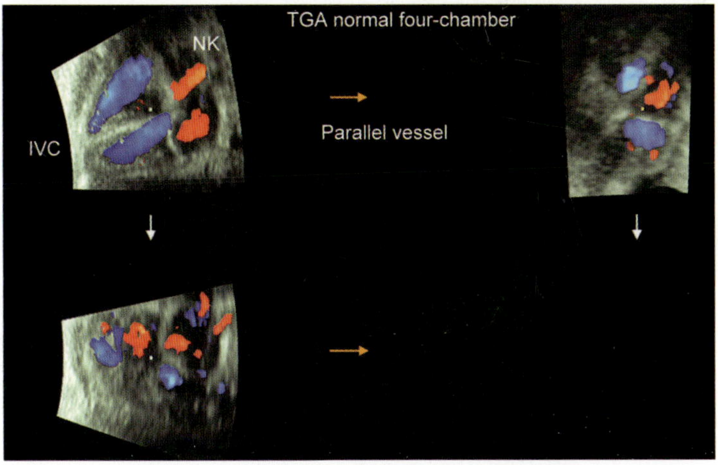

Figure 14.41 Both outflow tracts in same line

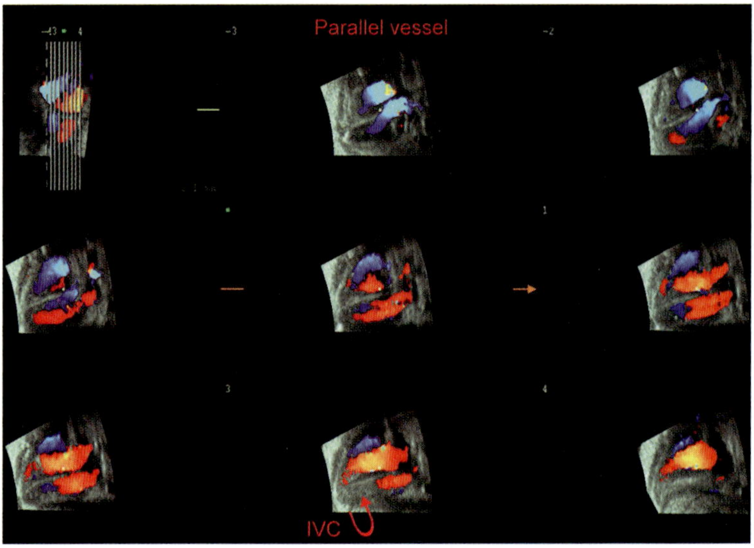

Figure 14.42 Both outflow tarcts in TGA in TUI

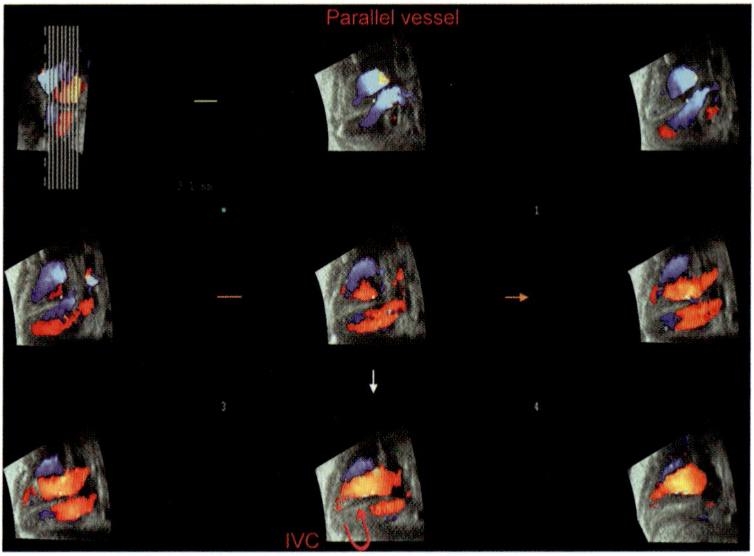

Figure 14.43 Both outflow tracts in same line in TUI

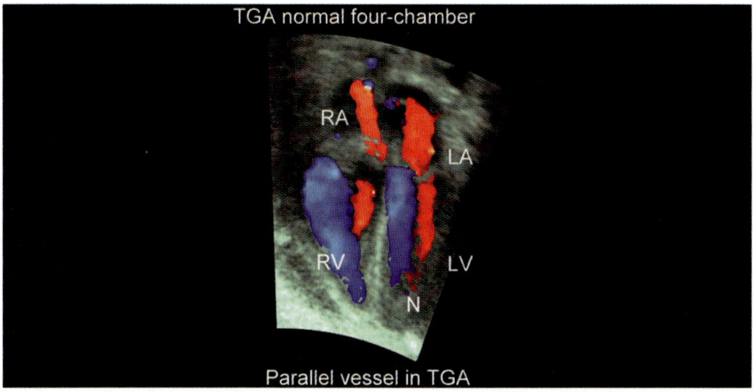

Figure 14.44 No corssing vessel in color in TGA

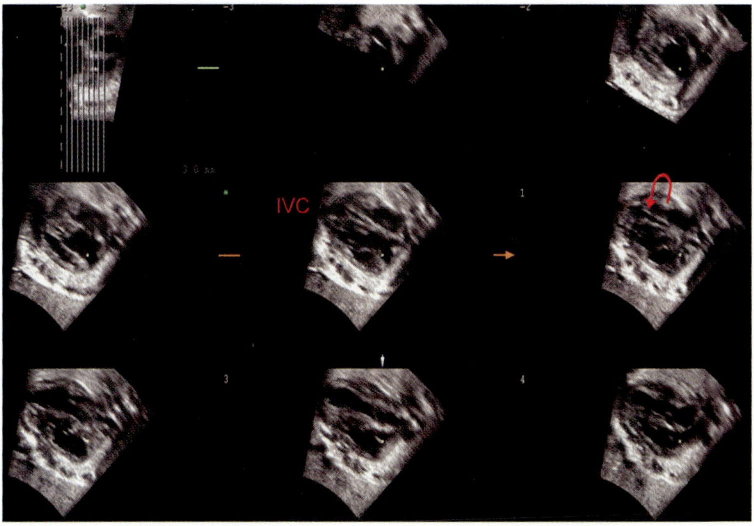

Figure 14.45 Normal four-chamber in TGA in TUI

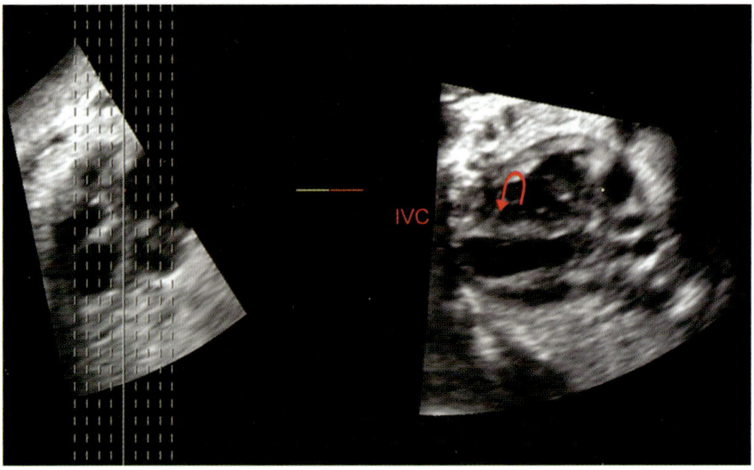

Figure 14.46 Normal four-chamber in TGA

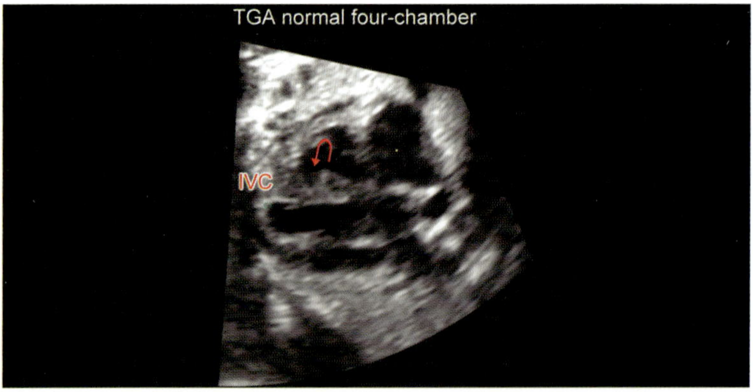

Figure 14.47 Normal four-chamber in TGA

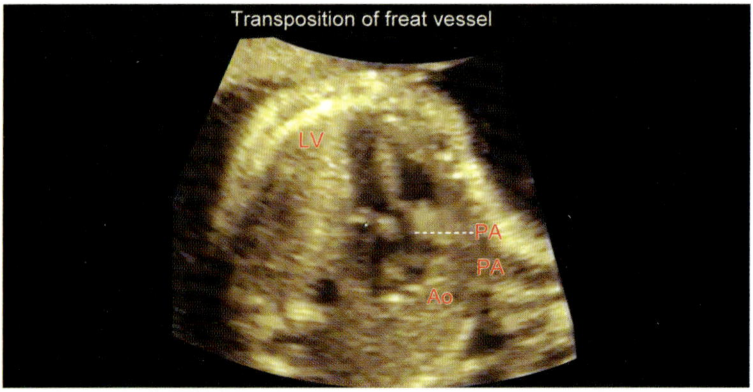

Figure 14.48 Aorta is arising from RV and pulmonary from LV

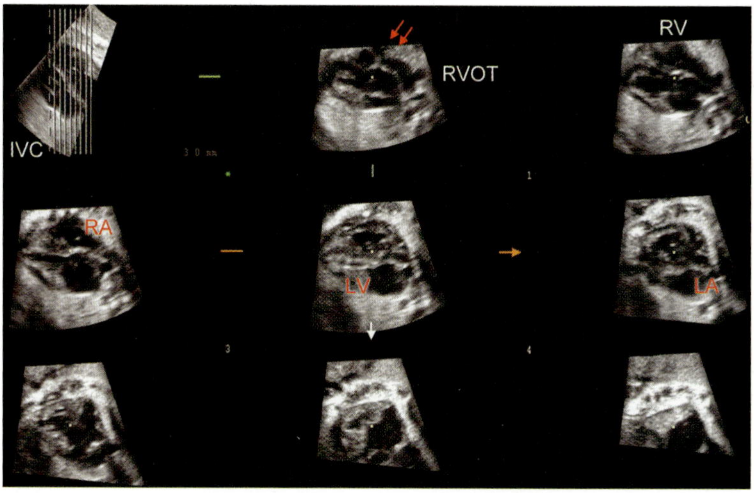

Figure 14.49 Right ventricular outflow tract (RVOT) in aorta in TGA

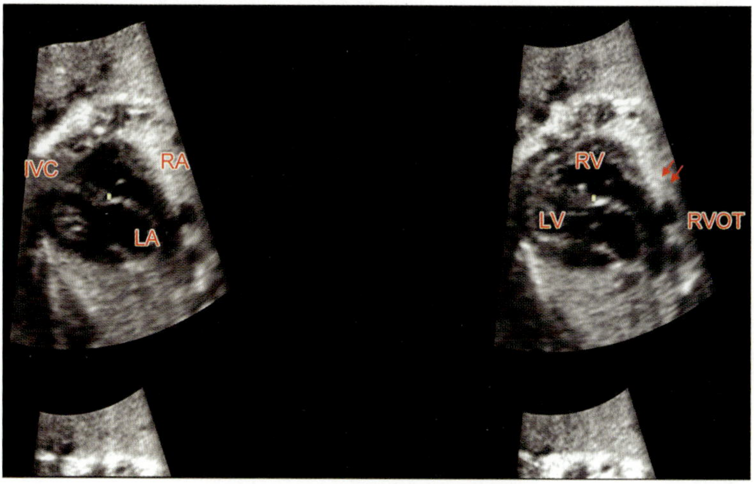

Figure 14.50 RVOT in aorta in TGA see arch of aorta

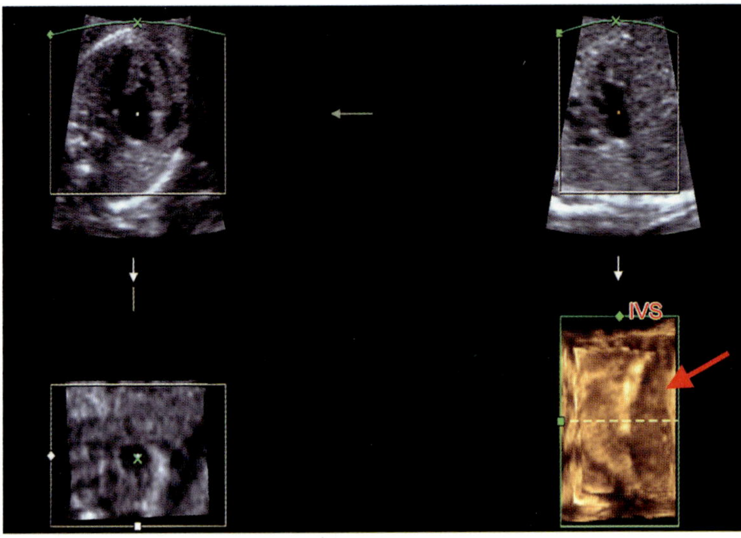

Figure 14.51 Abnormal four-chamber with right ventricular hypertrophy with 3D rendering image

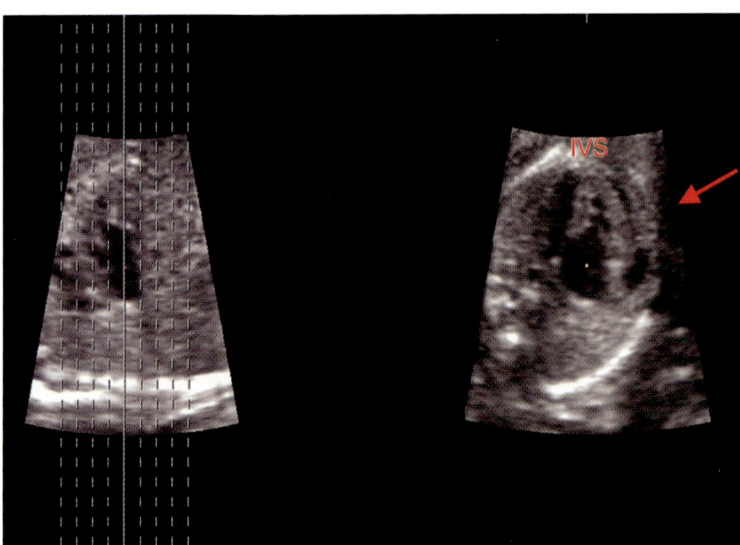

Figure 14.52 Abnormal four-chamber with right ventricular hypertrophy

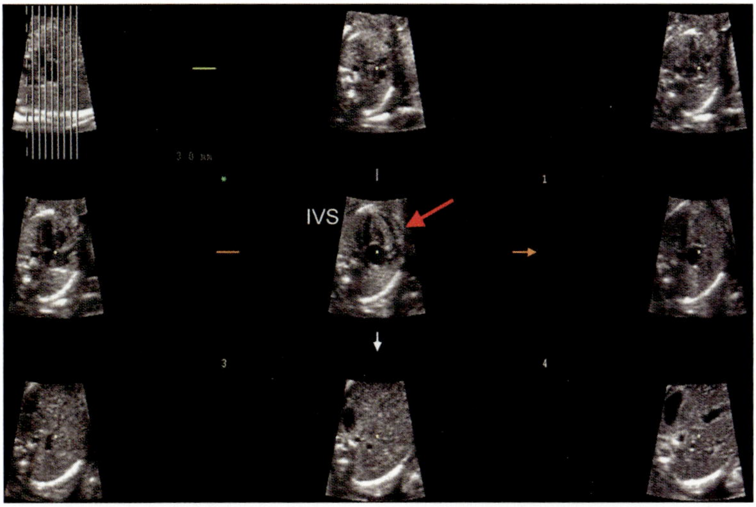

Figure 14.53 Abnormal four-chamber with right ventricular hypertrophy with TUI

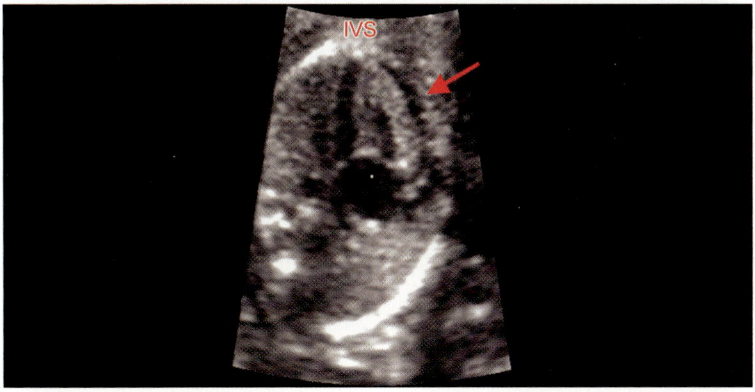

Figure 14.54 Abnormal four-chamber with right ventricular hypertrophy

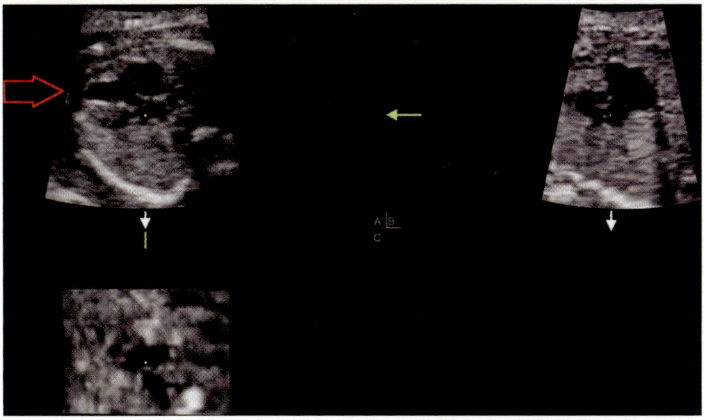

Figure 14.55 Right ventricular hypertrophy in 3D

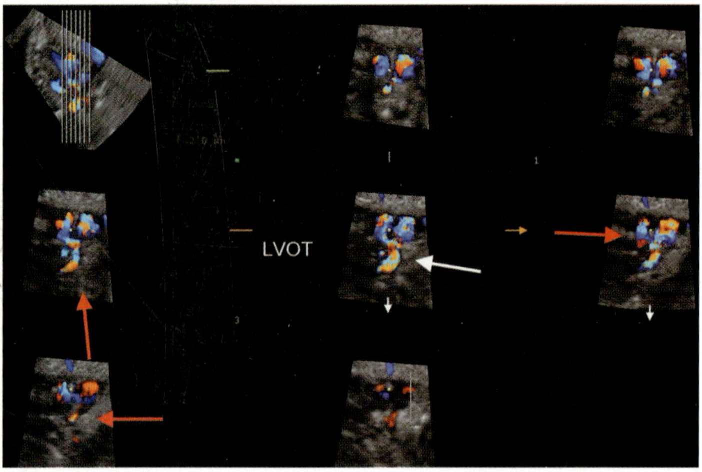

Figure 14.56 Over-riding of aorta in tetralogy of Fallot in TUI with LVOT

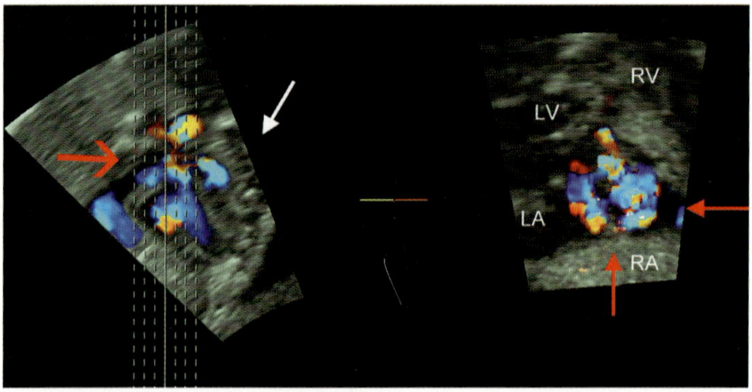

Figure 14.57 VSD with over-riding of aorta in TOF

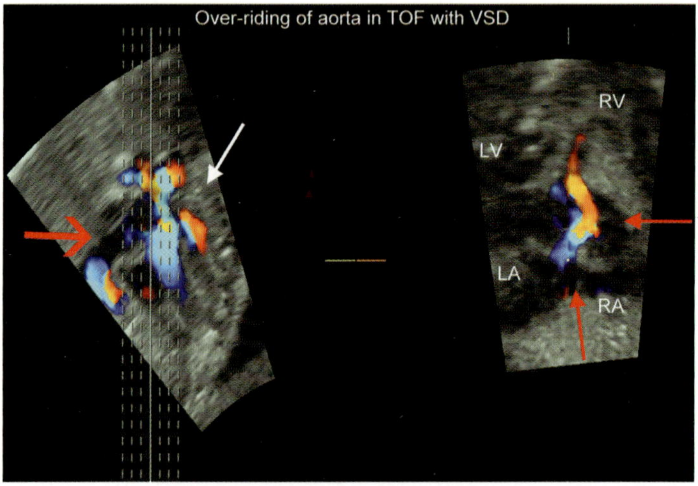

Figure 14.58 VSD in TOF with color aliasing

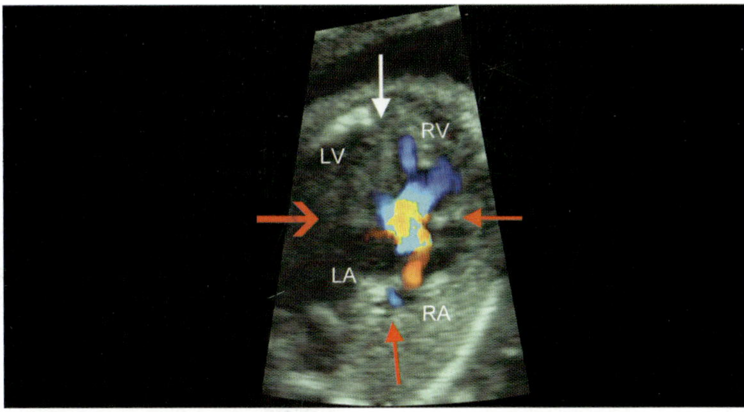

Figure 14.59 VSD and over-riding of aorta in TOF

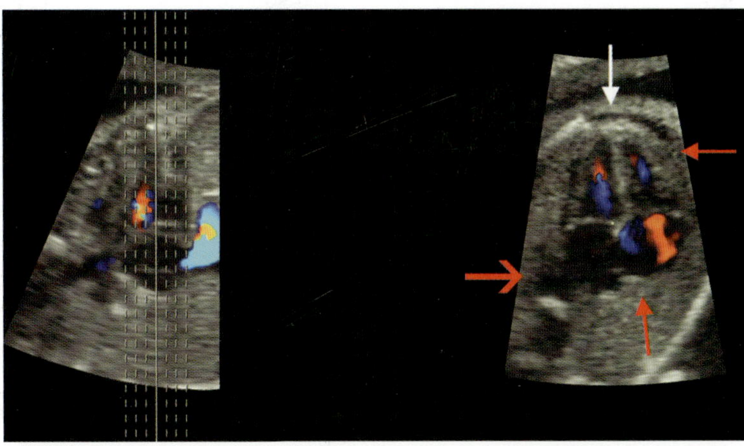

Figure 14.60 Normal four-chamber in TOF

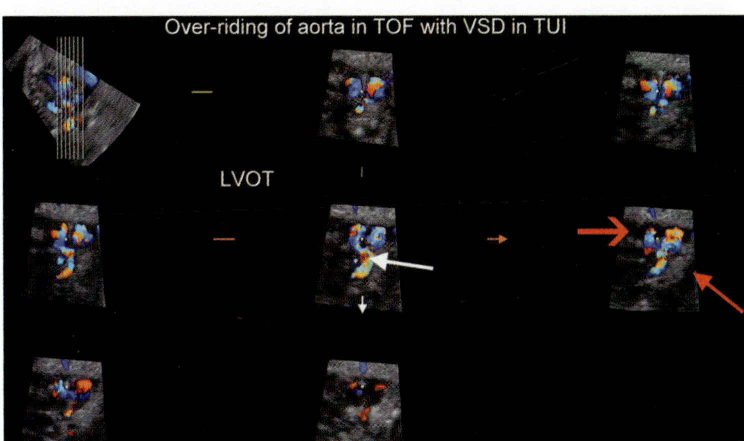

Figure 14.61 Left ventricular outflow tract (LVOT) and VSD in TOF

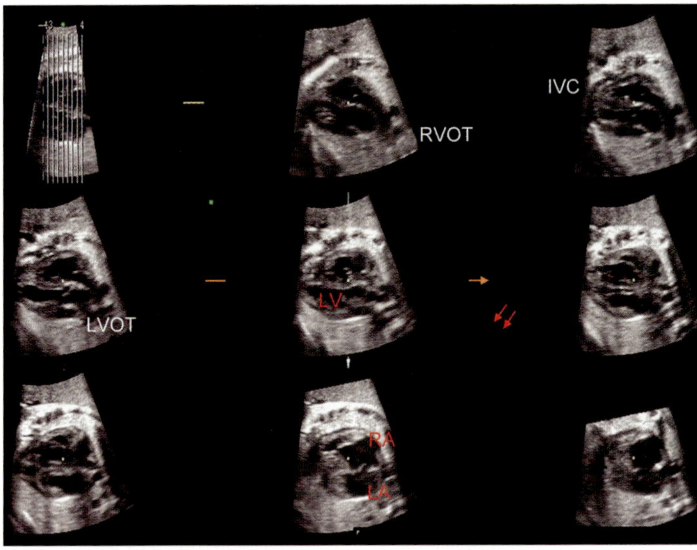

Figure 14.62 LVOT and RVOT in TGA in TUI

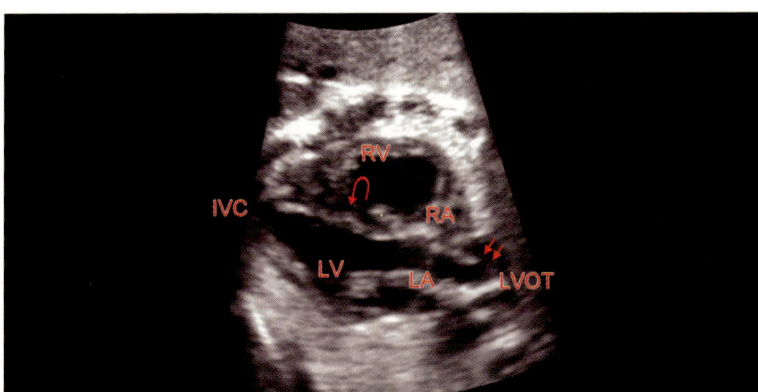

Figure 14.63 LVOT is pulmonary in TGA

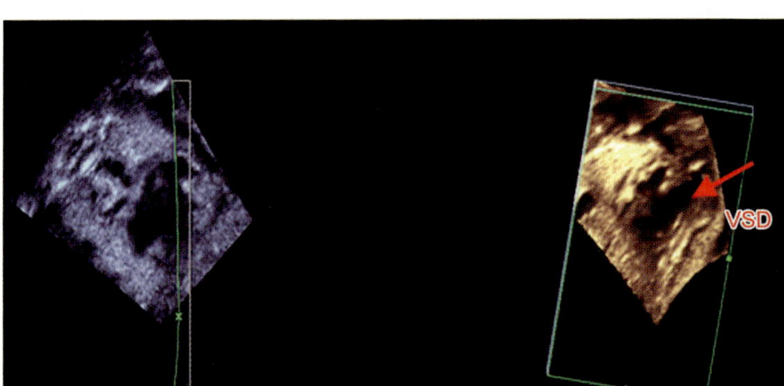

Figure 14.64 Abnormal four-chamber view with VSD in 3D reconstruction

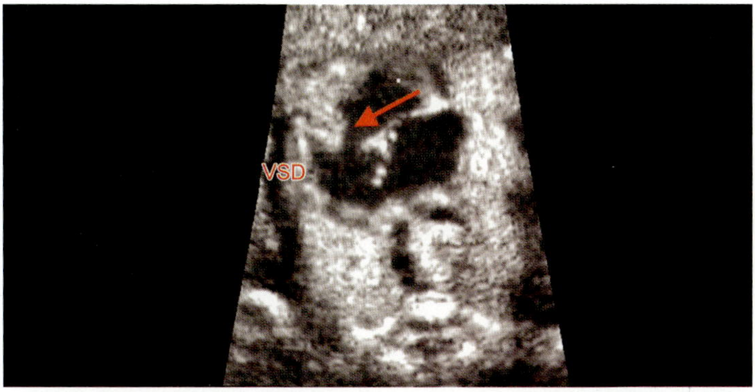

Figure 14.65 VSD seen in 2D with four-chamber view

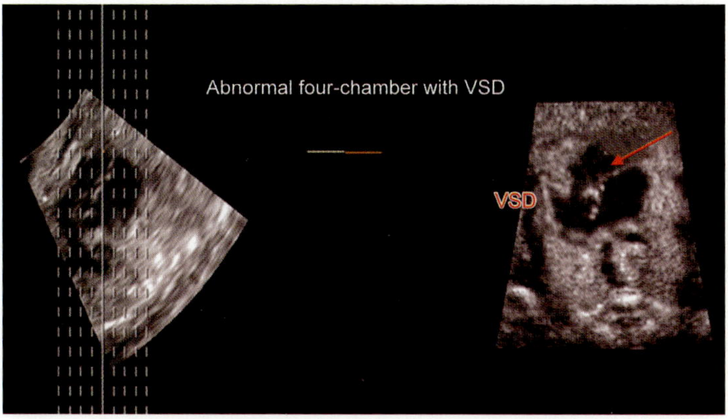

Figure 14.66 VSD seen with 2D with TUI

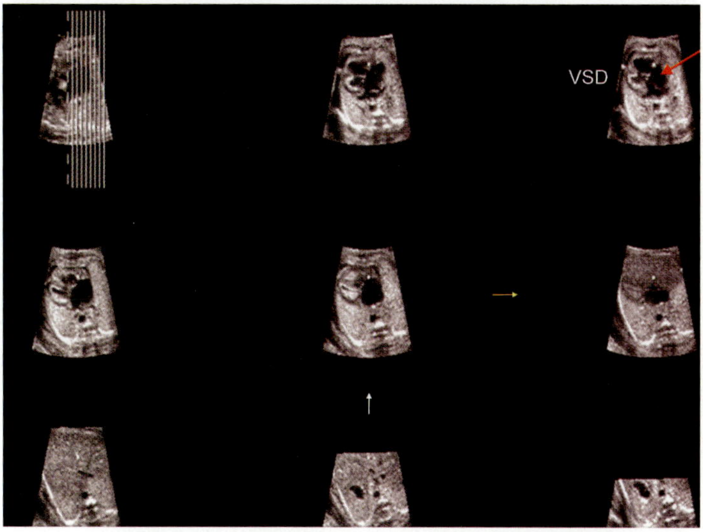

Figure 14.67 Abnormal four-chamber with VSD with TUI

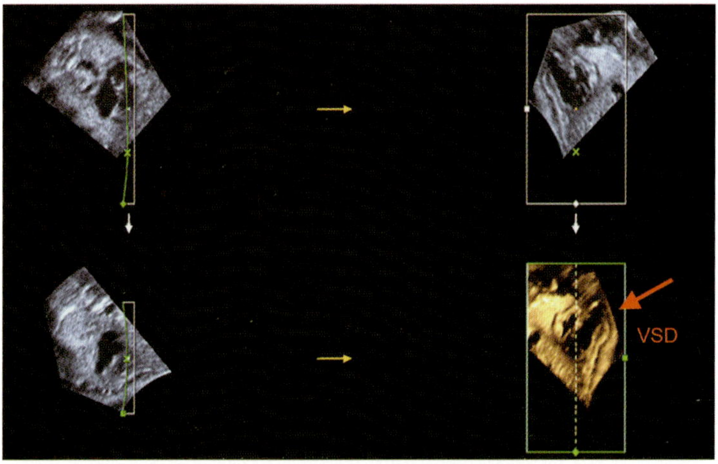

Figure 14.68 Abnormal four-chamber with VSD with X, Y and Z axis and 3D reconstruction (rendering image)

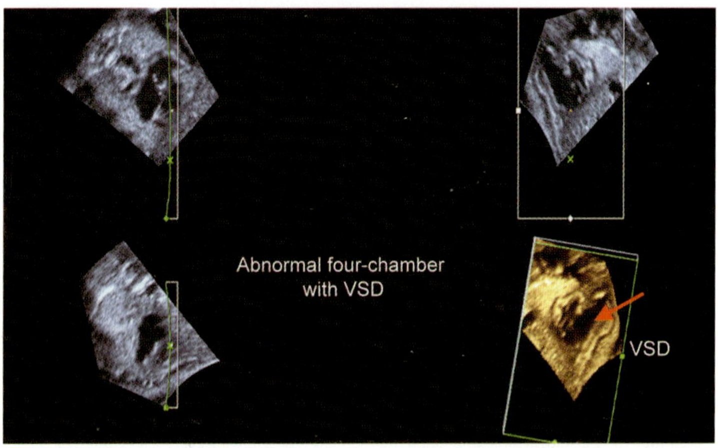

Figure 14.69 Four-chamber view in 3D with rendering image

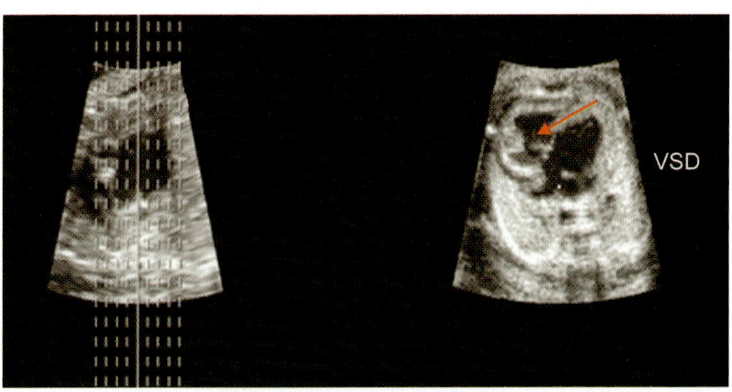

Figure 14.70 Abnormal four-chamber with VSD

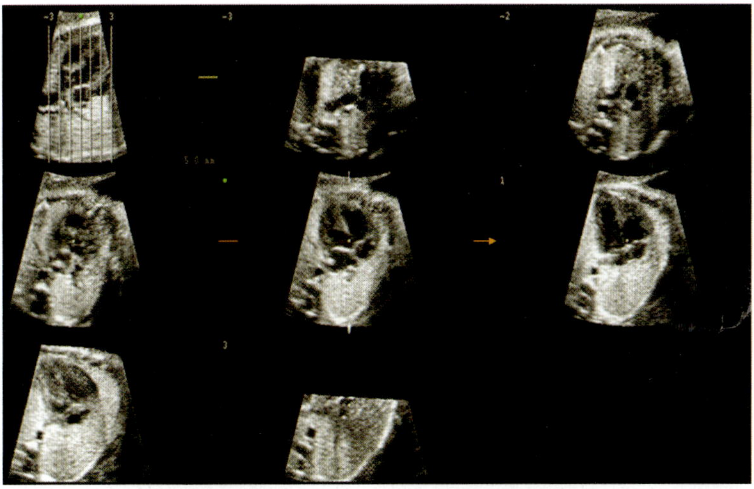

Figure 14.71 Abnormal outflow tract in TUI

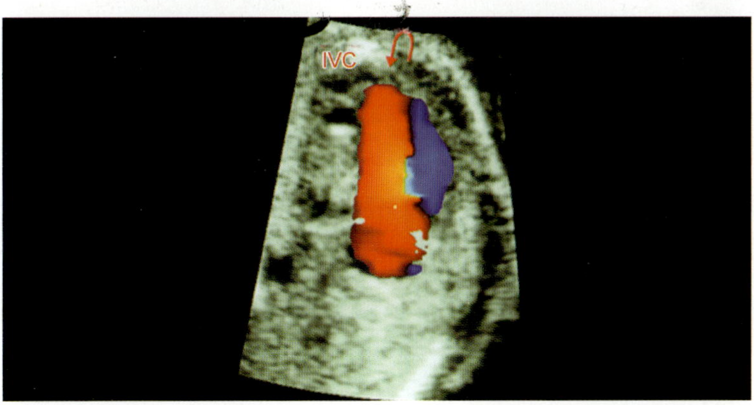

Figure 14.72 Abnormal tract shows absent color flow in left ventricle

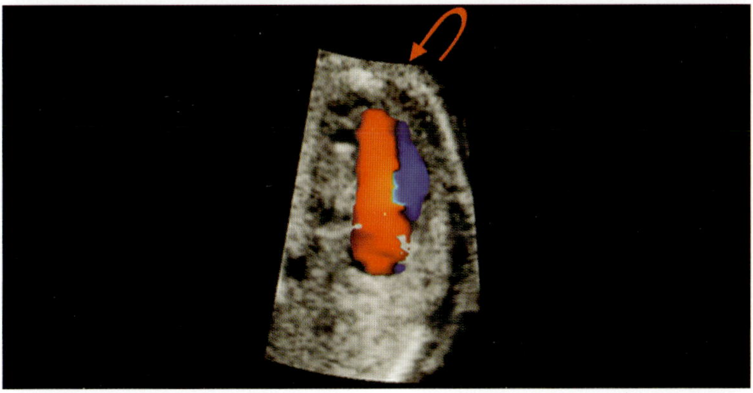

Figure 14.73 Absent color flow in LV with regurgitation in right ventricle

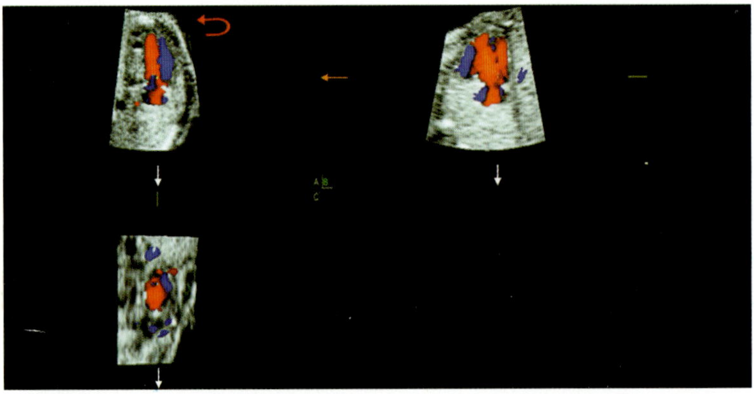

Figure 14.74 Abnormal outflow tract with no color flow in left ventricle

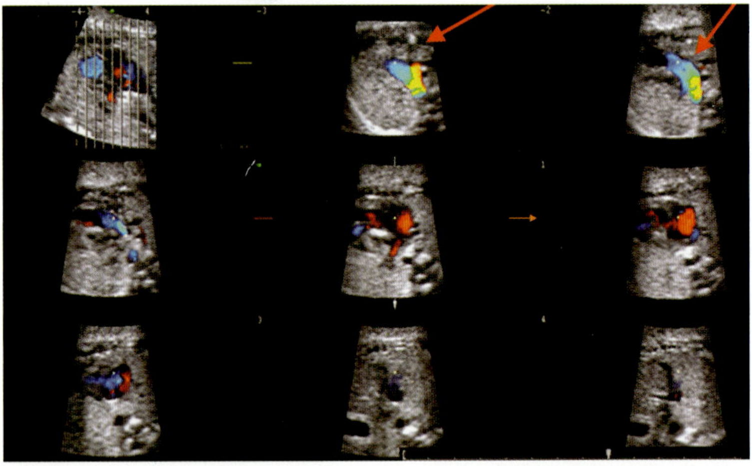

Figure 14.75 Abnormal tract with color regurgitation in right outflow tract

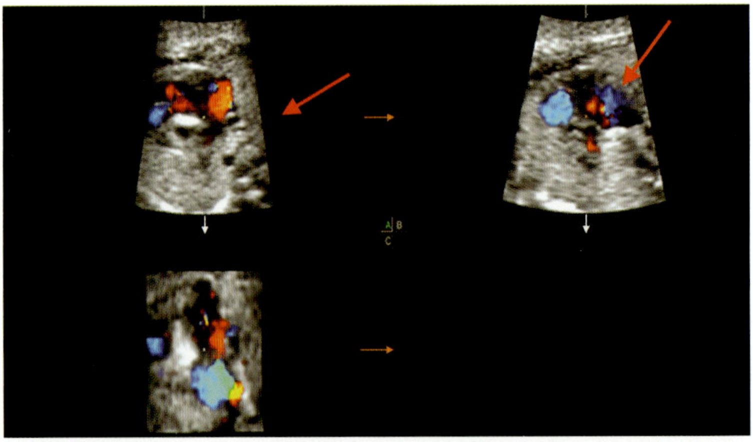

Figure 14.76 Abnormal tract with VSD

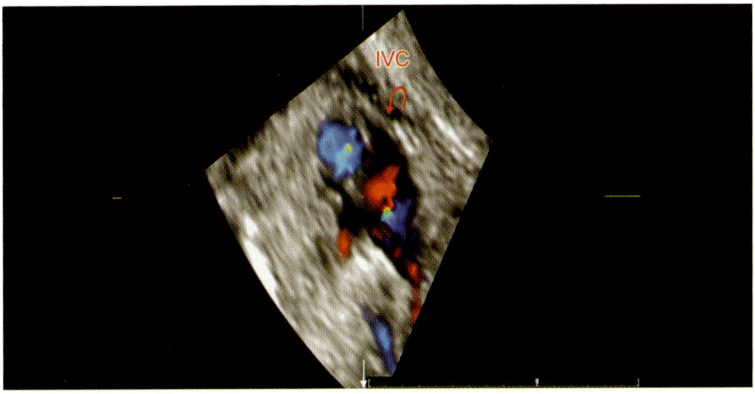

Figure 14.77 VSD seen with color

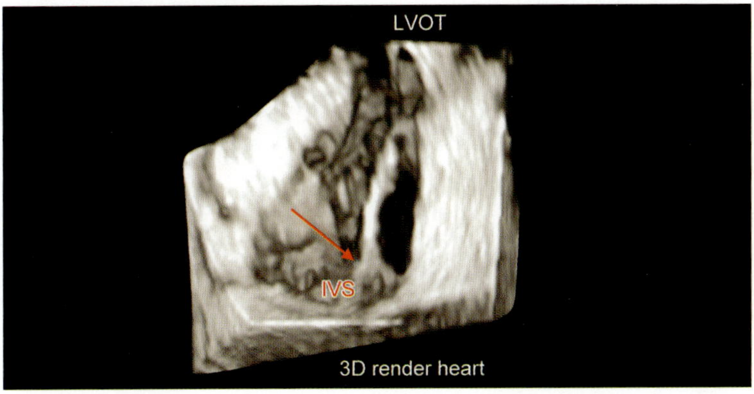

Figure 14.78 Abnormal tract with 3D rendering

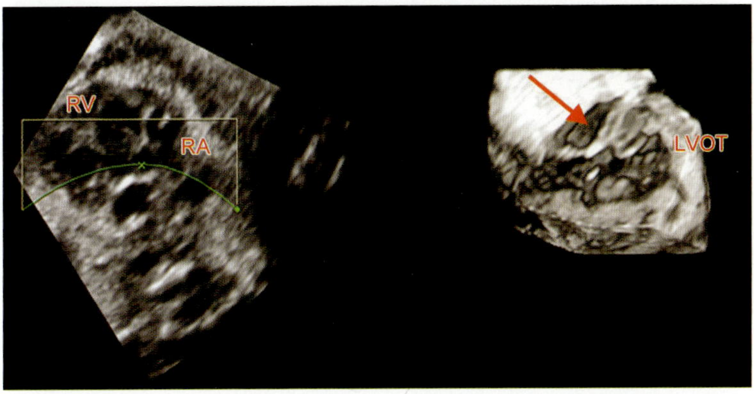

Figure 14.79 Abnormal tract with 3D heart reconstruction

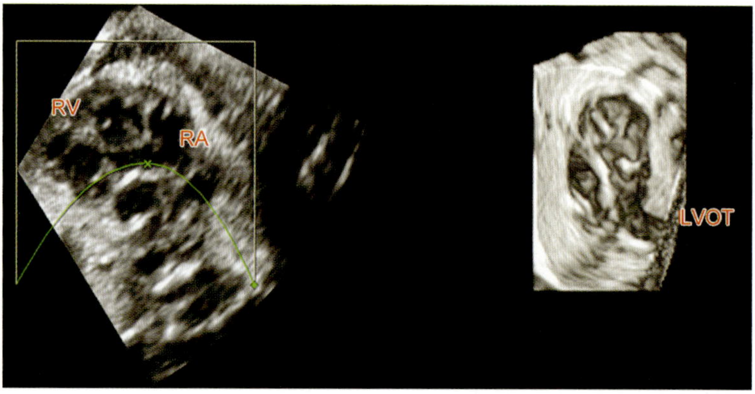

Figure 14.80 Abnormal tract with 3D rendering image

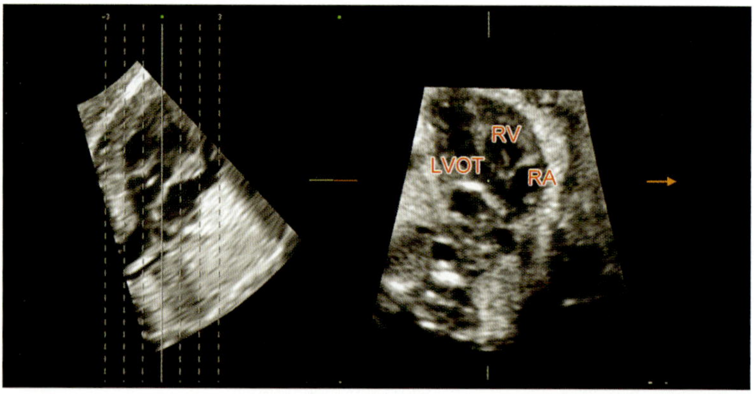

Figure 14.81 LVOT in abnormal tract image

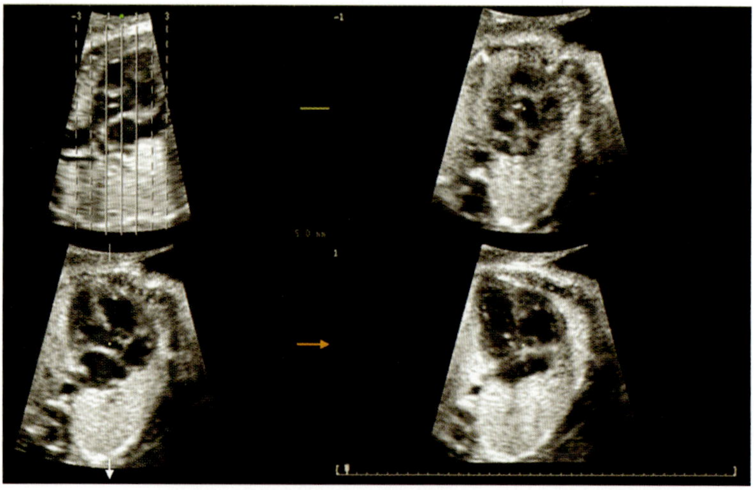

Figure 14.82 Abnormal tract with normal four-chamber view

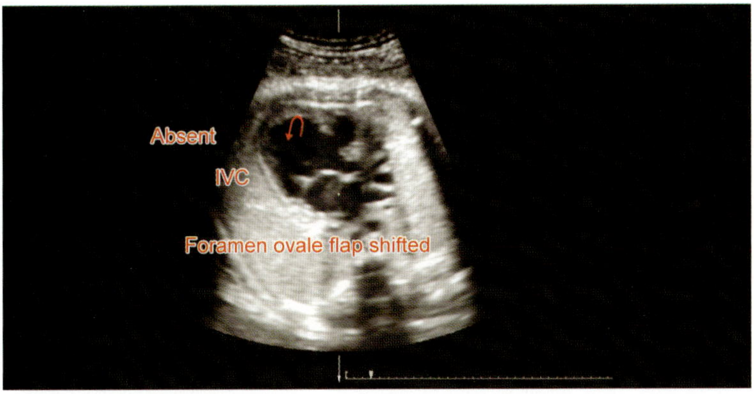

Figure 14.83 Absent interventricular septum

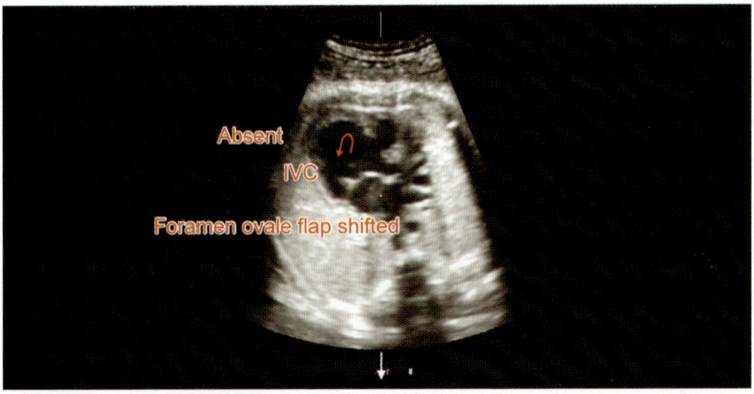

Figure 14.84 Interventricular septum in 2D

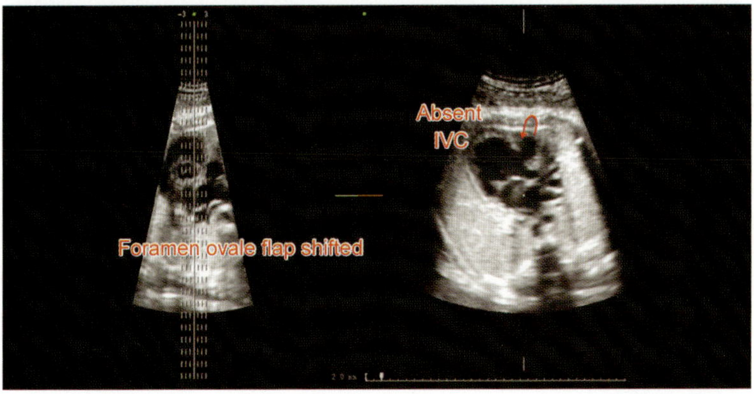

Figure 14.85 Absent interventricular septum with RVOT

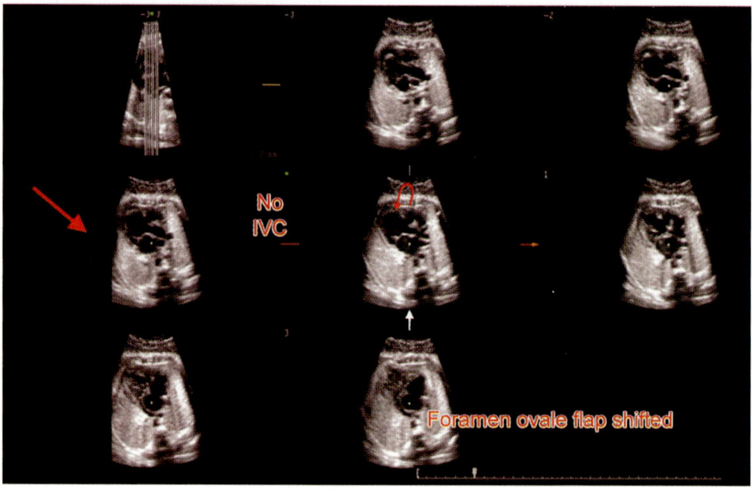

Figure 14.86 Absent IVS in TUI

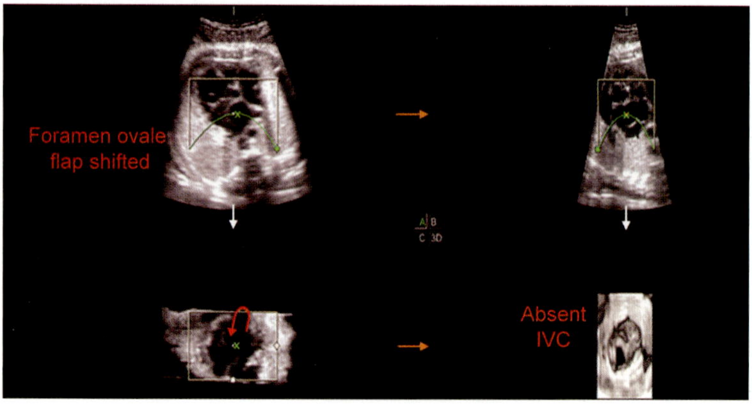

Figure 14.87 Absent IVC in 3D rendering image

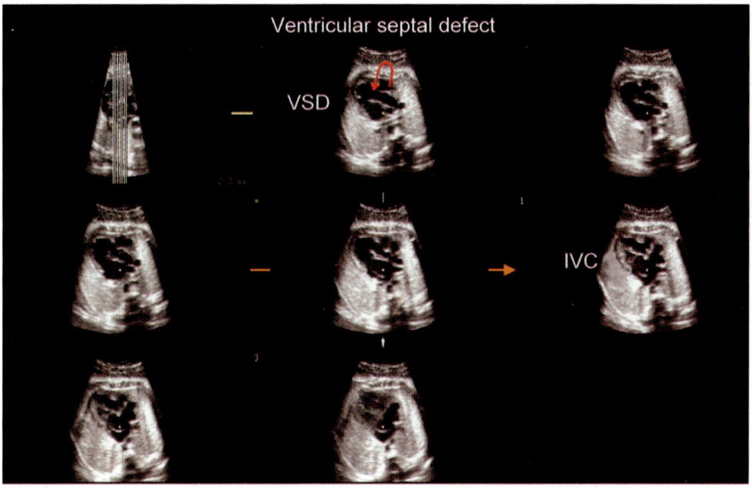

Figure 14.88 Ebstein anomaly

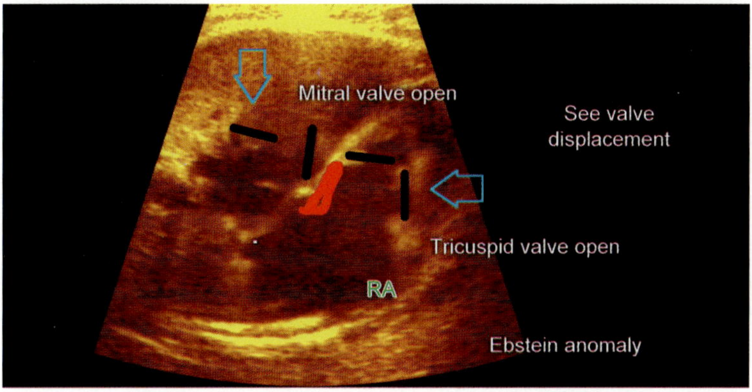

Figure 14.89 Ebstein anomaly with both valve open

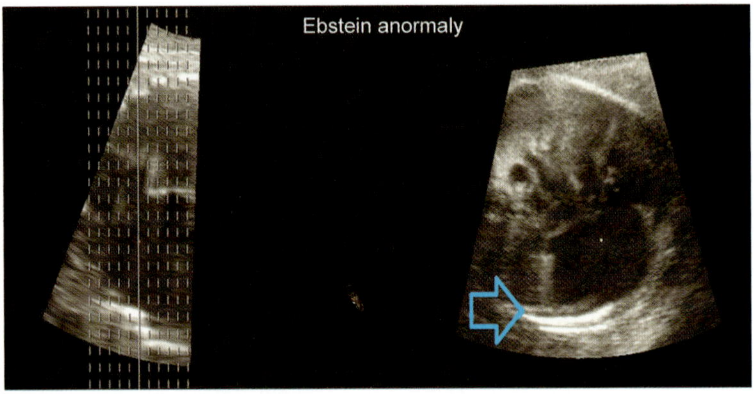

Figure 14.90 Ebstein anomaly shows large right atrium

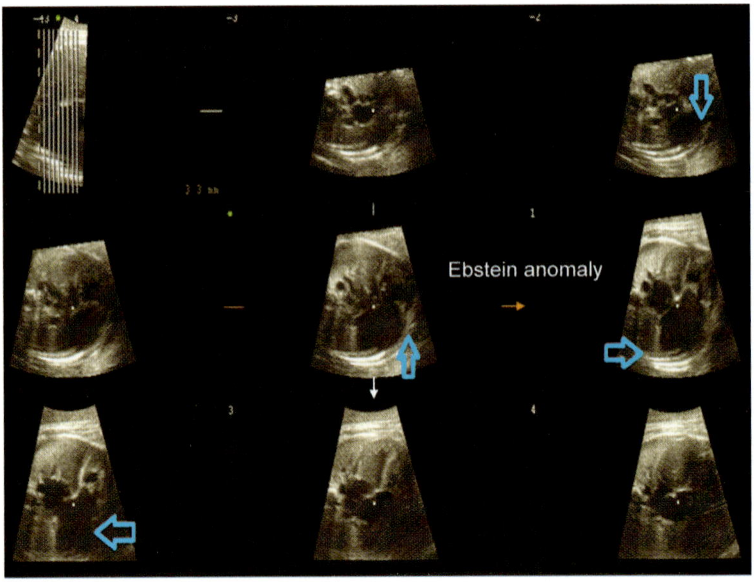

Figure 14.91 Ebstein anomaly with TUI shows atrialization of ventricle

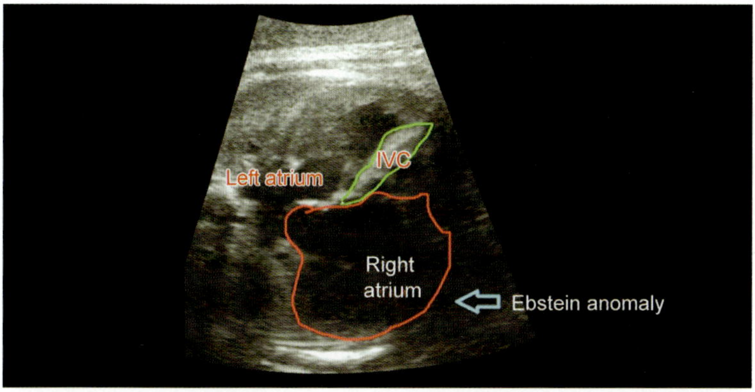

Figure 14.92 Ebstein anomaly labeled

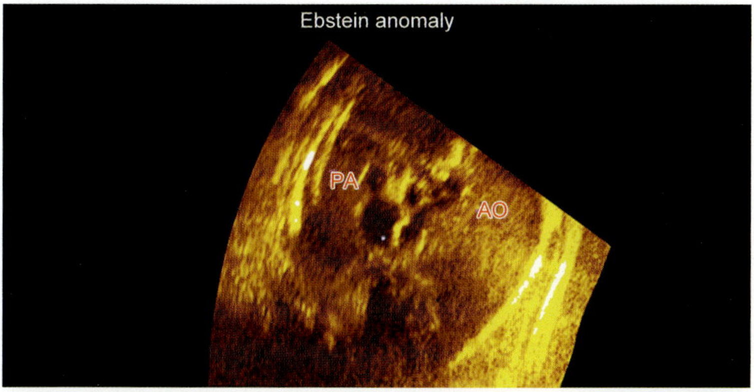

Figure 14.93 Ebstein anomaly with sepia shows abnormal outflow tract

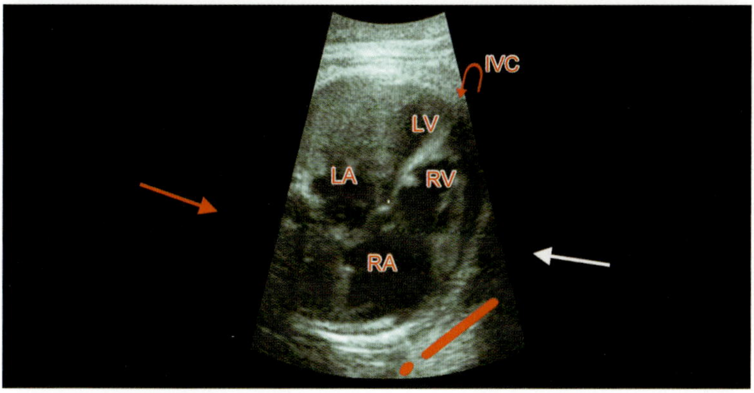

Figure 14.94 Ebstein anomaly with large right atrium

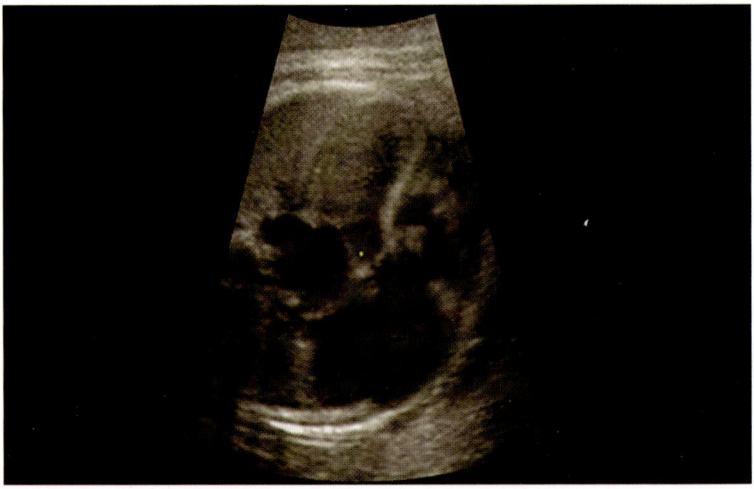

Figure 14.95 Ebstein anomaly in 2D

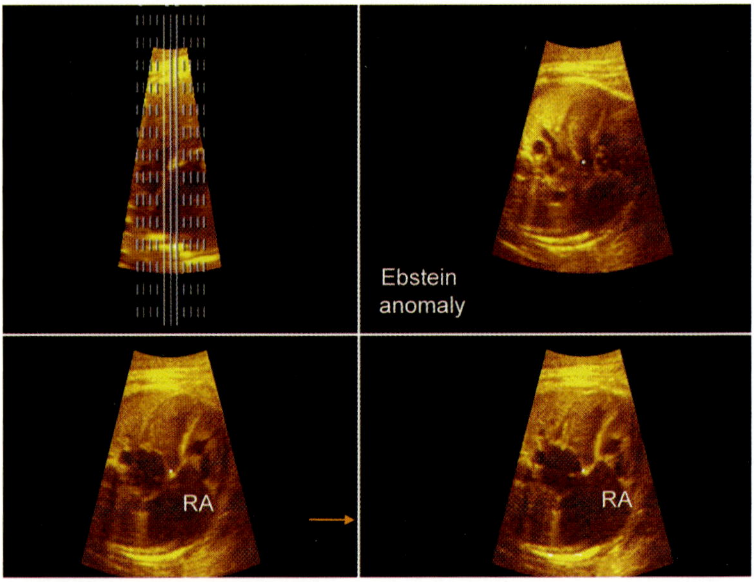

Figure 14.96 Ebstein anomaly with large RA in TUI

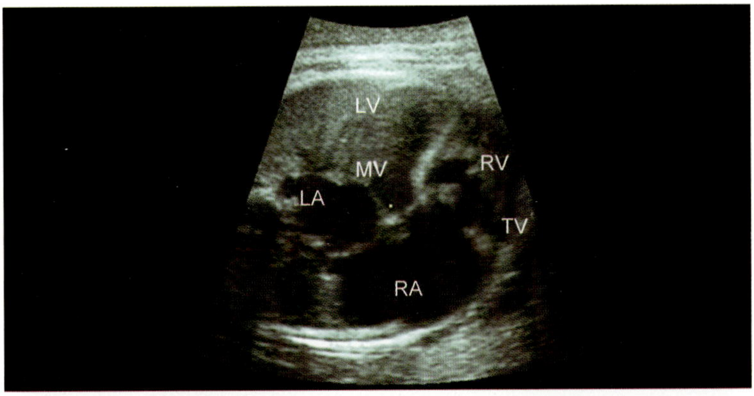

Figure 14.97 Ebstein anomaly with labeling

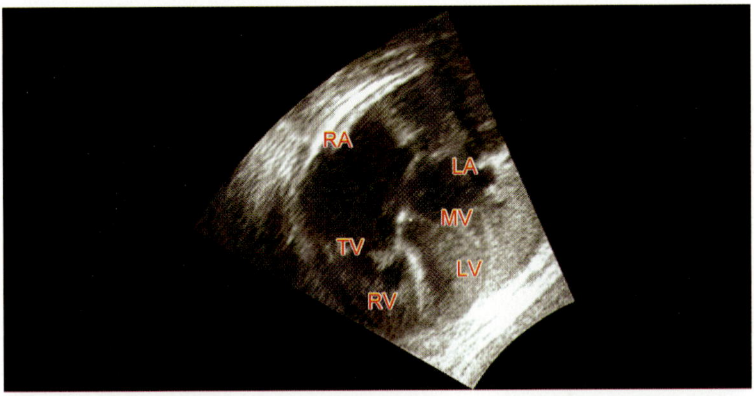

Figure 14.98 Ebstein anomaly with large RA and small RV

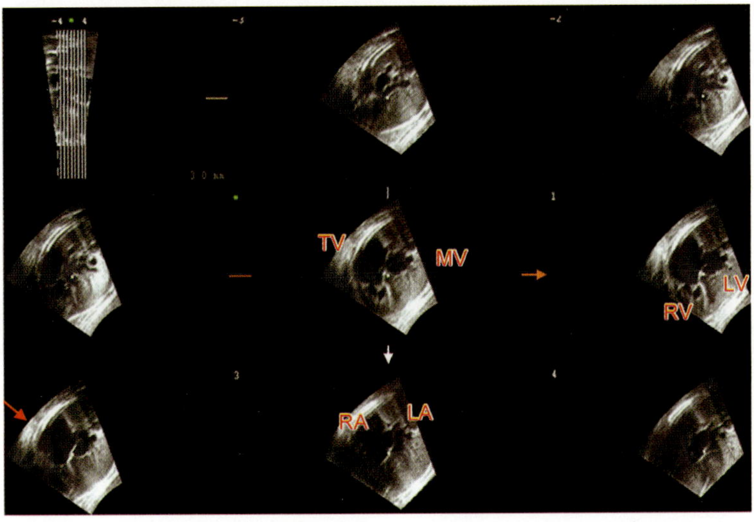

Figure 14.99 Ebstein anomaly with TUI

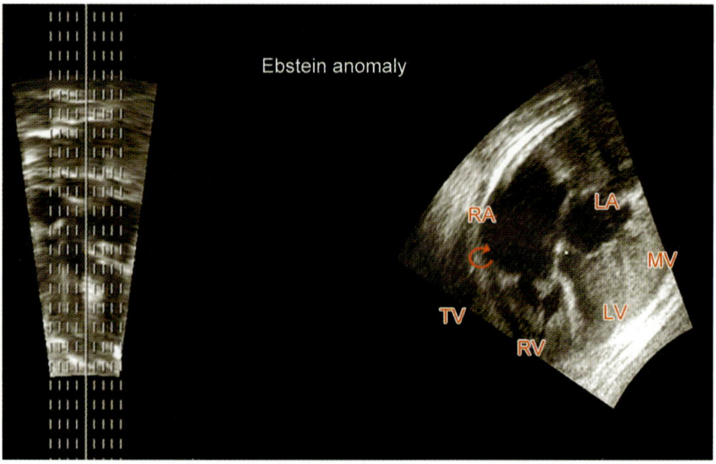

Figure 14.100 Ebstein anomaly with large RA

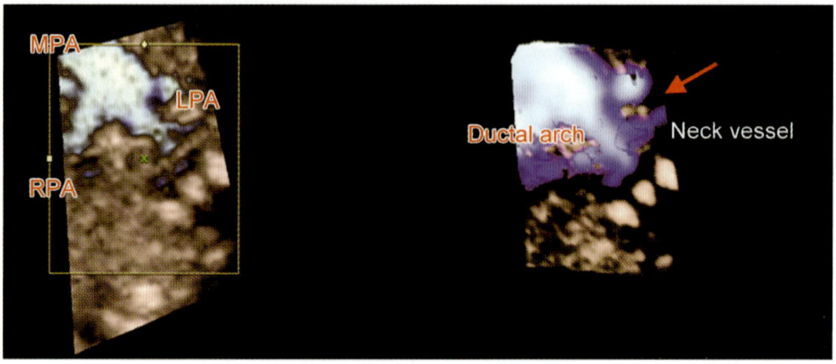

Figure 14.101 HD flow shows neck vessel

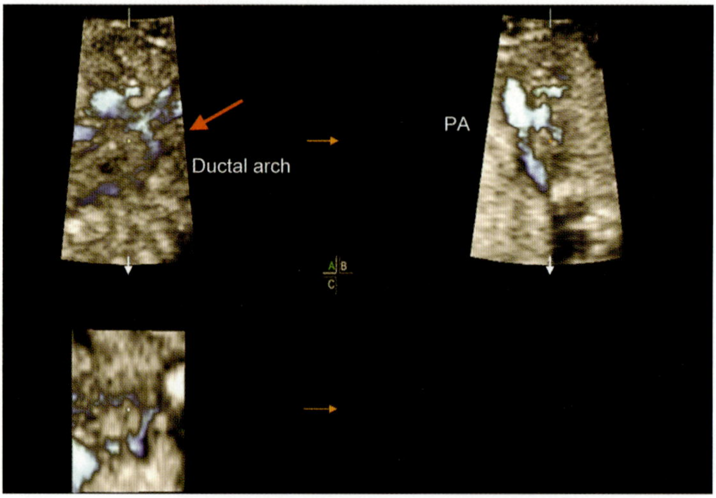

Figure 14.102 HD flow shows ductal arch

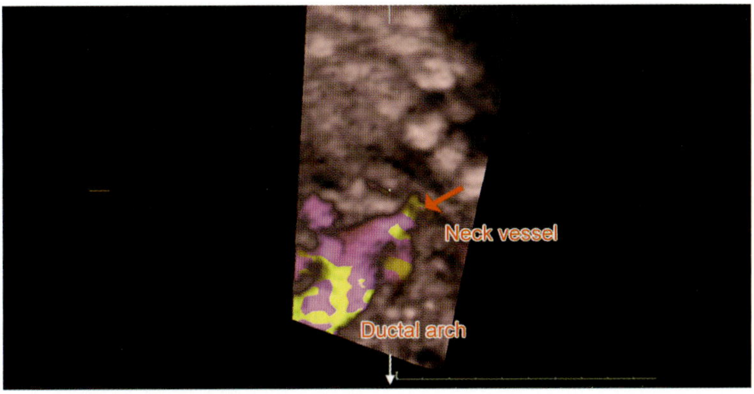

Figure 14.103 HD flow with neck vessel arising from arch of aorta

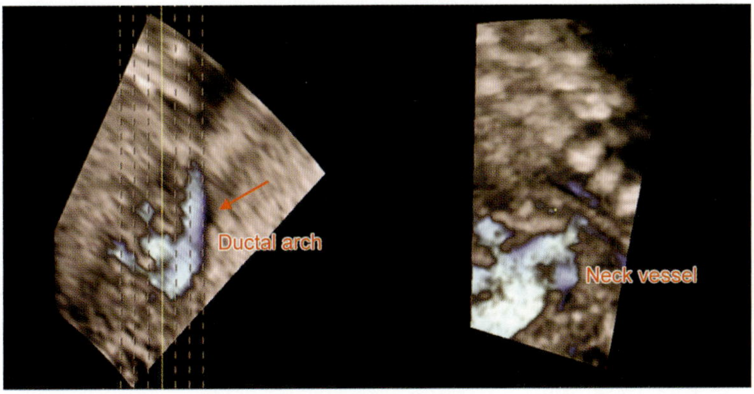

Figure 14.104 HD flow with ductal arch and neck veseel

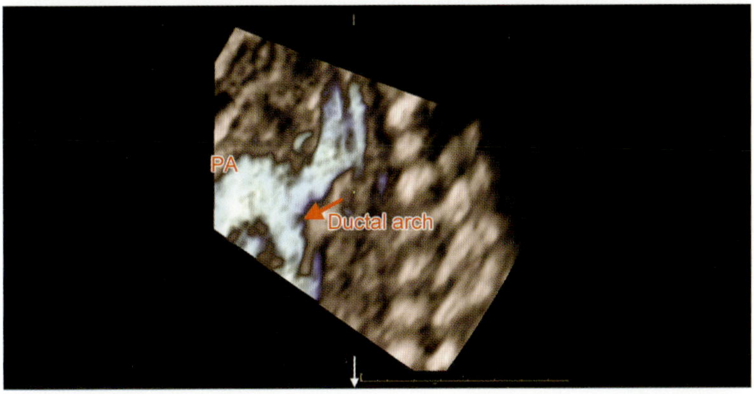

Figure 14.105 HD flow shows ductal arch with spatiotemporal image correlation (STIC) 4D

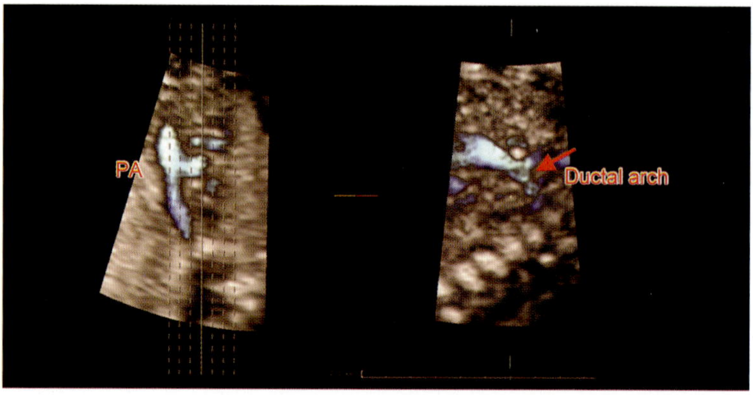

Figure 14.106 HD flow with RVOT and ductal arch

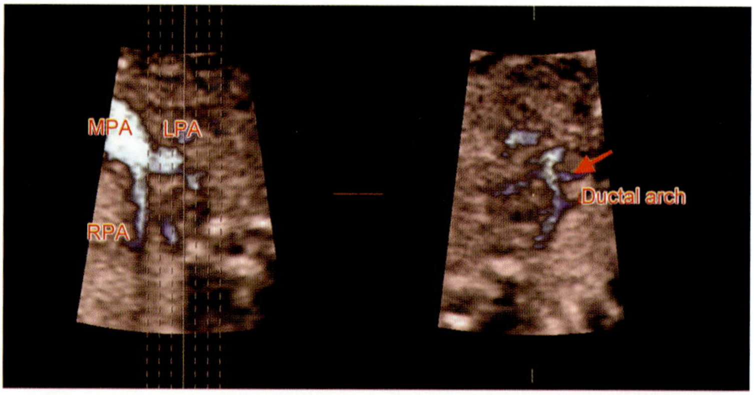

Figure 14.107 HD flow shows pulmonary conus RVOT and costal arch

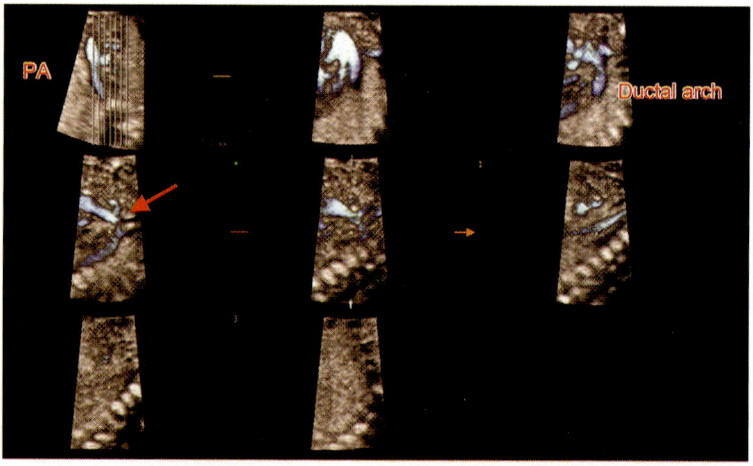

Figure 14.108 HD flow shows ductal arch in TUI

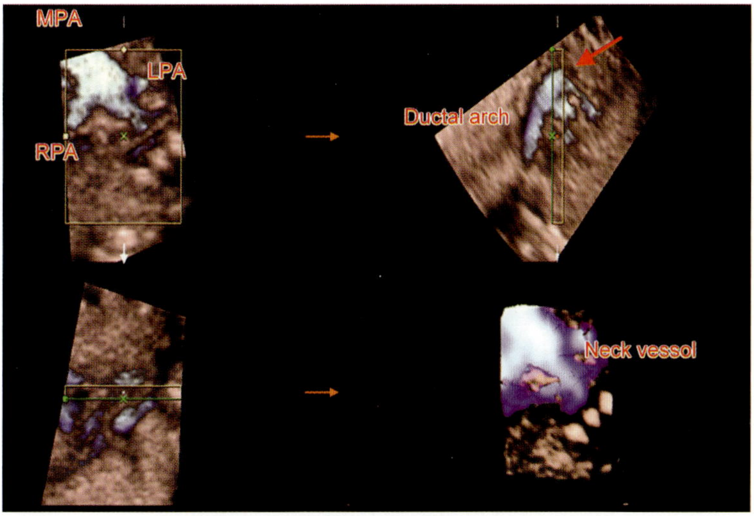

Figure 14.109 HD flow with neck vessel and RVOT

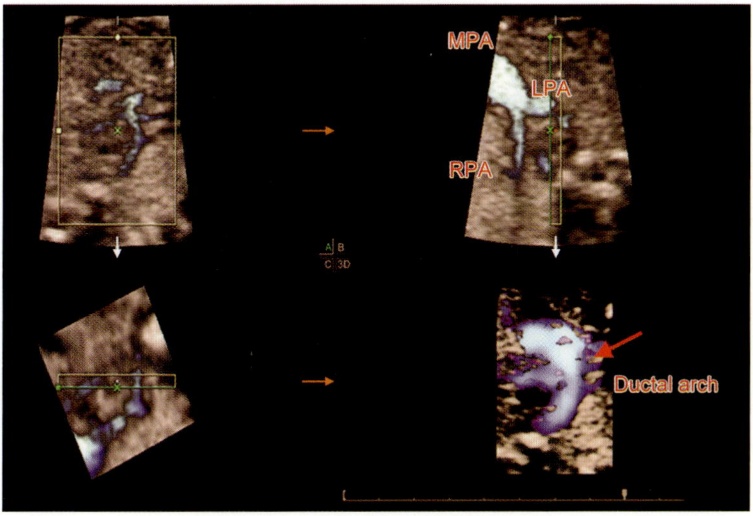

Figure 14.110 HD flow ductal arch RVOT

15

Frequently Asked Questions and their Answers

This chapter gives an incite of how to diagnose cardiac anomaly in fetal heart on one side, we will see normal image and we have to compare it and solve what is abnormal.

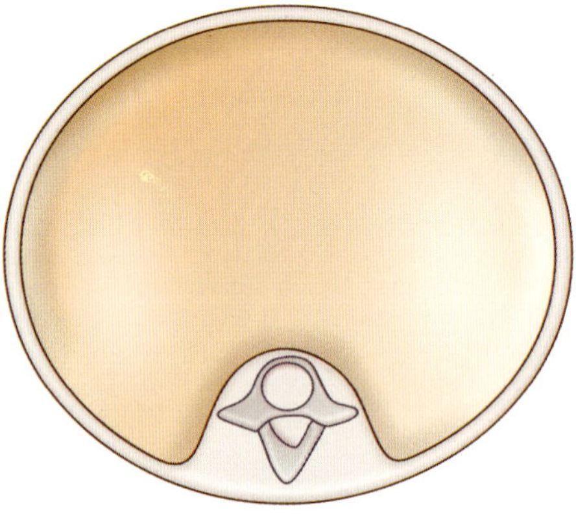

Figure 15.1 Base section of heart

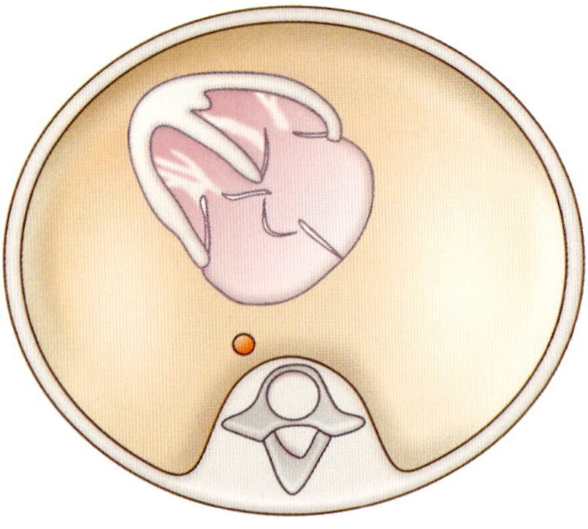

Figure 15.2 Four-chamber heart

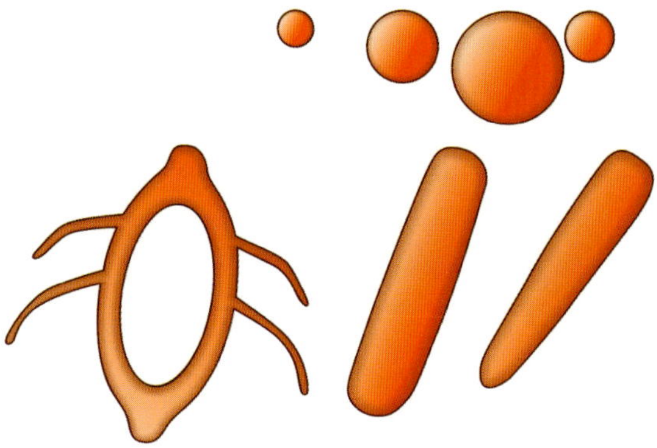

Figure 15.3 Aorta

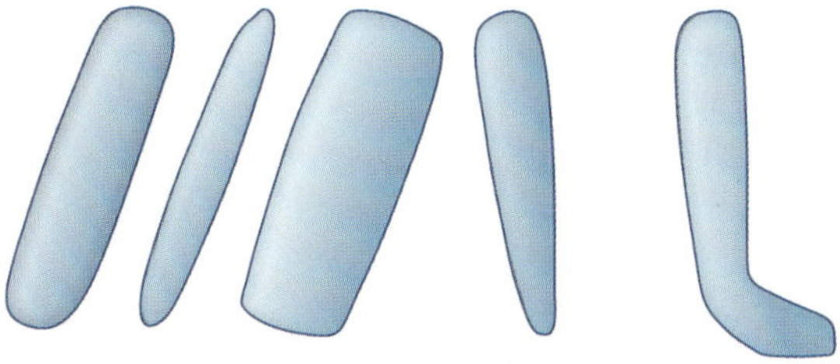

Figure 15.4 Pulmonary artery

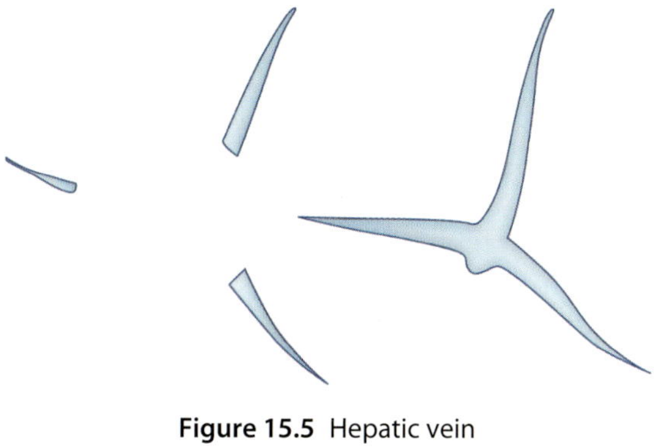

Figure 15.5 Hepatic vein

Figure 15.6 Fluid or stomach

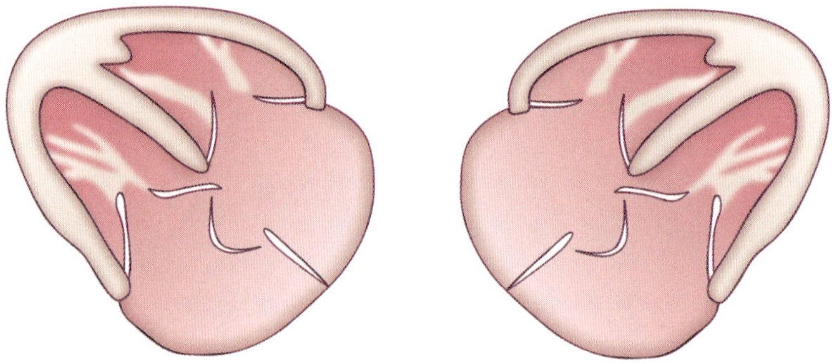

Figure 15.7 Four-chamber heart view

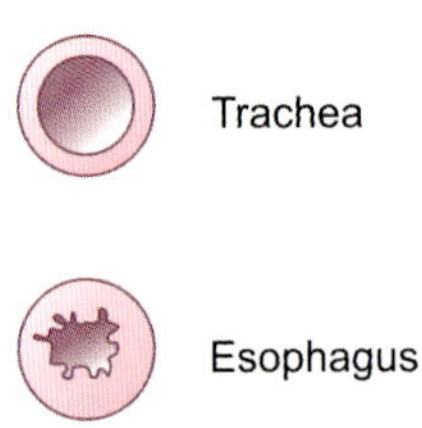

Figure 15.8 Symbols showing trachea and esophagus

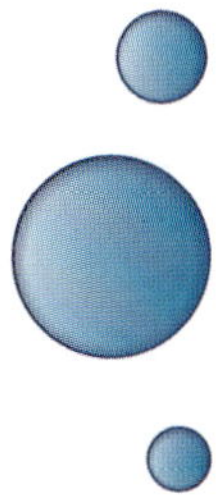

Figure 15.9 Symbols showing vena cava and azygos veins

Question 1: What does the Figure 15.10 show?

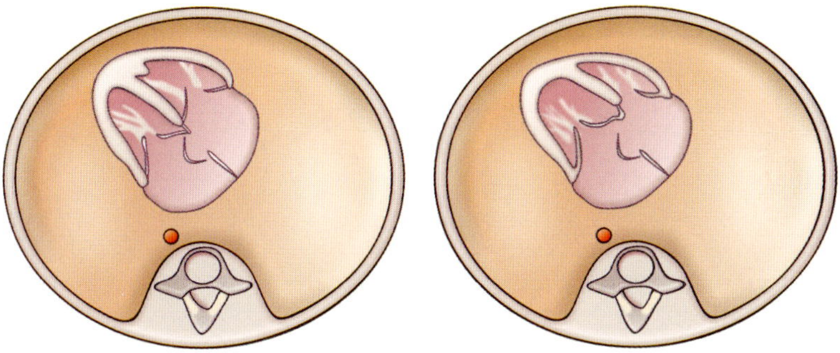

Figure 15.10

Ans: Small right heart

Possible Causes

- Hypoplastic right ventricle
- Early pulmonary stenosis
- Early tricuspid stenosis.

Question 2: What does the Figure 15.11 show?

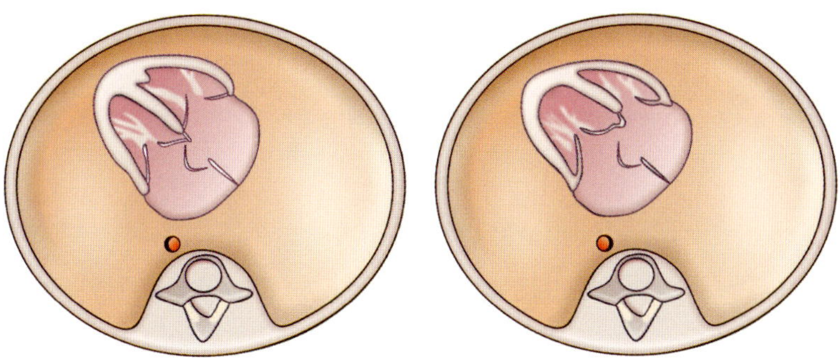

Figure 15.11

Ans: Enlarged left ventricle

Possible Causes

- Late aortic stenosis
- Some mitral regurgitation.

Question 3: What does the Figure 15.12 show?

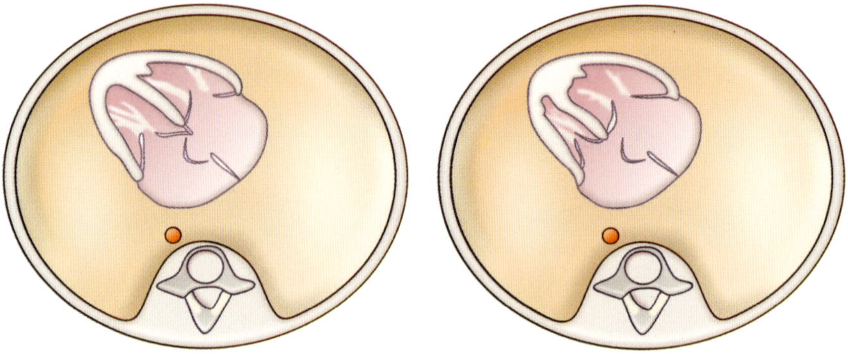

Figure 15.12

Ans: Small left heart ventricle

Possible Causes

- Hypoplastic left ventricle
- Early aortic stenosis
- Coarctation of aorta or interruption of the aorta
- Early mitral stenosis or regurgitation
- Premature closure of ductus arteriosus or foramen ovale.

Question 4: What does the Figure 15.13 show?

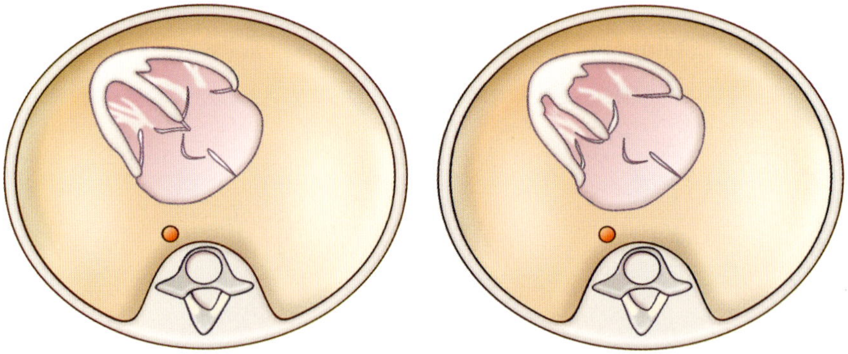

Figure 15.13

Ans: Enlarged right ventricle

Possible Causes

- Some late pulmonary stenosis
- Some late tricuspid regurgitation
- High flow situation such as:
  - Vein of galen aneurysm
  - Chorioangioma of the placenta
  - Hepatic angioma.

Question 5: What does the Figure 15.14 show?

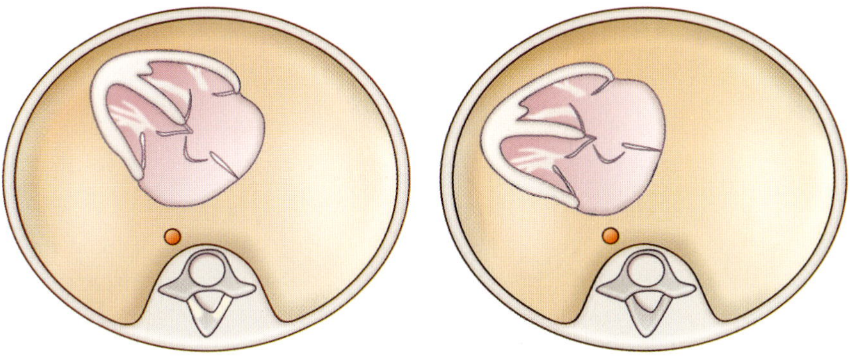

Figure 15.14

Ans: Left axis deviation (IVC at 90° anterior line)

Possible Causes

- Conotruncal anomalies
- Right-sided diaphragmatic hernia.

Question 6: What does the Figure 15.15 show?

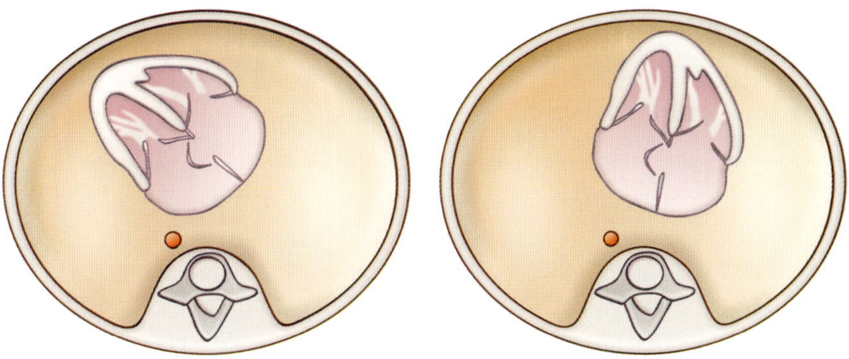

Figure 15.15

Ans: Right axis deviation [IVS parallel to the (anteroposterior) line]

Possible Causes

- Left-sided diaphragmatic hernia
- Isomerism and situs inversus
- Inversion of the ventricle
- Double outlet right ventricle
- Common atriums.

Question 7: What does the Figure 15.16 show?

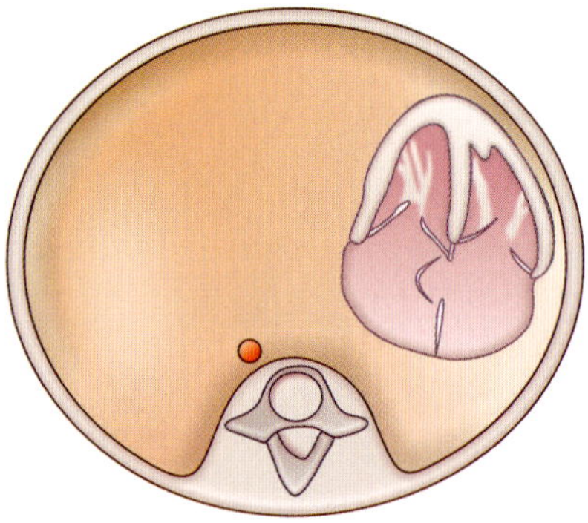

Figure 15.16

Ans: Dextroposition

Possible Causes

- Left diaphragmatic hernia
- Cystic adenomatoid malformation of the lungs
- Congenital lobar emphysema
- Left pleural infusion
- Chylothorax
- Right lung agenesis.

Question 8: What does the Figure 15.17 show?

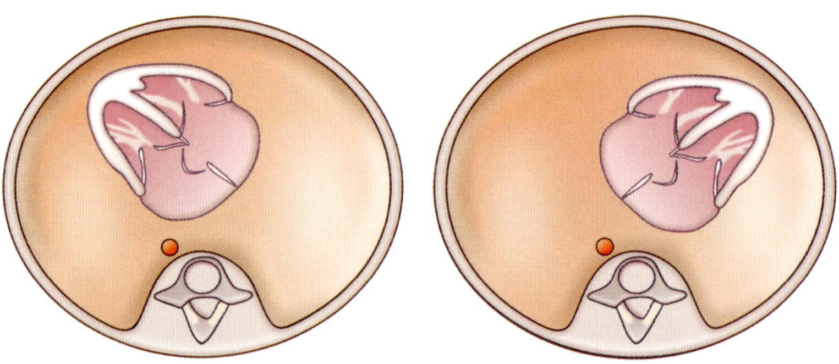

Figure 15.17

Ans: Dextrocardia

Possible Cause

Anomaly of embryological development.

Question 9: What does the Figure 15.18 show?

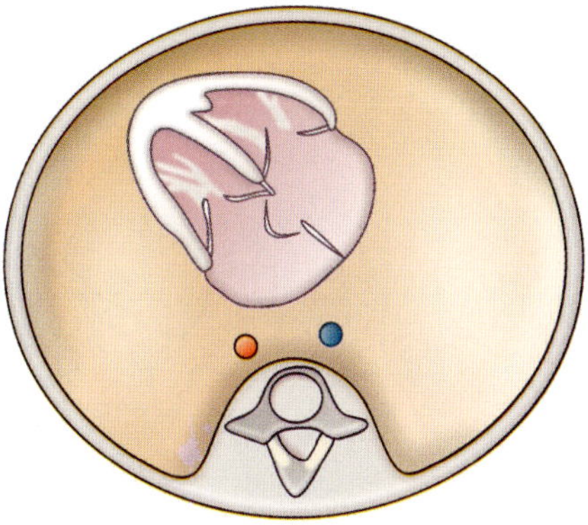

Figure 15.18

Ans: Vein behind the four-chamber view

Possible Cause

IVC interrupting with azygos or hemiazygos continuation.

Question 10: What does the Figure 15.19 show?

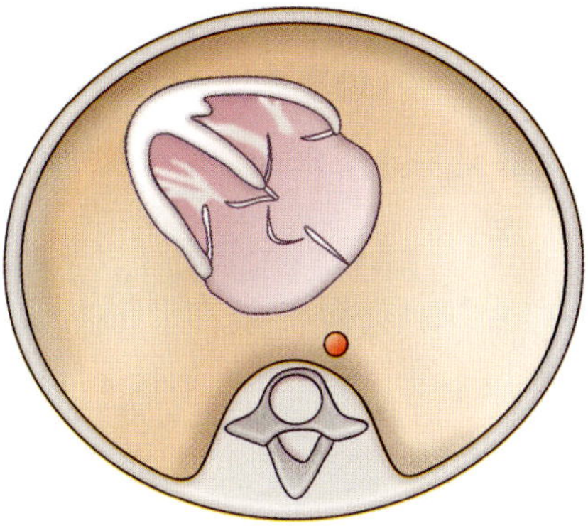

Figure 15.19

Ans: Right descending aorta

Possible Causes

- Tetralogy of Fallot
- Truncus arteriosus
- Transposition
- Interrupted aortic arch.

Question 11: What does the Figure 15.20 show?

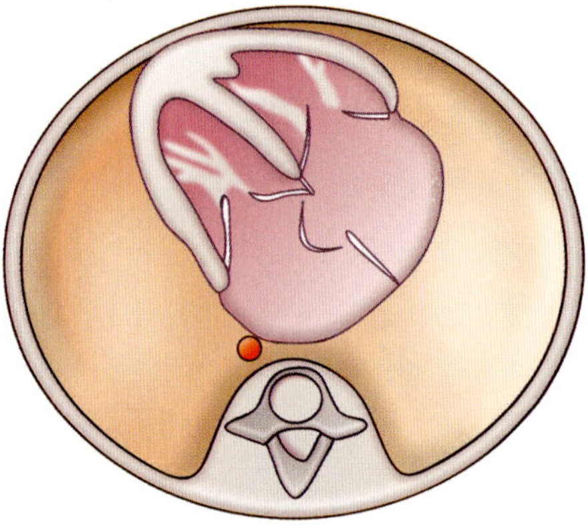

Figure 15.20

Ans: Global enlargement

Possible Causes

- Endocardial fibroelastosis
- Storage disorder
- Ischemia
- Infections
- Atrioventricular and semilunar valve regurgitation
- Extreme forms of shunts (vein of Galen "aneurysm", chorioangioma)
- Obstructive lesions (aortic stenosis, calcinosis, premature closure of the ducts, true knot of the cord, tumors in the outflow).
- Apparent enlargement (skeletal dysplasia, absent renal function).

Question 12: What does the Figure 15.21 show?

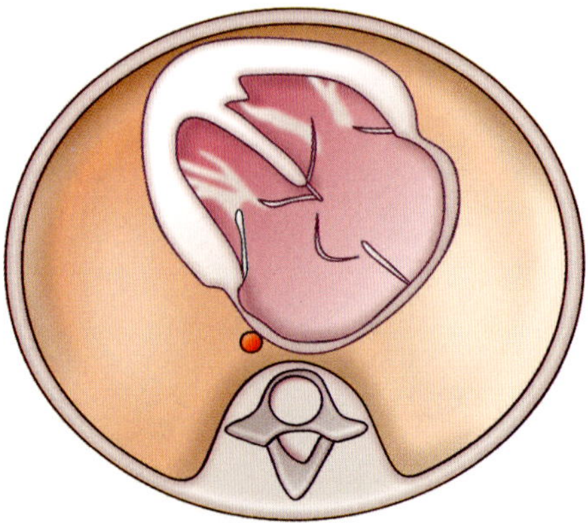

Figure 15.21

Ans: Thickened myocardium

Possible Causes

- Cardiomyopathies
- Univentricle heart
- Septal hypertrophy.

Question 13: What does the Figure 15.22 show?

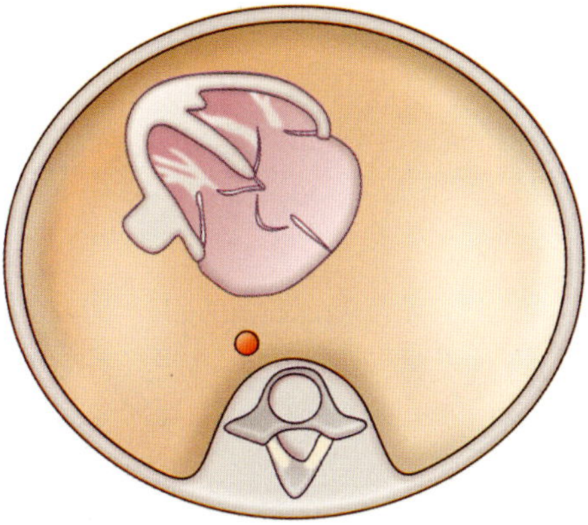

Figure 15.22

Ans: Localized enlargement

Possible Causes

- Diabetic cardiomyopathies
- Myocardial infarct
- Tumors.

Question 14: What does the Figure 15.23 show?

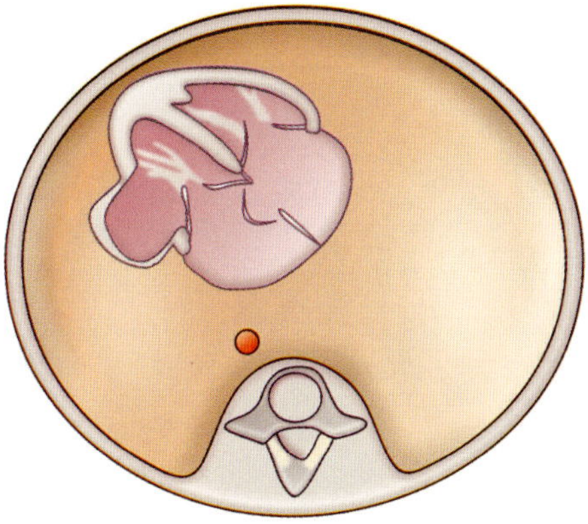

Figure 15.23

Ans: Localized dilatation

Possible Causes

- Diverticulum
- Aneurysmal dilatation
- Pericardial cyst.

Question 15: What does the Figure 15.24 show?

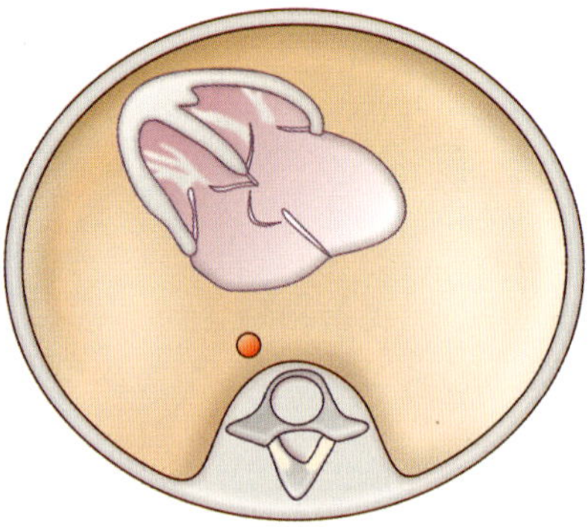

Figure 15.24

Ans: Enlarged right atrium

Possible Causes

- Tachyarrythmias
- Ebstein's and Uhl's anomalies
- Idiopathic right atrial enlargement
- Common atrium
- Tricuspid valve regurgitation
- Pulmonary stenosis with intact septum
- Premature closure of the foramen ovale or ductus arteriosus.

Question 16: What does the Figure 15.25 show?

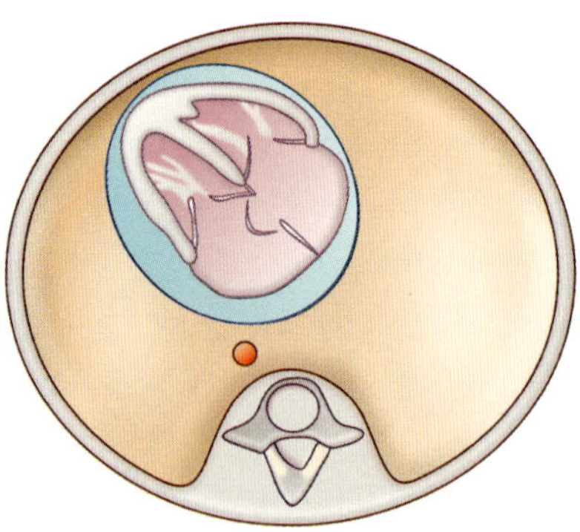

Figure 15.25

Ans: Pericardial fluid/effusion

Possible Causes

- Trisomy 21
- Hypoplastic left heart
- Teratoma
- Rhabdomyoma
- Hemangioma
- Tachyarrhythmia
- Chorioangioma
- Sacrococcygeal septal defect
- Cardiomyopathies
- Rh incompatibility disease
- Renal agenesis
- Posterior urethral valves
- Twin-to-twin transfusion.

Question 17: What does the Figure 15.26 show?

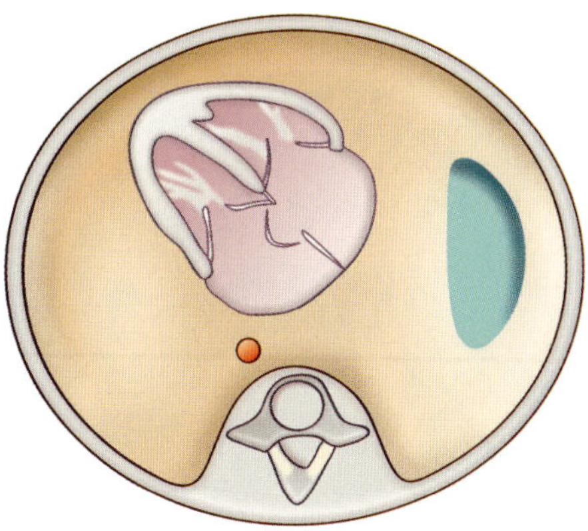

Figure 15.26

Ans: Right-sided stomach

Possible Cause

Visceral situs.

Question 18: What does the Figure 15.27 show?

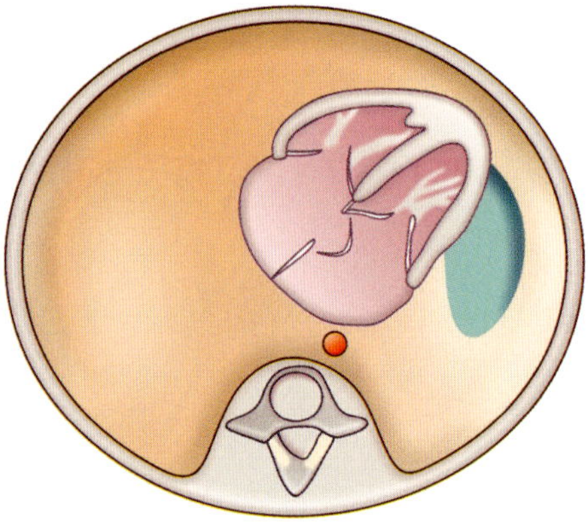

Figure 15.27

Ans: Stomach and heart on right side

Possible Cause

Situs inversus.

Question 19: What does the Figure 15.28 show?

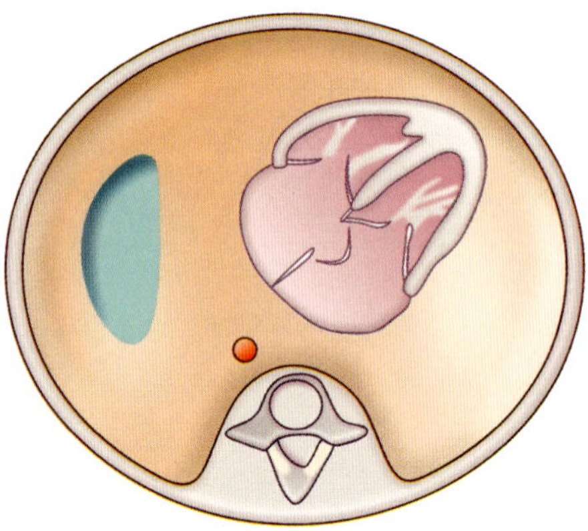

Figure 15.28

Ans: Dextrocardia

Possible Cause

Anomaly of embryological development.

Question 20: What does the Figure 15.29 show?

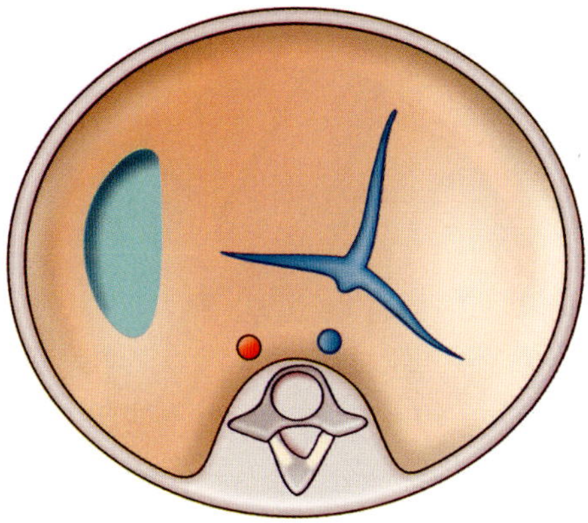

Figure 15.29

Ans: Vein next to the spine posterior to the hepatic veins

Possible Cause

IVC interruption with azygos or hemiazygos continuation.

Question 21: What does the Figure 15.30 show?

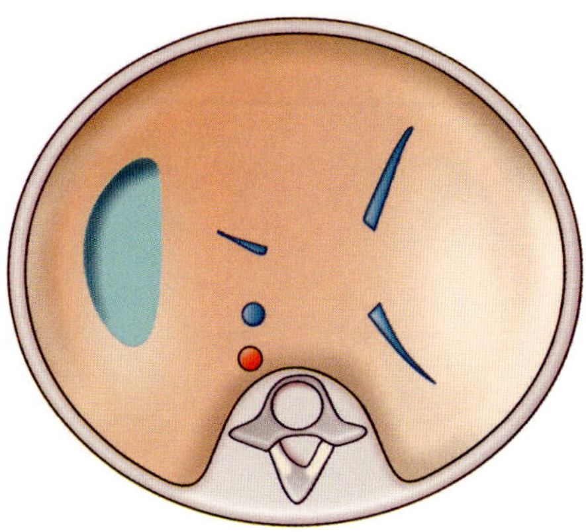

Figure 15.30

Ans: IVC anterior to aorta

Possible Cause

Left isomerism.

Question 22: What does the Figure 15.31 show?

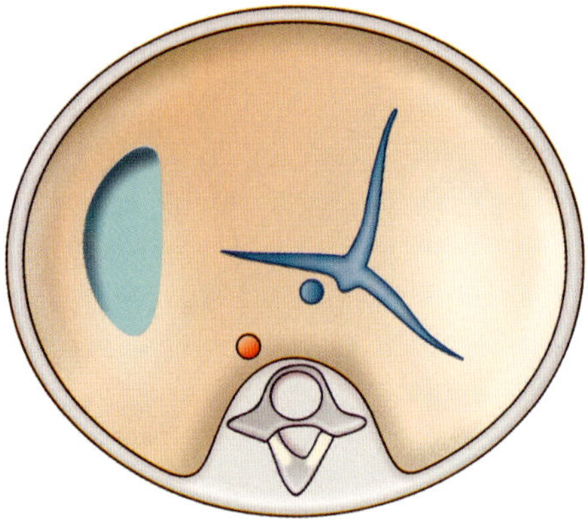

Figure 15.31

Ans: Vein flowing caudally posterior to hepatic veins

Possible Cause

Anomalous pulmonary venous return with infradiaphragmatic connection.

Question 23: What does the Figure 15.32 show?

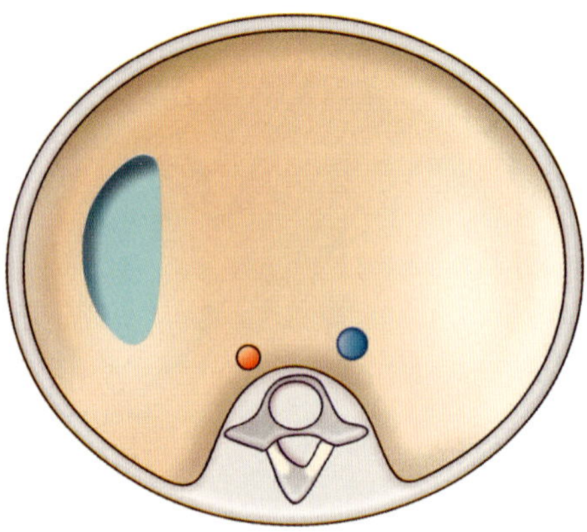

Figure 15.32

Ans: IVC larger than aorta

Possible Cause

Ductal agenesis with iliac connection.

Question 24: What does the Figure 15.33 show?

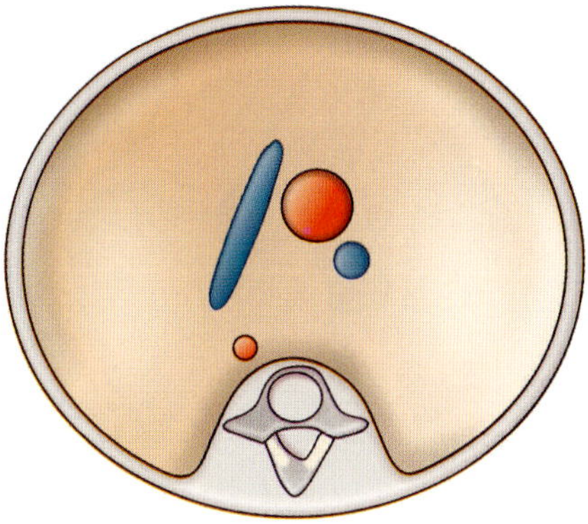

Figure 15.33

Ans: Thin pulmonary artery—large aorta

Possible Causes

- Tetralogy of Fallot
- Pulmonary atresia
- Pulmonary atresia with VSD
- Double outlet right ventricle
- Truncus arteriosus.

Question 25: What does the Figure 15.34 show?

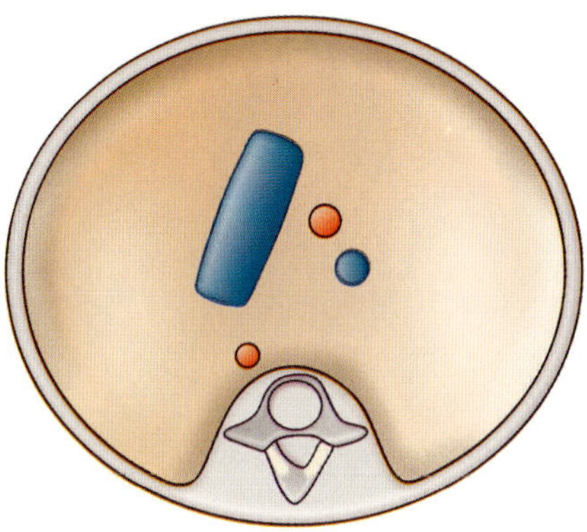

Figure 15.34

Ans: Thin aorta—large pulmonary artery

Possible Causes

- Aortic atresia/stenosis
- Mitral atresia/stenosis
- Double outlet right ventricle.

Question 26: What does the Figure 15.35 show?

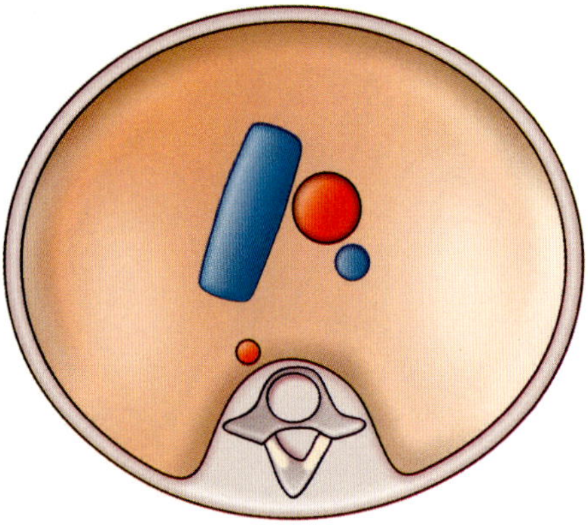

Figure 15.35

Ans: Thick aorta—large pulmonary artery

Possible Cause

Incompetent aortic and pulmonary valves.

Question 27: What does the Figure 15.36 show?

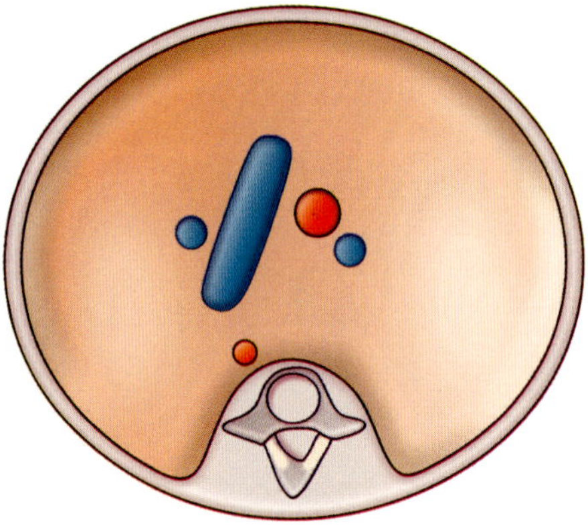

Figure 15.36

Ans: Abnormal aortic arch

Question 28: What does the Figure 15.37 show?

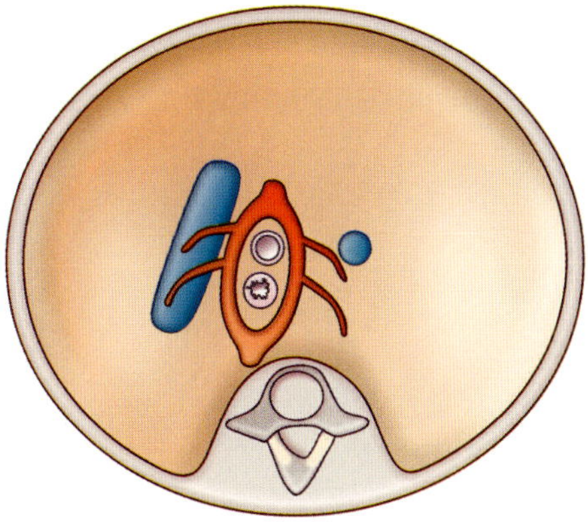

Figure 15.37

Ans: Double aortic arch

Question 29: What does the Figure 15.38 show?

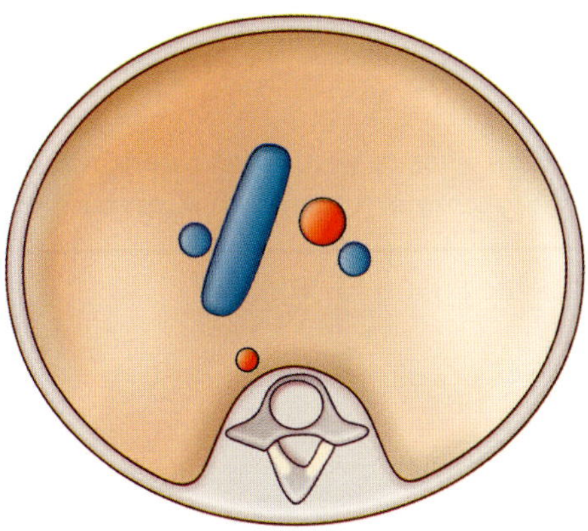

Figure 15.38

Ans: Vessel (vein) on the left of the pulmonary artery

Possible Cause

Persistent left superior vena cava.

Question 30: What does the Figure 15.39 show?

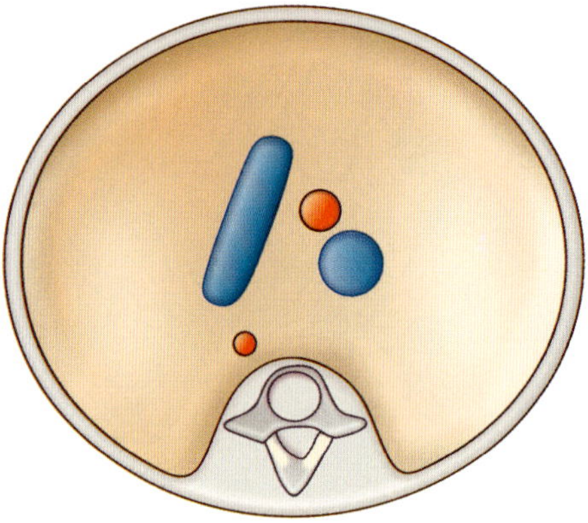

Figure 15.39

Ans: Large superior vena cava

Possible Causes

- IVC interruption with azygos or hemiazygos continuation
- Anomalous pulmonary venous return with supracardiac connection.

Question 31: What does the Figure 15.40 show?

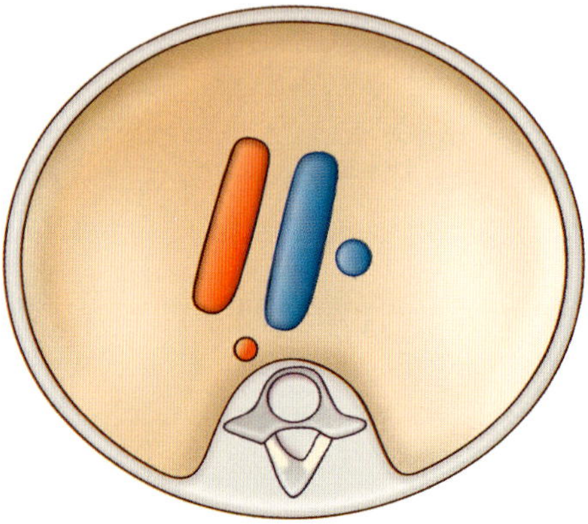

Figure 15.40

Ans: Great vessels in parallel (not necessarily in the same plane)

Possible Cause

Transposition of the great arteries.

Question 32: What does the Figure 15.41 show?

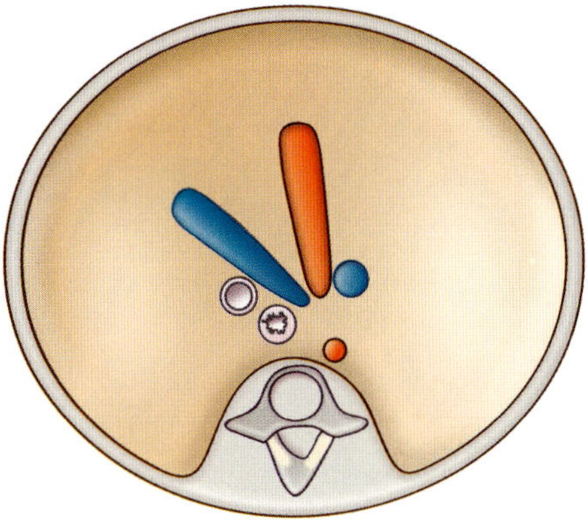

Figure 15.41

Ans: V-shaped confluence of aorta and ductus pointing to the right of the trachea

Possible Cause

Right aortic arch

Question 33: What does the Figure 15.42 show?

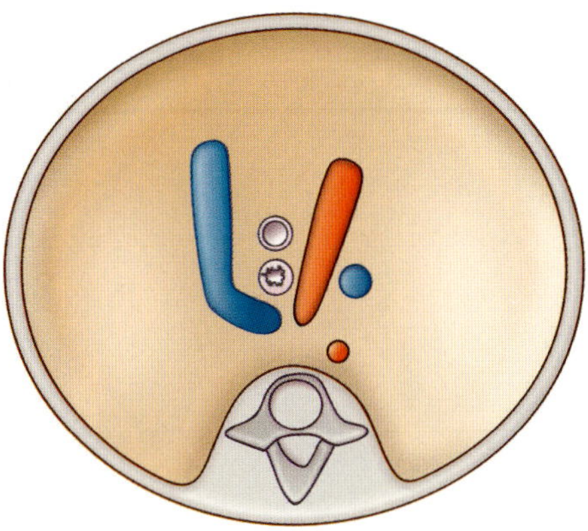

Figure 15.42

Ans: U-shaped confluence of aorta and ductus, encircling the trachea

Possible Cause

Right aortic arch.

NUTSHELL

1. 33 different questions and their answers for easy understanding.
2. Kindly see first all image and try to solve it

Index

Page numbers followed by *t* refer to table and *f* refer to figure